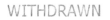

CARING FOR LESBIAN AND GAY PEOPLE: A CLINICAL GUIDE

Allan D. Peterkin, MD, and Cathy Risdon, MD

What should you say if your patient is struggling with her sexuality? How do you respond to your married patient when he discloses to you his same-sex sexual history? To which medical studies do you turn when you need to know more about club drugs? As physicians and health professionals, you want to provide the best possible care for your patients, but medical schools and other health care teaching institutions do not generally provide comprehensive information on how to approach caring for sexual-minority patients. *Caring for Lesbian and Gay People* is the first medical guide to offer busy clinicians practical, accessible, and evidence-based information to help in the care of lesbian and gay patients.

Allan D. Peterkin and Cathy Risdon begin with an overview of the history of medical relations with lesbian and gay patients, providing advice and guidelines for strengthening the doctor–patient relationship and raising the standard of care for all patients. The book then delves into a range of specific clinical issues, such as risk profiles for particular illnesses, screening for and managing sexually transmitted infections, and HIV treatment in the primary care setting. Subsequent chapters cover a wide range of topics such as mental health care and the effect of homophobia on relationships, same-sex parenting, the role that body image plays in health, and unique populations, such as lesbian and gay ethnoracial minorities, the transgendered, rural lesbian and gay people, and elders. Each chapter includes practical tips (advice on inclusive language, for example) and summaries, along with references of written and online resources. Comprehensive and detailed, this work covers physical and mental health throughout the life cycle, with equal emphasis on women's and men's health.

Based on more than twenty years of patient care and contributions to medical education and community development, this indispensable resource will greatly heighten the quality of care that clinicians, health care practitioners, and educators can provide to their patients, and will in turn provide patients and consumers with the means to take an active role in their own health care.

ALLAN D. PETERKIN, MD, is an assistant professor in the Department of Psychiatry and the Department of Community and Family Medicine at the University of Toronto.

CATHY RISDON, MD, is an associate professor and the David Braley and Nancy Gordon Chair in Family Medicine at McMaster University.

Caring for Lesbian and Gay People

A Clinical Guide

Allan Peterkin, MD, and Cathy Risdon, MD

UNIVERSITY OF TORONTO PRESS
Toronto Buffalo London

ISBN 0-8020-4857-9 (cloth)
ISBN 0-8020-8379-X (paper)

∞

Printed on acid-free paper

National Library of Canada Cataloguing in Publication

Peterkin, Allan D.
  Caring for lesbian and gay people : a clinical guide / Allan
Peterkin, Cathy Risdon.

  Includes bibliographical references and index.
  ISBN 0-8020-4857-9 (bound)   ISBN 0-8020-8379-X (pbk.)

  1. Gays – Medical care.   2. Lesbians – Medical care.   3. Gays –
Health and hygiene.   4. Lesbians – Health and hygiene.   I. Risdon,
Cathy.   II. Title.

  RA564.9.H65P48 2003   362.1'086'64   C2002-905194-0

University of Toronto Press acknowledges the financial assistance to
its publishing program of the Canada Council for the Arts and the
Ontario Arts Council.

University of Toronto Press acknowledges the financial support for
its publishing activities of the Government of Canada through the
Book Publishing Industry Development Program (BPIDP).

For Robert.
In memorium, Dr Ron Afanasiev and Dr Kelly McGinnis
– A.P.

For Lori, Gusto, Newton, and (in memorium) Alex.
Also to Pat Kimura, Lynn Andrews, and Dave Davis for being there
during the crucial turning points. My profound thanks for the depth
of your generosity and inspiration to me.
– C.R.

Contents

Online resources indexed at www.glbcare.com.

Foreword

The health of a nation, physically and emotionally, can only be as good as the health of its most vulnerable and stigmatized citizens. While culture, class, and religion are known to affect how illness may appear and be understood, sexual orientation has been less well researched or understood as a mediator of health and illness. Yet, as every gay, lesbian, or bisexual (GLB) person knows, developing a relationship with a medical or mental health provider that truly addresses the entire well-being of the person requires the provider not only to be tolerant but also knowledgeable about sexual orientation and its impact on psychological and physical health. Unfortunately, very little formal education or training in professional schools or clinical placements prepares clinicians with the knowledge and attitudes necessary to provide competent and compassionate care to lesbian, gay, or bisexual people.

Being open about one's sexuality to a medical provider is especially difficult if the patient perceives that sexuality in general, and same-sex orientation in particular, appears to make the provider uncomfortable. Even well-meaning providers can unwittingly create an atmosphere of discomfort for GLB people by assuming the patient is heterosexual and thereby forgoing the opportunity to ask the patient in a nonjudgmental way about his or her sexual orientation. Coming out as gay, lesbian, or bisexual over and over again in health care settings can be anxiety-provoking and difficult even for those people who have negotiated this process in other aspects of their lives. For young people particularly, health care providers can provide much-needed support for integrating sexual orientation into a positive self-image. Adolescence is an especially difficult time for GLB people, and finding a health care environment in which information and nonjudgmental care are offered can often help in avoiding dangerous and self-destructive behaviors.

   This book provides an excellent guide and reference for clinicians of all specialties who treat lesbian, gay, or bisexual patients, whether they are aware or not of which of their patients fit into which category. Indeed, many of the issues are relevant as well for heterosexual patients who may have GLB people in their lives. In covering general issues such as developing a clinical relationship with a GLB person, or providing specific knowledge about medical issues particular to lesbians, gay men, and bisexual men and women, this book uses case examples and strategic interventions to guide both the naive and experienced clinician in providing excellent medical and psychological care. The attention to how culture, race, ethnicity, age, and gender interface with sexual orientation distinguishes this volume from others and provides information and clinical suggestions that help providers become competent and caring professionals. In a world in which being part of a sexual minority remains highly stigmatized and outlawed in many lands, clinical settings can provide the safety and respect that is essential for people of all sexual orientations to have their psychological and physiological needs attended to and understood.

Marshall Forstein, MD
Assistant Professor of Psychiatry,
The Cambridge Hospital Department of Psychiatry,
Harvard Medical School
Medical Director of Mental Health and Addictions,
Fenway Community Health, Boston
Former President, Association of Gay and Lesbian Psychiatrists
(Affiliate of the American Psychiatric Association)

Introduction

Lesbian and gay health care concerns are now well recognized as an integral part of good medicine. There is, however, a dearth of information and teaching on the subject, and many providers have not been able to access information except for individual articles in journals. For that reason alone, this book is such a welcome and significant addition to the basic core of medical knowledge. Even more important, this text brings awareness of the lack of consistent, appropriate medical interactions between physicians and other health care providers and our patients and then concisely informs us how to overcome this lack to practice complete, inclusive medicine.

Sexual identity is an important aspect of patient information that health care practitioners need to provide optimum medical care. Yet a 2001 study showed that most health care providers do not ask about sexual identity (*Journal of the Gay and Lesbian Medical Association*, 2001, vol. 5, no. 1, p. 11). This, of course, means that many issues related to the patient's health are not addressed. As medicine matures, so grows the body of knowledge that physicians need to use competently. This text brings to the medical forefront another parameter of the person to consider, and a body of knowledge that goes along with that parameter. Addressing sexual identity and appropriately dealing with all the medical implications that accompany that information is the best management for achieving patient health and well-being, as the authors so appropriately demonstrate.

This book also gently allows us to confront our own prejudices and to deal with them in a positive manner – we all have them to more or lesser extents. The difficult aspect is to recognize them and act in a caring, sensitive manner toward our patients. This text shows us how to do that in a nonjudgmental way. In fact, the emphasis on harm reduction, as opposed to the moral and abstinence-focused approach, is in the forefront of current medical thinking, and the information contained here will be invaluable to anyone in the health care professions.

Medicine would do well to adopt this book as compulsory reading for all students in the field and those interested in updating their knowledge of lesbian and gay health care. This book should also serve as a very welcome reference guide for all other health care providers. As with all our patients, lesbian and gay clients deserve the best health care possible. This text aptly illustrates how to achieve that.

Ruth Simkin, MD, CCFP
Palliative Care Physician, Victoria Hospice Society, Victoria, BC
Certificant, American Board of Hospice and Palliative Medicine

Acknowledgments

There are many people who helped with the preparation and refinement of this book and to whom we owe deep thanks:

Jean Bacon and Wayne Herrington for editorial assistance; Amanda Miller for help with research; Jennifer Kelly for manuscript preparation; Melissa Pitts and the rest of the University of Toronto Press staff for tireless promotion of the project.

Volunteer reviewers included Dr Marshall Forstein, Dr Ruth Simkin, Dr Peter DeRoche, Charlotte Chagoya, RN, Dr Brian Cornelson, Dr Colin Kovacs, Dr Solomon Shapiro, and Farzana Doctor, MSW. Thanks to all organizations and groups who supported the book by allowing reprint of their own specific content.

We also want to express our gratitude to Dr Dale Guenter for lending his name and support to our efforts to obtain sponsorship as well as to Dr Cheryl Levitt and the McMaster University Department of Family Medicine for their generous support during manuscript preparation. Special thanks to our community and to all the friends, colleagues, and patients who have taught us along the way.

CARING FOR LESBIAN AND GAY PEOPLE:
A CLINICAL GUIDE

CHAPTER ONE

Why a Clinical Guide on Lesbian and Gay Health?

Sarah is a 25-year-old lesbian who was sent by her family doctor to a gynecologist for treatment of heavy menstrual bleeding secondary to fibroids. The male gynecologist took a medical history and asked Sarah whether she was sexually active and what form of birth control she used. When she revealed that she was sexually active but not using contraception, he reproached her for being irresponsible. Sarah chose not to come out to the gynecologist, but did inform her doctor of the unpleasant encounter. Sarah asked her doctor to refer her to a gay-affirmative specialist and to mention her sexual orientation in subsequent referral notes so that she would not have to come out to each new physician.

Phillip is a 40-year-old gay physician with glaucoma who was referred to an ophthalmologist for ocular pressure checks and fundii examination. When Phillip reveals on the standard intake form that he lives with a man, the specialist shifts his line of questioning to issues pertaining to STDs and HIV. Phillip tactfully reminds the ophthalmologist that such questioning is irrelevant to the clinical matter at hand.

At first glance, the health care needs of someone who is gay or lesbian appear to be no different from those of the general population. Everyone needs age-appropriate health education and treatment as well as the opportunity to explore preventive measures that can help maintain health. However, population health acknowledges that specific populations, such as gays, lesbians, and bisexuals, may have particular health needs that should be recognized and addressed. To date, surprisingly few guidelines exist for the clinician who wants to provide competent, sensitive care or for the teacher who hopes to help trainees examine their own attitudes toward sexuality.

The Health Needs of Lesbians, Gays, and Bisexuals

Two recent reviews of the international literature prepared for Health Canada – *Access to Care* (Brotman, Rowe, & Ryan, 2000) and *Gay Health: Current Knowledge and Future Actions* (Jalbert, 1999) – confirm that gays and lesbians have specific health risks. For men, these risks include specific gastrointestinal and sexually transmitted infections and colon, anal, and hepatocellular cancers. For women, breast, ovarian, endometrial, and colon cancer vulnerabilities are noted. At the same time, despite significant epidemiological trends, surveys of client satisfaction with care received by lesbians, gays, and bisexuals report high levels of dissatisfaction across health disciplines (Brotman et al., 2000; Jalbert, 1999). It appears that the comprehensive health needs of these populations are not being met. As a result, patients may fear and avoid traditional health care settings and may not be accessing appropriate care.

As will be explained fully in subsequent chapters, gay men and women may also be at higher risk of stroke, coronary artery disease, lung cancer, alcoholism, depression, suicide, and victimization by violent crime (see also Appendix A). Regrettably, the medical literature on the specific health concerns of bisexuals and transgendered individuals is scant. Often, such concerns are subsumed under overlapping trends noted in studies of gay and lesbian health. Clinical guidelines for working with these populations are reviewed in Chapter 12.

Who Constitutes the Lesbian, Gay, and Bisexual Populations?

In his 1940s study, Alfred Kinsey estimated that 10% of the American population was homosexual (Brotman et al., 2000). However, many researchers now question that figure's accuracy and estimate that in the United States between 1.4% and 4.3% of women are lesbian or bisexual and between 2.8% and 9.1% of men are gay or bisexual (Friedman & Downey, 1994). Although the proportion of the population that is homosexual is smaller than originally thought, physicians and other health care providers continue to underestimate the number of gay, lesbian, and bisexual patients they see in professional practice. This may be due in part to the ongoing lack of conceptual clarity in the definitions of 'gay' and 'lesbian' (Rankow, 1995).

When estimating the incidence of gays and lesbians in the population, individuals can be categorized in three ways: by identity, by behavior, and by attraction (Dean et al., 2000):

- *Identity* constitutes how individuals define themselves with respect to sexual orientation in the context of a social group with whom they share particular values.
- *Behavior* refers to an individual's same-sex activity.
- *Attraction* refers to an individual's same-sex arousal fantasy with or without creative activity.

Based on these categories, 1% to 4% of the population self-identify as gay or lesbian, 2% to 6% report some same-sex behavior during the previous five years, and 21% report at least one incidence of same-sex behavior in adulthood (Sell et al., 1995).

1.1 Terms and Definitions

Bisexual: A person who is attracted to members of both sexes. Bisexual identities are not homogeneous – each person may be attracted in differing degrees to men and women over periods of time and within changing contexts. Although bisexuals may be attracted to both women and men, do not presume nonmonogamy.

Coming out: The process of disclosing to others one's lesbian, gay, or bisexual sexual orientation. This process may occur over a short, intense period of time, or it may be a gradual process wherein a person takes into confidence only a close friend. Coming out is a highly individualized transition, governed by one's own comfort level and internal and external influences.

Gay: A man whose primary interest, sexually and intimately, is in his own gender. Although the term is often used when referring to both homosexual men and women, many women feel that this is similar to using masculine pronouns as inclusive terms and that 'gay' does not satisfactorily establish their identity as distinct from men.

Gender: Behavioral, cultural, or psychological traits commonly associated with one sex. Unlike sex, which is biologically determined, gender is considered to be a social construct.

Heterosexism: The promotion and perpetuation of the superiority of heterosexuality, and the assumption that everyone is heterosexual. Heterosexism awards privileges to the dominant group while denying nonheterosexuals access to similar rights and privileges (legal, financial, and social). Examples of heterosexism in practice include the assumption that a person's partner is of the opposite sex or the denial of survivor benefits to a lesbian because she was not a legal 'spouse' of the deceased.

Homophobia: An irrational fear of, aversion to, or discrimination against homosexuality or homosexuals, which can be expressed through social ostracism, religious and legal interdiction, and verbal or physical violence.

Homosexual: An outmoded term used primarily for diagnostic purposes, meaning 'same-sexual'; use 'gay' or 'lesbian.'

Internalized homophobia: Internalized fear or shame of and for one's own sexuality. Such feelings are often evoked by external messages that one's innate way of being is disgusting, sick, or unnatural, and may be expressed by feelings that this is true of one's self.

Lesbigay: A generic term incorporating lesbian, bisexual, and gay concerns.

Queer: A previously derogatory term for gays and lesbians now reappropriated by lesbigays, especially those born after 1970.

Sexual identity: A chosen mode of self-presentation, based on social identity, sexual behavior, or both. A person may choose to publicly identify using a term that does not strictly conform to his or her sexual behavior (e.g., a man who identifies as a heterosexual may engage in sex with other men, or a bisexual woman may be intimate only with women). How one identifies one's self is a personal choice.

Sexual orientation: The basis of one's innate sexual desires and attractions. This term is preferred over 'sexual preference,' which implies that one's desires are a matter of choice rather than an inherent part of one's nature. Sexual orientation is recognized as encompassing heterosexuality, homosexuality, bisexuality, and asexuality.

Adapted from Canadian AIDS Society. (1991). *Homophobia, heterosexism and AIDS: Creating a more effective response to AIDS.* Ottawa, pp. 64–6.

Factors that Affect Professional Care for Lesbians, Gays, and Bisexuals

Lack of Knowledge and Education

Although gays and lesbians have specific health needs and risks, health care providers across disciplines may be unaware of or indifferent to these needs and may have had minimal training in identifying or addressing them. In a preliminary questionnaire sample of family physicians conducted at the 2000 Annual Meeting of the College of Family Physicians of Canada (Brotman, Peterkin, & Risdon, 2000), most physicians estimated that 5% to 10% of the people in their practice were gay or lesbian. The same sample indicated that most physicians were 'somewhat to very interested' in gay and lesbian health issues and did not automatically refer gay and lesbian patients out of their practice. While the majority of physicians surveyed listed openness, lack of judgment, and acceptance as the most important needs for physicians treating gay and lesbian patients, most also reported that they worked in clinics where forms did not include questions on same-sex identity, relationships, or alternative families. They noted that the main barriers to care for lesbians and gay men were the physician's own lack of information and awkwardness in asking questions about sexual orientation and practices. In terms of information and education about gay and lesbian issues, physicians reported:

- Their primary sources of information/education were reading journals, accessing the Internet, and discussing cases with gay-affirmative colleagues.
- Their preferred methods for learning more about gay and lesbian health were attending interactive workshops and having access to up-to-date websites and local community resources, as well as textbooks written for a medical audience.

Lack of Standards of Care for Gay and Lesbian Patients

The lack of information on lesbian and gay health issues on the part of individual physicians is compounded by the nonexistence of up-to-date standards of care for gay and lesbian patients, including appropriate modifications of the periodic health exam. This is due to the limited number or poor quality of gay-specific research studies and the lack of relevant research to guide clinical practice and policy making. Lesbians and gay men in North America are noticeably absent from reported research in clinical and public health and program evaluation literature, and there is very little research to inform our understanding about health care delivery and access.

A variety of factors affect the gay and lesbian health research agenda; see also the GLMA–Columbia University White Paper, *LGBT Health: Findings and Concerns*, available online (www.glma.org/policy/whitepaper):

- Clinical trials, longitudinal cohorts, and population health studies fail to recognize and record sexual orientation as a unit of analysis. In fact, until the recent past, studies in the United States that attempted to do so were denied federal funding.
- Fear of stigmatization prevents many people from identifying themselves as gay, lesbian, or transgendered. Hidden or 'invisible' populations are difficult to access for research purposes.
- Lesbians are a difficult cohort to study because poverty or past unpleasant experiences lead them to avoid clinical contact, and fear of seeking health care may result in their exclusion from health studies.
- Methodological challenges affect the ability to define homosexual identity and to recruit and compare study participants. For example, standard definitions of the terms 'gay' or 'lesbian' are not universally applied and may differ significantly between studies.
- Research about people who identify as gay or lesbian often fails to consider other variables such as socioeconomic status, race, or ethnicity.
- There is no coordinating public health infrastructure in either Canada or the United States to direct and fund gay and lesbian health research initiatives.
- Over the last fifteen years, the bulk of research related to the concerns of gay men has focused on HIV/AIDS to the exclusion of other health concerns.

These and other social trends are summarized in 1.2. With no high-quality research on gay and lesbian health issues, public health researchers have had to rely on studies that use 'convenience sampling' and relatively small numbers, which do not support accurate policy planning or health analysis.

Negative Social Attitudes: Homophobia and Heterosexism

The physician's lack of information and standards of care for gay and lesbian patients is further compounded by social or cultural attitudes. All health care is provided within a general cultural context and reflects prevailing social norms, such as homophobic and heterosexist attitudes, which can create specific barriers to care for gay and lesbian patients.

O'Hanlan et al. (1997) link homophobia to all aspects of health and health care for gays, lesbians, or bisexuals and suggest that homophobia poses a major public health risk. Misinformation and negative stereotypes about gays and lesbians, their lack of civil rights, and the invisibility of this minority population all lead to chronic stress. Gays and lesbians may face discrimination in housing, the workplace and career advancement, as well as the threat of physical violence. Stigmatization in family, church, and educational settings can complicate interpersonal, family, and spousal relations. Efforts to conceal their identity may lead to chronic social isolation and low self-esteem. O'Hanlan et al. argue that these factors often result in poor health habits, including not accessing screening and appropriate care or presenting late in the course of illness.

Specific population health risks, such as unsafe sex, suicide attempts, and substance abuse, can be linked to both internal and external homophobia. O'Hanlan et al. conclude that homophobia is a chronic environmental and social stressor that affects individuals' coping styles and their vulnerability to disease. Gay, lesbian, and bisexual patients frequently do not come out about their sexuality to their health care providers, thereby allowing specific physical and mental health risks and concerns to go unaddressed. This has led the American Medical Association (1996), in its statement paper 'Health Care Needs of Gay Men and Lesbians in the United States,' to conclude: 'The AMA believes that the physician's nonjudgmental recognition of sexual orientation and behavior enhances the ability to render optimal patient care in health as well as in illness. In the case of the homosexual patient, this is

1.2 Social Origins of Gay, Lesbian, and Bisexual Health Concerns

Infection and disease risk related to sexual behavior	Cultural factors	Disclosure of sexual orientation, gender identity	Prejudice and discrimination	Concealed sexual identity
HIV/AIDS	Body culture: eating disorders	Psychological adjustment, depression, anxiety, suicide	Provider bias, lack of sensitivity	Reluctance to seek preventive care
Hepatitis A and B	Socialization through bars: drug, alcohol, and tobacco use	Conflicts with family of origins, lack of social support	Harassment and discrimination in medical encounters, employment, housing, and child custody	Delayed medical treatment
Enteritis (e.g., giardia, amoeba)				Incomplete medical history (e.g., concealed risks, sexually related complications, social factors)
Human Papillomavirus (and associated anal cancer)	Nulliparity or pregnancy later in life: breast cancer	Physical/economic dislocation		
Bacterial Vaginosis	Parenting: mental health concerns, questions on insemination methods		Limited access to care or insurance coverage	
Anal cancer			Pathologizing of gender-variant behavior	
Other STDs	Gender polarity in dominant culture: conflicts for transgender and inter-sex persons		Violence against LGBT population	

Adapted from GLMA–Columbia University White Paper. (2000). *LGBT health: Findings and concerns.* New York. Available online (www.glma.org/policy/whitepaper).

especially true since unrecognized homosexuality by the physician or the patient's reluctance to report his or her sexual orientation and behavior can lead to failure to screen, diagnose or treat important medical problems. With the help of the gay and lesbian community and through a cooperative effort between the physician and the homosexual patient, effective progress can be made in treating the medical needs of this particular segment of the population.'

1.3 Toward More Comprehensive Care for Lesbian and Gay Patients: Some Working Assumptions

The clinician or teacher who wants to learn more about providing sensitive, holistic care to lesbian and gay individuals might begin by considering the following key themes, as they underscore the cultural determinants of both identity and health.

1. Intolerance based on sexual orientation is still largely accepted in our society.
2. All of us have been exposed to homophobic attitudes and heterosexist assumptions, and we have each incorporated aspects of these attitudes into our ways of thinking, feeling, and relating in the world.
3. Health care practitioners are committed to creating an open, comfortable, and empowering environment for staff and clients. Health practitioners play a leadership role in providing education on issues such as homophobia.
4. There are lesbian, gay, bisexual, and transgendered staff and clients involved in most health care agencies. There are also many people who may be in varying stages of exploring their sexual orientation. The terms 'gay,' 'lesbian,' and 'bisexual' are labels used to describe general categories. Some people move in and out of these categories during their lives. Others refuse to acknowledge labels. We can only gain a full understanding of what these labels mean when we hear them explained by people who are living that experience.
5. Heterosexism/homophobia, sexism, and racism are interrelated. An individual's experience of homophobia is usually different depending upon race, class, culture, gender, and ability.

6. Oppression hurts everyone. It diminishes and deeply damages those targeted for marginalization or hatred, and it robs those doing the hating of their full humanity. While we as individuals may not be personally responsible for oppression, we can take responsibility for ending it. Reading a handbook such as this one and discussing it with colleagues represents a significant initial step.

Adapted from various pamphlets with permission from Pink Triangle Services, Ottawa.

A comprehensive selection of online resources used throughout this book has been indexed by the authors and is available at www.glbcare.com.

CHAPTER TWO

Improving the Doctor–Patient / Provider–Client Relationship

Verendra is a 37-year-old paralegal who has chosen to live alone and main-tain a long-term committed relationship with Mohit, her partner for the past eight years. When Verendra was 17, her mother found a love letter she had written to a female friend. Verendra was taken immediately to the family physician, who assured her mother that they 'had caught it in time' and sent her to a psychiatrist who specialized in 'curing homosexuals.'

It has been sixteen years since Verendra has seen a physician, but the nurse who did her insurance physical referred her for a blood pressure check. She overcomes her terror to make an appointment with a nearby practice. Her fear is calmed by a waiting room decorated with images of singles, families, and couples – including two women hugging. She notices the intake form asks her to name significant supports and whether she is in a 'committed relationship' rather than her marital status. By the time her name is called, she has decided to share her past experience with her new physician.

Craig is a 55-year-old married man, awaiting his turn for a routine blood pressure check. He is happily married to his wife of thirty-five years and has three grown children. Over the past several years, he has had trouble achiev-ing and maintaining erections, but he has been too embarrassed to discuss it with his physician. In the waiting room, he notices several pamphlets that make frank reference to sexual issues, including same-sex relationships. Pictures and posters on the wall show a variety of people and sexual orientations.

Although Craig comfortably identifies as heterosexual, the office's open atmosphere regarding sexuality is reassuring to him. He decides to share his concerns about his erections with his doctor.

Homophobia is the most significant health risk facing lesbians and gay men (see Chapter 1). Fear of homophobia and discrimination – often based on past experience – can prevent gays and lesbians from seeking health care. It is up to health care professionals and the health care system to regain the trust of patients with diverse sexual orientations and behaviors. This chapter briefly examines some of the literature on the relationship between lesbian and gay patients and the medical profession and suggests concrete ways to improve the provider–client relationship (O'Hanlan et al., 1997).

Professional Homophobia

Surveys of attitudes of health professionals indicate a significant proportion are homophobic, or that professional attitudes about homosexuality affect quality of care. For example:

- A 1987 survey of faculty members at a bachelor-degree-granting nursing school in the American Midwest found that 17% believed lesbianism was a disease, 23% thought it was immoral, 34% found lesbianism disgusting, and 52% thought it unnatural (Randall, 1989).
- In a survey conducted in Canada, one-third of psychiatric and family practice residents and psychiatry faculty were found to be homophobic (Chaimowitz, 1991).
- 40% of physicians surveyed in San Diego reported they were sometimes or often uncomfortable providing care to lesbian or gay patients, and 40% also said they would stop referring patients to a colleague who was known to be homosexual (Mathews et al., 1986).
- 58% of 6,500 psychologists surveyed by the American Psychological Association knew of negative incidents involving gay and lesbian patients, including cases in which practitioners defined lesbians or gay men as sick and in need of change and instances when a client's sexual orientation distracted a therapist from treating the person's central problem (Goodchilds & Peplau, 1991).
- Of 711 gay and lesbian physicians from the United States and Canada surveyed in 1994 by the American Association of Physicians for Human Rights (which later became the Gay and Lesbian Medical Association), 88% had heard physician colleagues disparage gay or lesbian patients because of their sexual orientation, and 52% had observed lesbian and gay patients being denied care or given less or suboptimal care. Although almost all physicians (98%) believed knowl-

edge of sexual orientation was critical to optimal care, 64% believed that patients who disclosed their sexual orientation risked receiving substandard care (Schatz & O'Hanlan, 1994).

Patients' Experience of Homophobia

According to lesbian and gay patients, the process of coming out and disclosing their sexual orientation is the most difficult part of seeking treatment or consulting with health professionals (Brotman et al., 2000). For example:

- Nearly 75% of lesbian respondents in a 1990 study reported negative experiences coming out to a health care provider (Stevens & Hall, 1988).
- As a result of past negative experiences, lesbians report feeling uncomfortable and fearful during subsequent appointments once their sexual orientation is disclosed (White & Dull, 1998).
- Lesbians identify family planning counseling, pelvic exams, and psychological consultations as the most stressful medical appointments and attribute the stress to disclosing sexual orientation and heterosexist assumptions (Reagan, 1981).

Fear of homophobia also affects the care-seeking behavior of gay men (Owen, 1996). In general, urban, well-educated, affluent, 'out' gay men tend to have access to gay-positive providers and to be most satisfied with the care they receive, while lower-income, nonurban gay men are more likely to report delays in treatment and lack of regular checkups (Ernst & Houts, 1985). In one study (Kass et al., 1992), fears of contagion and stigma on the part of care providers were cited as factors by gay men who were refused care because they were HIV-positive.

In general, homosexual patients report that heterosexual practitioners are often inadequately informed about gay and lesbian relationships, social dynamics, and the realities of heterosexism and homophobia (Bradford & Dye, n.d.). They also report that their doctors lack sensitivity and adequate knowledge about their particular health risks and needs and fail to disclose essential treatment or prevention information (Gambrill et al., 1984).

Practitioners who are sympathetic to the health care needs of lesbians and gay men report that they feel ill equipped to provide culturally competent care to this group and would welcome additional training

(Schatz & O'Hanlan, 1994). However, clinical training programs have been slow to address the needs of lesbian and gay patients or their dissatisfaction with care. In 1998, only half of the family medicine programs surveyed in the United States spent any curricular time addressing the care of gay and lesbian patients (Tesar & Rovi, 1998). A national U.S. survey of eighty-two medical schools reported similar results: a mean of 3 hours, 26 minutes of education about lesbian and gay patients' health needs over the four-year curriculum (Wallik et al., 1992); there are no Canadian data.

Improving Care for Gay and Lesbian Patients

Most physicians and care providers don't set out to provide substandard care. In most cases they simply lack the attitudes, skills, or working environment to provide appropriate care and meet patients' health needs.

Assessing Provider Attitudes

Although attitudes may be difficult to change, it's essential that health care providers reflect upon and name their own personal beliefs about gay and lesbian people and take an honest inventory of how those beliefs may affect the care they provide. Traditional medical education doesn't usually give clinicians much opportunity to understand the nuances of any human sexuality – let alone minority sexual orientations. If they want to provide full care, including sexual health care, to gay, lesbian, and bisexual patients, clinicians must examine their own degree of comfort and willingness to learn.

A self-inventory may help physicians identify learning needs around lesbian or gay sexuality. For example, questions in a self-inventory could include the following: Do you feel comfortable talking about sex? Do you have a range of terminology and language that will allow you to communicate with patients who prefer either clinical or slang language? Will your discomfort with such issues as multiple sex partners, anal sex, or bondage and domination keep you from caring for patients without imposing your own values?

Two tools are available to help professionals assess their attitudes toward lesbians and gays: the Riddle Scale (Riddle, 1994), outlined in 2.1, and the validated, 25-item Wright, Adams, and Bernat Homophobia Scale (Wright, Adams, & Bernat, 2000). The Riddle Scale was designed to help people understand the continuum of attitude toward gays and lesbians. The scale can also be used to assess the educational or institutional culture in which health providers work (for example, What level of the scale are you at now? At what level are your learners? At what level would you like to be? At what level is the organization for which you work?). See also 2.2 for examples of homophobia and heterosexism in the medical setting.

Any professional who finds that his or her beliefs reside largely at the negative end of the continuum is probably not ready to provide truly effective care to lesbian and gay patients. Lesbians and gay men deserve much more than continued willful ignorance or judgment. For physicians who really aren't comfortable with issues of sexuality – with either gay or straight patients – it is important for them to cultivate other referral sources to augment the care they are able to provide.

2.1 The Riddle Scale of Homophobia

Negative (Homophobic) Levels of Attitude

1. *Repulsion* – Homosexuality is seen as a 'crime against nature.' Lesbian, gay, and bisexual (LGB) people are sick, crazy, immoral, sinful, or wicked. Anything is justified to change them, including: prison, hospitalization, negative behavior therapy, and electroshock therapy.
2. *Pity* – Heterosexual chauvinism. Heterosexuality is more mature and certainly preferred. Any possibility of 'becoming straight' should be reinforced, and those who seem to be born 'that way' should be pitied, 'the poor dears.'
3. *Tolerance* – Homosexuality is just a phase of adolescent development that many people go through and most people 'outgrow.' Therefore, LGB persons are less mature than 'straights' and should be treated with the protectiveness and indulgence used with children. LGB persons should not be given positions of authority because they are still working through their adolescent behavior.
4. *Acceptance* – Still implies there is something to accept. Characterized by such statements as 'You're not lesbian to me, you're a person!' or 'What you do in bed is your own business' or 'That's fine with me as long as you don't flaunt it!'

Positive Levels of Attitude

1. *Support* – The basic ACLU position. Work to safeguard the rights of lesbians, gays, and bisexuals. People at this level may be uncomfortable themselves, but they are aware of the homophobic climate and irrational unfairness.
2. *Admiration* – Acknowledges that being LGB in our society takes strength. People at this level are willing to truly examine their homophobia, attitudes, values, and behaviors.
3. *Appreciation* – Value the diversity of people and see LGB persons as a valid part of that diversity. These people are willing to combat homophobia in themselves and others.
4. *Nurturance* – Assumes that LGB persons are indispensable in our society. They view them with genuine affection and delight and are willing to be allies and advocates.

From Riddle, Dorothy. (1994). The Riddle scale. In *Alone no more: Developing a school support system for gay, lesbian, and bisexual youth.* St Paul: Minnesota State Department.

2.2 Homophobia and Heterosexism in the Medical Setting: Some Examples

Homophobia

- A doctor emphasizes HIV/AIDS when treating gay men to the exclusion of all other health concerns.
- A religious doctor refers a lesbian patient for reparative therapy and provides resources on the ex-gay movement.
- A clinic administrator refuses to place pamphlets on gay and lesbian health in the waiting room so as not to offend other clients.
- A physician jokes to a young male patient about how unpleasant the rectal examination is going to be.
- A doctor refers a child of lesbian parents for preventive counseling.
- A doctor assumes that gay males are promiscuous and orders unnecessary STD tests.

- The local psychoanalytic institute refuses to accept a gay trainee for advanced psychotherapy study.
- A male emergency room nurse repeats a homophobic joke to a male patient in triage.
- A gay or lesbian spouse is refused access to the bedside of an ill partner and is not permitted to participate in treatment decisions.
- A receptionist reveals to her son that a classmate of his, treated in the clinic where she works, is gay.
- A clinic counselor asks two women to stop holding hands in the hospital outpatient waiting room.

Heterosexism

- A clinician doesn't ask about sexual orientation during intake or the initial patient interview.
- A doctor assumes contraception is a priority before establishing the gender of the patient's partner.
- A nurse practitioner assumes that all perpetrators of domestic violence are male.
- All photographic images and illustrations in the clinic room feature traditional families and heterosexual couples.
- A physician does not ask gay or lesbian patients about plans to have children.
- A physician insists on annual Pap smears for all adult female patients regardless of sexual orientation or sexual practices.
- In a medical education setting a preceptor jokes with a medical student about his or her attractiveness to the opposite sex.
- A doctor does not book a series of grief sessions for a gay male patient after the breakup of the patient's relationship.
- When a lesbian patient is diagnosed with new onset diabetes, the doctor does not invite her partner to attend educational sessions.

Enhancing Provider Skills

Arguably, the most important skill set in the care of lesbian and gay patients is the ability to conduct inclusive, open interviews and histories. Patients size up their physicians very early in their encounters with them, and the language physicians use is a powerful signal (Beckman & Frankel, 1984). Language and dialogue that invites patients to tell their story in their own words allows physicians to gather more accurate data, and the process itself will have an important impact on the outcome of the clinical encounter (Kaplan et al., 1989). See 2.3 for specific language to use when caring for lesbians or gay men.

2.3 Lesbian and Gay Friendly Language for Patient Interviews and Histories

Sexual Activity

- Are you sexually active?
- Do you have a partner or partners? What do you know about the sexual behaviors of your partner(s)?
- Is your partner a man or a woman?
- When you have sex, do you have sex with men, women, or both?

Sexual Identity

- Many people identify themselves with certain groups. In terms of your sexual identity or orientation, do you see yourself as:
  Gay/lesbian/homosexual?
  Bisexual?
  Heterosexual?
  Other or none of the above?

Risk for STDs and Unplanned Pregnancy

- Many women who identify themselves as lesbian occasionally have sex with men. Do you have, or have you ever had, sex with men? It would be important for me to know about this so that I can assess your health accurately.
- Some men who (are married and) think of themselves as heterosexual occasionally have sex with other men. In order to provide you with proper care, I need to know if you've ever (or recently) had sex with men or women other than your wife (spouse, partner).

Confidentiality

- I usually write down significant relationships in a patient's life. Do you feel comfortable with having me write down that you're gay? (Or: that you are in a relationship/having sex with someone of the same gender?) How would you prefer I worded it? Would you rather I use some type of symbol?

Significant Relationships and/or Family

- Do you have a significant other? Who do you include in your family?
- Who do you live with? Tell me about your family? Tell me about the supports in your life?

Adapted from Harrison, A. (1996). Primary care of lesbian and gay patients: Educating ourselves and our students. *Family Medicine, 28*, 10–23.

Creating a Nonhomophobic Environment

Physicians' efforts to create a safe and welcoming atmosphere during the clinical encounter may be undermined by other aspects of the health care setting. See 2.4 for ways to ensure gay and lesbian patients feel comfortable and safe in seeking and receiving health care.

2.4 How to Welcome Gay and Lesbian Patients in Your Practice

- Display general charters or statements of principle that explicitly include a commitment to equal treatment for all irrespective of sexual orientation.
- Include material oriented to lesbian, gay, bisexual, and transgendered people (e.g., posters, pamphlets, and reading materials) in the waiting area and in the examination room.
- Develop confidentiality guidelines. Discuss them with patients. Ensure your staff are aware of these guidelines and respect them.
- Ask patients for feedback about how they experience your care setting.

- Familiarize yourself with local and national resources (e.g., networks, support, care facilities) and, when appropriate, refer patients to them. Relevant online resources are available at www.glbcare.com.
- Avoid referring patients to colleagues, practitioners, and facilities or services that are known to be unsupportive or homophobic.
- Clarify whether the patient wants his or her sexual orientation documented on the chart. (*Note:* This information could affect the patient's insurance coverage.)
- Consider identifying your clinic as an accepting environment by displaying a 'Lesbian, Gay, Bisexual, Transgendered Positive / Safe Space' sticker on the door.

Lesbian and gay patients use a variety of techniques to find skilled, supportive providers. 'Word of mouth' is the most common technique. Local AIDS service providers, women's shelters, women's services, lesbian and gay community centers, or gay-owned businesses often maintain a list of gay- and lesbian-friendly providers who are accepting patients. (The same groups also may keep an informal 'blacklist' of providers who are perceived as a 'health risk.') Because of past negative experiences and the perception that the health care system is relatively hostile and unsupportive, gay and lesbian patients are often anxious when they meet a new clinician for the first time. See 2.5 for a guide for patients, which outlines the attitudes and skills that gay and lesbian patients should look for in a physician. A checklist that physicians can use to help determine their progress in creating an effective care environment for gay and lesbian patients is provided in 2.6.

2.5 Lesbian and Gay Guide to Evaluating a Prospective Physician

When choosing a physician, gay and lesbian patients should evaluate the doctor's receptiveness to questions, his or her attitude toward homosexuality, the doctor's responsiveness to patient concerns, and the degree of trust that he or she elicits. Patients should also assess potential physicians on the basis of

their knowledge and experience in dealing with gay and lesbian health concerns. Asking a physician questions does not
indicate mistrust, and patients are not obligated to justify any
questions.

When evaluating a doctor, patients should consider whether
or not the physician is experienced in treating gay men and
lesbians and in other clinical treatment that may be of personal
significance, such as HIV/AIDS, substance use, depression, or
with patients who live with 'chosen' rather than biological family members. Questions to ask prospective physicians include the
following:

- Do you have experience treating gay/lesbian/transgendered/
  transsexual persons?
- Do you believe homosexuality is curable?
- Do you currently employ any gay, lesbian, or transgendered
  persons?
- Are you affiliated with a gay-positive hospital?
- Do you have a group of lesbian and gay-positive specialists to
  whom you can refer?

To determine whether or not a practitioner respects and can
ensure confidentiality, patients may have to ask highly specific
questions about the degree of privacy a doctor can offer, particularly with regard to disclosing information to employers or in-
surers (e.g., Are you required to release any information to
insurance companies? What if my employer calls for information?).

Patients may also wish to gauge the level of sex-positive care a
doctor is willing to provide by asking about his or her position
on nonmonogamous sexual relationships, masturbation, and un-
conventional sexual behaviors, including sadomasochism (S/M).
Dismissive or judgmental responses (e.g., the use of words such
as 'promiscuity') or avoidance may indicate doctor/patient in-
compatibility. Patients who are uncomfortable asking a doctor
questions should examine whether this discomfort is due to
internal barriers or a response to an unreceptive environment.
Patients can also learn a great deal about their health care
provider and facility without asking questions. For example,
material either displayed in or absent from the waiting area and

examination room as well as the attitudes of support staff reflect the quality of care a gay or lesbian patient may expect to receive.

From Penn, R.E. (1997). *The gay men's wellness guide.* New York: Henry Holt.

2.6 Are You a Gay and Lesbian-Affirmative Health Care Provider?

- My staff is welcoming and comfortable with gay and lesbian issues.
- The environment we work in is sensitive and inclusive.
- When taking a medical history, I use inclusive (i.e., non-heterosexist) questions about sexual history and relationship status.
- I feel comfortable and knowledgeable about anal health and can approach anal examinations in a sensitive manner.
- As for all patients, when outlining treatment guidelines, I provide information about treatment options, explain the choices for treatment or no treatment of a patient's condition, and encourage patients to take an active role in their care, including being receptive to patients' personal research into treatments.
- I am comfortable initiating and responding to concerns that may embarrass patients. My patients are able to ask questions about treatment guidelines and ensure they have received complete information. They are also able to discuss their fears and physical pain with me.
- I have a working knowledge of gay-affirming resources and facilities in my community.
- I am careful to refer my gay and lesbian patients to colleagues who will provide sensitive care. If not, I will let my patient know.

CHAPTER THREE

Lesbians' Physical and Sexual Health

Julie, an otherwise healthy 66-year-old woman, presents to her doctor with a three-month history of weight loss, sleep disturbance, and loss of appetite. The exchange with the busy physician is brief:

    'Do you live alone?'

    'Yes.'

    'What about your husband?'

    'He died twenty years ago.'

    The physician diagnoses depression and prescribes an antidepressant with follow-up in two weeks. When Julie returns, a different doctor is covering that day.

    'Who do you live with?'

    'No one – I'm alone.'

    'Is that a change for you?'

    'Yes.'

    'Tell me about what has happened recently.'

    'Sheila died.'

    'Sheila ... did she live with you?'

    'Yes.'

    'How long did the two of you live together?'

    'Eighteen years.'

    'Were the two of you close?'

    'Yes. Very.' (patient in tears ...)

    In addition to the antidepressant, the physician offers Julie bereavement counseling. In future follow-up, Julie reveals a relationship with Sheila that the two women had hidden from their children and community, all of whom assumed they were 'just roommates.'

Although diseases and morbidities do not occur more frequently in lesbians than in women in general (in fact, lesbians may be at lower risk for genital tract disease than heterosexual women), lesbians do have distinct health risks and needs. This chapter briefly discusses the relationships between sexual identity, behavior, and health care and explores the unique physical and sexual health care needs of lesbians.

The Relationship between Sexual Identity, Behavior, and Health Care

Lesbians make up an estimated 1.4% to 4.3% of the female population; yet very few clinicians realize that, during an average day, they will provide care for one or two lesbian women. Physicians simply assume that the women they see are heterosexual, and will ask them first whether they are sexually active, and then what form of birth control they use. Because of this assumption and past negative experiences with the health care system, many women who have sex with women or who identify themselves as lesbian do not voluntarily disclose their sexual orientation to physicians – although most would prefer to do so (Geddes, 1994).

When considering the health care needs of lesbians, clinicians face an interesting paradox: sometimes the invisibility of the patient's sexual orientation and heterosexist assumptions can significantly interfere with the effectiveness of the doctor–patient relationship or cause physicians to miss or lose crucial data during a clinical encounter (see Chapter 2); at other times, the physician's knowledge of the patient's lesbian identity leads to other assumptions, which also interfere with care. For example, upon learning a patient is 'lesbian,' clinicians may make a series of incorrect assumptions:

- She doesn't have sex/intercourse with men.
- She doesn't want to become pregnant or have children.
- She hates men.
- She will always be a lesbian.

These kinds of assumptions often result in missed screening opportunities (e.g., Pap smears, STD screening, abusive relationships) and lack of anticipatory care (e.g., folic acid, alternative insemination, STD prevention).

The most effective way for clinicians to counter erroneous assumptions is to remember two key factors:

- Lesbian identity is fluid and may change any time and over time.
- Lesbian identity and behavior are two entirely different things and may or may not overlap.

There is often very little correlation between *identity* and *behavior*. Good medicine depends on developing strategies to elicit both types of information from patients – and on understanding the significance of each.

As a general rule, in situations where an ongoing relationship between clinician and patient is unlikely, where encounters tend to be problem-focused, and where the problem is acute (i.e., emergency rooms, STD clinics), behavior takes precedence over identity. If the practitioner is trying to rule out an ectopic pregnancy in the ER, it's more helpful to know when a woman last had intercourse with a man (with or without birth control) than whether she considers herself to be gay, lesbian, straight, or bisexual. However, in other areas of medicine, an understanding of the patient's identity is essential to developing a successful relationship over time. For example, family physicians need to explore both identity and behavior in order to understand the nuances of the worlds our patients travel.

Lesbians' Use of Health Services

In general, lesbians visit the doctor less often than heterosexual women. This underuse of health services may be related in part to their lower need for prenatal and contraceptive care, but it also reflects the fact that lesbians tend to avoid regular medical examinations (Harrison & Silenzia, 1996) and postpone seeking treatment longer than heterosexual women (Carroll, 1999). This avoidance may be due to their belief – and corresponding emotional stress – that a symptom or illness is linked to sexual practices (Harrison & Silenzia, 1996). It may also be due to the fact that the health care system, with its institutional and cultural homophobia, often fails to provide appropriate services for women who fall outside the white, heterosexual, middle-class 'norm' and has not always been a safe place for gay and lesbian people. The most significant risk to lesbians' health is their interaction with a health care system that is at best indifferent and at worst hostile to their needs and identity. For example:

- In one study of lesbian health care experiences, 72% of respondents reported experiencing ostracism and rough treatment, overhearing antigay remarks, and having their life partner excluded from discussions by their practitioner (Stevens & Hall, 1988).
- Lesbian patients' negative experiences generally begin immediately after they disclose their sexual orientation (Smith et al., 1985). Fear of negative repercussions leads the majority to choose not to reveal their homosexuality or same-sex sexual behavior to practitioners (Cochran & Mays, 1988).
- Lesbians continue to be excluded from medical research studies and are rarely visually portrayed in textbooks (Whatley, 1992).

While lesbians may avoid the medical health care system, they tend to seek treatment from complementary or alternative health care practitioners more frequently than nonlesbian Canadian women (Moran, 1996).

Preventive Health Care Needs

Many researchers assume that lesbians' health needs are synonymous with the collective homosexual population (Simkin, 1991), so little research has been done on lesbian health issues. Despite the lack of research, we do know that lesbians have a similar incidence of common chronic illnesses as heterosexual women (Moran, 1996) and that some biological factors (e.g., higher body mass index) and behavioral factors (e.g., higher rates of smoking, excessive alcohol consumption, and excessive coffee consumption) (Moran, 1996) may increase their risk of developing cardiovascular diseases as well as lung, cervical, uterine, and colon cancers. These risks may be compounded by the fact that lesbians receive less frequent medical examinations and often avoid screening tests (White & Dull, 1998). They may also be exacerbated by the lack of understanding of lesbians' health care needs and the failure of the health care system to provide appropriate preventive and treatment services.

Coronary Health Issues

Coronary artery disease (CAD) is the number one killer of North American women, so it stands to reason that it is also the leading cause of death for lesbians (Ulstad, 1999). Based on currently available data, it is impossible to draw any specific conclusions about the risk of CAD in a lesbian population (Solarz, 1999). On the one hand, lesbians have higher rates of smoking and a higher body mass index (BMI) than hetero-sexual women – two factors associated with CAD. On the other hand, lesbians use fewer oral contraceptives, which may reduce their risk. Until more is known about the risk of CAD in lesbians, all women should be offered heart disease and stroke prevention information, screening tests, and services – based on age and other risks and regard-less of sexual identity.

Cancer

Cervical Cancer

Most medical practitioners believe that lesbians do not require regular Pap tests as part of their routine physical examinations (Ferris et al., 1996). As a result, lesbians undergo fewer cervicovaginal smears than other Canadian women (Moran, 1996). In one study of women attend-ing the same clinic, the mean interval between routine Pap smears for lesbians was twenty-one months compared to eight months for hetero-sexual women (Johnson et al., 1987). This statistical outcome might be explained in that lesbian women are less likely to receive Pap smear screening appropriately as medical practitioners make assumptions about their relative risk for cervical dysplasia and cancer. Not surpris-ingly, there is a correlation between a practitioner's awareness of and sensitivity to lesbian issues and the likelihood of lesbian patients re-ceiving regular Pap tests (Rankow & Tessero, 1998). As well, lesbian women are less likely to seek Pap smear screening because of their own distrust of the medical community.

Are lesbians at risk of acquiring human papillomavirus (HPV), which is associated with cervical cancer? Do lesbians need Pap smears? Risk factors for HPV include:

- age – being between 25 and 30 years old
- smoking
- a history of abnormal Pap smears
- more than ten lifetime male sexual partners
- engaging in sex with a male partner within the past two years.

According to the research, there is no significant correlation between the presence of HPV DNA and annual income, a history of sexual partners with genital warts, a history of nongenital warts, or use of insertive sex toys (Marrazzo et al., 1998). Although lesbians might not appear, based on these risk factors, to be at high risk for HPV, it is important for clinicians to note that the majority of women (80%) who describe themselves as lesbian have also engaged in unprotected sexual intercourse with a man and may be at risk for cervical neoplasia (Lemp et al., 1995). A 1999 survey (Diamant et al., 1999) of 6,935 self-identified lesbians indicated:

- 70% had a lifetime history of penile-vaginal intercourse (64% without a condom)
- 17.2% had a lifetime history of anal intercourse
- 17.2% had a lifetime history of a sexually transmitted disease
- 5.7% reported having had a male sexual partner within the past year
- 17% reported a history of an abnormal Pap smear (including 10% of respondents who had never had sex with men).

What about the women who have never had penile-vaginal penetration? Are they at risk of HPV or cervical cancer? In a word, yes. A study of 149 women who reported having sex with another woman in the past year found HPV in the genital tracts of 30% of these women. Of the 21 subjects who reported never having had sex with men, 19% were infected with HPV. Little is known about how HPV is transmitted from one woman to another, or the incidence and prevalence of same-sex HPV transmission. However, it is clear that HPV can be transmitted from woman to woman (Berger et al., 1995), and women who have sex only with other women are at risk of acquiring HPV and cervical cancer.

Breast Cancer
According to the research, lesbians perform breast self-exams less frequently than other women and are less likely to benefit from early screening and detection programs (Lemp et al., 1995). Is this a problem?

Many lesbians were upset by a well-publicized paper in the early 1990s, which reported that lesbians' risk of acquiring breast cancer was two to three times as high as the risk for women as a whole. However, the study was an epidemiologic extrapolation that was taken out of context and caused misunderstanding. Prospective studies are currently underway comparing rates of breast cancer in lesbians and closely matched controls. To date, no data confirm a higher risk. When a woman chooses or discovers a lesbian identity, she is not increasing her risk of breast cancer. The primary risk factor for breast cancer is *age*, regardless of sexual identity. The risk of breast cancer is also associated with higher consumption of alcohol, body mass (obesity), and nulliparity (Haynes, 1995).

Other Cancers

Lung cancer is the number one cause of cancer deaths in women. A significant proportion of women also develop ovarian cancer. As with other population groups, the prognosis is significantly better when these cancers are detected early. Cancer risk factors are generally well known: smoking, age, family history, exposure to radiation and toxins, diet, reproductive history, and socioeconomic factors that impact screening behaviors. The factors that may have an impact on lesbians are smoking, reproductive history, and screening behaviors:

- According to data from the 1998 Women's Health Initiative (an ongoing study), about twice as many lesbians as heterosexual women reported being 'heavy' smokers (6.8% to 7.4% of lesbians compared to 3.5% of heterosexual women). Almost 50% of the heterosexual women surveyed reported never smoking, while only 25% to 33% of lesbians reported never smoking (National Heart, Lung and Blood Institute; see Solarz, 1999). According to the 1988 National Lesbian Survey, the rate of smoking among lesbians increases with age, whereas rates of smoking among women in the general population decline with age (Ryan & Bradford, 1993).
- Women who have never had children have a higher risk of developing ovarian cancers. Lesbians are more likely to fall into this category than heterosexual women – although it is dangerous to generalize among extremely heterogeneous groups.
- As noted earlier, lesbians are less likely to be routinely screened for cancer, in part because of their avoidance of the health care system and in part because of misunderstandings and misconceptions on the part of providers.

The bottom line for good clinical practice in cancer prevention: *Cancer prevention for lesbians involves the same preventive measures recommended for all women:*

- All women, regardless of sexual identity, should receive cervical screening at appropriate intervals.

- All women, regardless of sexual identity, should have an annual breast exam.
- All women between the ages of 50 and 69 should receive breast screening, including mammography, every two years, or according to current guidelines.
- All women should also be encouraged to stop smoking, eat a diet rich in fruits and vegetables, reduce their exposure to the sun, and use sunscreen.

Successful, ongoing prevention efforts also depend on an open and trusting relationship with a health care provider.

Reproductive Health Issues

Up to one-third of lesbians are also mothers (Hall, 1978). Many may have conceived and borne children during heterosexual relationships, while others desire and plan pregnancies within same-sex relationships. When asked their reasons for becoming a mother within a same-sex relationship, lesbians cite the following factors:

- the desire to experience pregnancy and motherhood
- the importance of mother–child bonds
- the desire to raise a newborn
- barriers to adoption.

Most lesbian mothers conceive through alternative insemination; more than half use anonymous donors (Harvey et al., 1989).

In choosing to conceive and bear children, lesbians have the right to informed, supportive prenatal, intrapartum, and postnatal care. However, the traditional health care system tends to expect heterosexual unions. It will tolerate single mothers, but it rarely considers the possibility of pregnancy as part of a same-sex relationship. A sensitive provider will demonstrate skill and understanding of some of the unique dilemmas facing lesbians who wish to become mothers.

Planning and Conception

Lesbians who choose to become biological parents must give a great deal of forethought and planning to conceiving. With few societal and cultural models of 'dual-mother' families, lesbians must often weigh a number of social, lifestyle, and relationship factors. At this point, some may choose not to become parents because of fears about how their families or social groups may react. Those who choose to seek pregnancy must make two key decisions:

- Whether to use known or anonymous donors.
- Whether to use alternative insemination or sexual intercourse. (Alternative insemination is now the accepted term for artificial insemination.)

See 3.1 for a summary of the advantages and disadvantages of each option and Chapter 14 for an outline of the issues governing sperm donation arrangements.

3.1 Conception Options for Lesbians Who Desire Pregnancy

Artificial / Alternative Insemination (with Unknown Donor)

Pros:
- Usually obtained from accredited labs/institutions with measures to ensure sperm is free of transmittable disease
- Assures confidentiality, avoids potential complications related to co-parenting
- Does not require sexual intercourse (may be considered a pro, depending on personal preference)
- With sensitive providers, potential exists for the couple to participate in conception process together

Cons:
- Expensive – each cycle can cost up to $500 depending on setting and method used
- Requires significant interaction with health care system; common barriers may include ineligibility for service because of 'unmarried' status, difficulty finding providers who support their concept of family, homophobic or judgmental attitudes, and a lack of sensitivity to the lesbian couple's needs
- Procedure becomes 'medicalized,' control shifts from the couple desiring conception to the medical system
- Some fears related to unknown donor's health history

Coitus / Known Donor

Pros:
- Less expensive
- May offer chance to know more about donor characteristics
- If desired, may offer opportunity for ongoing relationship between child and donor
- Conception rates may be higher with fresh sperm

Cons:
- Potential for custody complications
- Higher risk of disease transmission
- May be unacceptable to women who prefer not to have sex with men

Adapted from Kenney, J., & Tash, D. (1992). Lesbian childbearing couples' dilemmas and decisions. *Health Care for Women International, 13,* 209–19.

Pregnancy and Prenatal Care

Once a woman or a same-sex couple have conceived, she or they must decide where to have the baby and who will deliver it. Finding a practitioner who is comfortable and values lesbian parenting is often difficult. In one study (Hall, 1978), 11% of lesbians seeking prenatal and intrapartum care were initially refused care based on their sexual orientation. It is interesting to note that lesbians are more likely than heterosexual women to choose midwives (Hall, 1978). Home births may be one way for them to avoid perceived homophobia within the hospital setting (Harvey et al., 1989; Kenney & Tash, 1992).

Infertility Issues

If 20% of lesbians seek to have children (a conservative estimate) and 20% of those women experience fertility difficulties (comparable to the rate in the general population), there could be between 150,000 and 300,000 North American lesbians with infertility problems who need help to become pregnant.

Infertile lesbians are an invisible minority. While much has been written and researched about a heterosexual woman's infertility experience, little is known about lesbians who become pregnant, let alone those who wish to but cannot. Lesbians have several challenges in becoming pregnant that may be different from heterosexual women (Jussim, 2000). For example:

- Lesbians usually make the decision to have children later in their lives than their nonlesbian sisters, and age is the number one risk factor for infertility.
- During the time it takes to discover their fertility problems, it is unlikely lesbians will 'accidentally' become pregnant – unless they are having regular sexual intercourse with men.
- Frozen donor sperm is less potent than fresh sperm. Freezing sperm reduces the rate of conception by half.
- Lesbians have higher rates of untreated endometriosis, which can interfere with fertility. (The years that heterosexual women spend on oral contraceptives may have the 'hidden' benefit of treating mild endometriosis.)

Community resources designed to support women through the emotional devastation and grief associated with infertility are unlikely to acknowledge or understand how infertility affects lesbians and their female partners. Lesbians dealing with infertility may have to work harder to push beyond insensitivity and their invisibility to the health care system in order to receive standard quality care.

Adoption

In many jurisdictions, lesbians who want to adopt often face ambiguous adoption policies and barriers (Reilly, 1996), which are often the result of systemic discrimination (Brotman et al., 2000). Although most Canadian provinces and American states do not specifically prohibit adoption by lesbians and gay men, their applications to adopt are often neglected, assessed based on different (higher) standards, or given low priority (Reilly, 1996). To overcome these barriers, adoption agencies in many regions routinely advise gay men and lesbians to pursue adoption or foster parenting as single parents rather than as a couple (Patterson, 1996).

Sexual Issues

Lesbian Desire / Sexual Dysfunction

Research published in the mid-1980s by Blumstein and Schwarz (1983) suggested that lesbian couples have less sex than gay men or heterosexual couples. The phrase 'lesbian bed death' has since been coined to describe the phenomenon of diminishing sexual activity in long-term lesbian relationships. Is it true, or is this another example of complex relationship and intimacy issues distilled into glib, descriptive phrases?

At issue is the way in which sexual desire and sexual activity are defined. In the study in question, researchers asked gay, lesbian, and heterosexual couples how often during the last year they had sexual relations. Most heterosexual couples interpret 'sexual relations' to mean only 'sexual intercourse.' However, 'sexual relations' between two women is more difficult to define. There is some evidence to suggest that, although important, genital contact does not account for the sum total of lesbian sexuality.

To understand issues of desire and sexuality among lesbian couples, it's important for clinicians to move away from measures such as 'how often' and 'how much' when assessing sexual dysfunction. For couples who are satisfied with the amount and frequency of genital contact, the clinician's role may simply be to help them feel a sense of ownership and choice about what feels right for them. However, when partners have different levels of sexual desire, they may need therapy to explore the issues underlying the discordance.

When diagnosing sexual dysfunction, clinicians should be aware that lesbians experience differences in sexual desire for many of the same reasons as busy, stressed heterosexuals and gay men. However, some lesbians' level of sexual desire may also be affected by other issues, such as body image, past history of sexual abuse, internalized homophobia, and undiagnosed mood disorders. It may be important to refer these patients to lesbian-aware and supportive clinicians who provide sexual counseling.

Polyamory

Not all lesbians are in monogamous relationships. Polyamory is a term often used in lesbian communities to describe simultaneous intimate relationships with more than one partner. Another commonly used term is nonmonogamy. To provide appropriate care for a lesbian who is polyamorous, clinicians should try to understand the patient's support system: Who will be involved if the patient needs hospitalization? Who will be responsible for surrogate decision making? If the patient's relationships involve sexual contact, clinicians should discuss issues of safer sex and screening for sexually transmitted diseases. For a more detailed discussion of lesbian relationships, see Chapter 11, and for more information on lesbian sexuality, see *The Whole Lesbian Sex Book* by Felice Newman (1999), which includes an excellent multimedia bibliography.

Gynecological Health

When providing gynecological care for lesbians, clinicians should be aware of the following:

- Serious gynecological or pathological conditions do not occur more frequently in lesbians than in heterosexual or bisexual women (Simkin, 1998).
- Although the overall incidence of vaginal infections in lesbians does not differ significantly from that of heterosexual women, bacterial vaginosis does seem to occur more frequently in lesbians (Skinner et al., 1996).

Sexually Transmitted Diseases

Lesbians are less vulnerable to many sexually transmitted diseases than heterosexual women. Among women who have had sex only with women, chlamydia and herpes infections are rare (Johnson et al., 1987), the incidence of syphilis and gonorrhea is lower than in any other sexually active group of people, the incidence of hepatitis A is rare, and hepatitis B and C occur only in the presence of other risk factors (Walter & Rector, 1986). However, lesbians can develop candidiasis and trichomonas vaginalis – both of which they can transmit to their female partners (Degen & Waitkevicz, 1982).

Women who identify as lesbians may acquire HIV in a number of ways, including sharing needles, receiving tainted blood products, having sex with an infected male, using contaminated donor sperm, occupational exposure, or having sex with an HIV-infected woman. The Centers for Disease Control in Atlanta has published a series of case reports confirming probable woman-to-woman transmission (for a summary, see White, 1997).

Until recently, information on woman-to-woman sexual behaviors was not collected as part of routine HIV surveillance, so it is difficult to know the exact risk of woman-to-woman transmission of HIV or which behaviors are riskier than others. In 1999, the Centers for Disease Control began funding a formal study of lesbians in four major cities to follow their risk behavior and HIV status. To help women who have sex with other women assess their risk of acquiring a sexually transmitted disease and take steps to reduce that risk, clinicians must be able to take an accurate history of the woman's past and current sexual practices and injection drug use. The history should focus on behaviors, not identity.

3.2 Sexual Practices, Risks, and Risk Reduction

The following table lists sexual activities or behaviors, the risks associated with them, and suggestions for safer sex practices. See 3.3 for lesbian safer sex guidelines that can be given to patients and 3.4 for a patient guide to using dental dams.

Activity	Risk of sexually transmitted diseases	Safer sex suggestions
Oral Sex Oral-vaginal sex (cunnilingus, eating out, eating pussy) Oral-anal sex (analingus, 'rimming') For some lesbian women, oral sex may also involve going down on their partner wearing a strapped-on dildo.	Oral sex can transmit HPV and herpes. If blood is present, risk of hepatitis B, hepatitis C, and HIV increases considerably. Analingus can transmit hepatitis A, anal herpes, anal warts, and parasites.	Use of a barrier is strongly encouraged. Plain and flavored dental dams are available. Plastic wrap also provides an acceptable barrier to bacteria and viruses. Alternatively, a condom may be cut along its length and opened to provide barrier protection.

Activity	Risk of sexually transmitted diseases	Safer sex suggestions
		Women who engage in unprotected ana-lingus are strongly advised to be vac-cinated against hepatitis A.
Vaginal Penetration Clitoral tissue cradles the urethra and ex-tends back to the vag-inal walls. During penetration, the clit-oris is stimulated in-directly through the walls of the vagina. The outer third of the vagina contains the most nerve endings and is the most sen-sitive to stimulation. The 'G' spot or ure-thral sponge is an area of concentrated sexual pleasure for some women and is located on the front wall of the vagina, fairly close to the opening. Penetration may in-volve fingers, hands, fists, dildos ('strap-ons'), or vibrators.	Herpes, HPV, chlamydia, bacterial vaginosis, and candi-diasis have been transmitted during penetrative sex. Risks increase with ungloved hands (fingernails can cause microscopic vaginal trauma for receptive partner; cuts on cut-icles or fingers pose a risk for insertive partner), and when sharing sex toys and/ or body fluids.	Use latex gloves during manual penetration. Change gloves if practicing vaginal penetration after anal penetration. If sharing sex toys, use a new latex condom for each new episode of penetration be-tween partners or wash toy with soap and water between uses. Make generous use of a water-based lubricant to protect mucosal surfaces from trauma dur-ing penetration.
Anal Penetration The anus is richly enervated and a source of sexual pleasure for many. Unlike the vagina, however, the rectum is not self-lubricating.	Similar to risks for vaginal penetrative sex. However, rectal tissue is more vulner-able to trauma during penetration and there-fore offers a more likely portal to the bloodstream.	If it hurts, stop! Use plenty of lubri-cant. Use latex gloves to protect receptive partner from fing-ernail injuries and

Activity	Risk of sexually transmitted diseases	Safer sex suggestions
The tissue of the rectum, although elastic, is fragile and easily torn. Anal stimulation and sexual play shouldn't hurt. Successful anal eroticism usually depends on the use of lots of lubrication, good communication, and relaxation.		insertive partner from naturally occurring bowel flora, which can cause vaginal or enteric infections. Use condoms on insertive sex toys. Wash sex toys thoroughly with antibacterial soap or with boiling water between uses. See also the patient's guide to more comfortable anal penetration in Chapter 4.
Bondage, Dominance, Submission, and Sadomasochism (BDSM) Involves the consensual exchange of power between sexual partners. BDSM practices vary widely. For devotees of BDSM, pushing the boundaries of their own sexual comfort may be scary or overwhelming, but it also offers the opportunity for sexual intensity that may not be obtained in any other way. BDSM may be hard for the uninitiated to	Any activity that involves blood or body fluids carries the risk of transmitting HIV and other sexually transmitted diseases. To assess the risk, the clinician should take a careful sexual history for patients involved in BDSM.	See precautions listed above.

Activity	Risk of sexually transmitted diseases	Safer sex suggestions

understand. Doctors may equate it with physical or psychological abuse. However, by definition, activities in BDSM sexual play are mutually negotiated and consensual, have built-in safety rules, and can be stopped by either partner at any time. Patients who describe sexual activities without these parameters may well be in an abusive situation and may require appropriate support or psychotherapy.

Conversely, if practitioners detect bruises during a physical exam that a patient reports are the result of consensual sexual play with a partner and don't represent unwanted trauma, it may not be appropriate to intervene.

Consent and negotiation require the full presence of both partners. If BDSM activity occurs in the context of mind-altering alcohol or drug use, the questions of safety and abuse may be legitimate.

3.3 Lesbian Safer Sex Guidelines

Not Risky

Massage
Hugging
Fantasy
Voyeurism
Exhibitionism
Masturbation (touching yourself)
Vibrators or other sex toys (not shared)
Dry kissing
Body-to-body rubbing or 'tribadism' when fluids are not
   involved

Possibly Risky

Wet (French) kissing
Shared hand and genital contact with a barrier such as a
   fingercot, glove, or latex dam (a square piece of latex)
Cunnilingus (oral-genital contact) using a barrier
Fisting using a barrier

Probably Risky

Shared hand, finger, and genital contact with cuts or sores
Cunnilingus (oral or tongue to genital contact) without a
   barrier

Very Risky

Cunnilingus without a barrier during menstruation
Female or male ejaculate in the mouth, vagina, or anus
Rimming without a barrier
Fisting without a barrier such as a glove
Sharing sex toys without a barrier
Sharing needles of any kind (e.g., to shoot drugs, pierce or
   tattoo the skin)

3.4 Patient Guide to Using Dental Dams

Dental dams are pieces of latex originally designed to isolate a tooth during dental procedures. However, they also provide effective barrier protection during oral/vaginal or oral/anal sex. When using a dental dam:

- Add lubricant to the 'lickee's' side to help increase sensation.
- Avoid accidentially reversing the dam by marking one side with a pen.
- To hold the dam in place for hands-free pleasure, purchase a holder from a specialty shop.

If you find dams too small, you can use long sheets of plastic kitchen wrap. (Although there are no studies to prove that plastic wrap is an effective barrier to viruses and bacteria, it's likely safer than no protection at all.) You can also cut the tip off a condom and cut along one side to make a prelubricated latex barrier.

CHAPTER FOUR

Gay Men's Physical and Sexual Health

Ramon is a 55-year-old single teacher, working in a rural community, who presents to his doctor with a history of nocturia, frequency, and intermittent dysuria over the last several months. He sees his doctor rarely, preferring to touch base with a gay doctor in Toronto when he gets there. After discussing diagnostic possibilities, the doctor makes a remark about the 'dreaded' prostate exam and asks Ramon if he would like 'a bullet to bite on.' Ramon feels angry, but also worries that his doctor might notice a looser sphincter tone and figure out that he is gay. He declines the exam, and his doctor expresses irritation at his 'cowardice' and for obstructing medical care.

Greg is a 35-year-old construction worker who has just ended a five-year relationship and is feeling low. He has put on weight and is feeling unattractive and 'old.' His doctor, who is out as a gay man, asks about Greg's sexual life and safe sex practices. With some anxiety, Greg tells the doctor that he was at the bathhouse on the weekend and met 'a cute guy with a great body' who insisted on unprotected intercourse. Greg's doctor expresses concern about possible acute exposure to HIV or other STDs. He asks for Greg's take on what happened, and Greg tearfully describes his sense of loss over his relationship, his loneliness, and his fear of never finding another partner. Greg's doctor explains health options, including acute testing and post-exposure medication protocols, while incorporating pretest counseling. They agree to meet again the next day to implement Greg's decision. Greg is encouraged to bring a friend along for support, and his doctor signals that some counseling sessions on grief and self-esteem would be helpful when the concerns about STDs have been addressed.

Although gay and heterosexual men are physically and anatomically identical, the life expectancy of gay men is twenty to thirty years shorter. The current average age of mortality in gay men is under 50 (Jalbert, 1999). Although AIDS-related mortality is a factor in the shorter life span of gay men, it is not the only threat to their health. Gay men are also vulnerable to cancers, cardiovascular disease, and other sexually transmitted diseases.

With the AIDS epidemic, gay male health has focused primarily on sexually transmitted diseases, particularly HIV (Jalbert, 1999), and prevention and treatment of other diseases has been neglected. This chapter discusses the incidence of cardiovascular disease, cancer, and sexually transmitted diseases in gay men and suggests protocols for standardized, age-appropriate care. It also includes a detailed discussion of gay men's genitourinary, anal, and sexual health, including sexual dysfunction.

Providing Care for Men Who Have Sex with Men

When providing care for gay patients, clinicians should recognize that heterosexual patients indulge in the same spectrum of activities. Care and treatment should focus on behavior and prevention, rather than sexual orientation. This is particularly important, given that some men who engage in same-sex activity do not identify as gay or bisexual (Dean et al., 2000). Even those who do identify themselves as gay may be reluctant to disclose their identity to care providers or to identify with a gay community. This may be due to fear of HIV infection or to negative stereotypes of gay men (Ungvarski & Grossman, 1999). Men who do not identify as homosexual may then have difficulty accessing certain care and supportive services, such as HIV services, where identification with a gay community can increase access to a greater number of supportive networks (Dean et al., 2000).

Preventive Health Care Needs

Cardiovascular Disease

Gay men have a higher risk of stroke, coronary artery disease (CAD), and myocardial infarction than heterosexual men, which is linked to the increased incidence of smoking and decreased access to screening exams among gay men (Jalbert, 1999).

Cancer

Studies of the incidence of cancer among gay men are usually based on urban, self-identified, highly sexually active men, so it is difficult to know to what extent results are applicable to the broader gay population (Dean et al., 2000). Having acknowledged that:

- Gay men are at an increased risk for anal cancer and Hodgkin's disease (Koblin et al., 1996). Gay men's higher risk of anal cancer is associated with a history of sexually transmitted diseases and anal intercourse (Daling et al., 1987).
- Gay men have higher rates of human papillomavirus (HPV) than heterosexual men. According to research results reported by Dr Stephen Goldstone at the International Symposium on HIV in Human Pathology in Paris in April 2000, 60% of HIV-negative men carry the HPV virus, and 90% to 95% of HIV-positive men carry the HPV virus. Although HPV occurs in both HIV-positive and HIV-negative men, it is most prevalent in men in the advanced stages of HIV disease (Palefsky et al., 1998). HPV virus has been shown to be a risk factor for the development of anal cancer. The incidence of anal cancer in gay men is 70 per 100,000 in HIV-positive men, and 35 per 100,000 in HIV-negative men, compared to 0.8 per 100,000 in heterosexual men (Goldstone, 1999). Risk factors for HPV include unprotected receptive anal intercourse, rectal administration of recreational drugs, and a higher number of lifetime sexual partners (Breese et al., 1995).
- Gay men may have a greater risk of lung and colon cancer than heterosexual men, which is due to higher rates of smoking and lower rates of preventive screening for these cancers (Jalbert, 1999).
- Men who have sex with men have a higher incidence of hepatitis B (HBV) infection and, therefore, a higher risk of liver cancer (hepatocellular carcinoma) (Jalbert, 1999).
- Gay men are also at a moderately elevated risk for HIV-related non-Hodgkin's lymphoma (Koblin et al., 1996).
- Gay men have higher rates of Kaposi's sarcoma (KS) than heterosexual men. This is due to the fact that the herpes virus associated with KS is transmitted sexually, as well as the fact than an HIV-

weakened immune system is more vulnerable to KS (Martin et al., 1998). However, the development of KS in gay men has been significantly reduced by highly active antiretroviral therapies. Before the emergence of these therapies, incidence of KS among gay men was dramatically higher than in the general population (Buchbinder et al., 1999).

- The comparatively low survival time among gay men with cancer is attributed to HIV/AIDS comorbidity as well as to delays in detection and treatment, which may be due to barriers gay men face accessing care and poor communication with health care providers (Koblin et al., 1996).

Providing Appropriate Preventive Care

To provide appropriate preventive care for men who have sex with men, physicians should see healthy HIV-negative men under age 40 every two to five years. (Care for HIV-positive men is described in Chapter 7.) After 40, clinicians should review standard age-related health/periodic health exam protocols, including vaccinations, for adult men. (Diet and exercise guidelines are described in Chapter 10.)

Digital rectal exam has been suggested as a method for screening for both prostate and anal cancer. However, screening for prostate cancer remains controversial. The U.S. Preventive Services Task Force gave the digital rectal exam, PSA testing, and ultrasound all 'level D' recommendations. In its view, there is fair evidence to *exclude* screening asymptomatic men for prostate cancer during the annual health exam. The corresponding Canadian agency gave these methods a 'C' grade, indicating no good evidence one way or another. Adding to the confusion are the specialists. The American Urological Association supports screening, as do many urological associations worldwide. There have also been a number of public figures who have encountered prostate cancer and have spoken in favor of screening. One of the potential harms of prostate screening is the high proportion of false positives, including the tendency of the screen to detect minute cancers whose surgical or chemical 'cure' does more damage than the cancer would. An excellent overview of the issues can be found online (www.prostatepointers.org).

Because of the association between HPV and anal cancer, cytology is a more effective screening method for anal cancer in gay men. Some preventive health specialists also suggest that gay men examine their anus and rectum themselves, looking and feeling for irregularities within the anal canal or the prostate, and encourage their partners to report any irregularities noticed during digital anal sexual play. Dr Stephen Goldstone (1999), who reported on the incidence of HPV and anal cancer in gay men, recommends the use of the anal Pap smear as a way of detecting early cytological changes related to HPV virus in the anus.

Although no standard protocol for anal Pap screening exists at this time, a recent study from the Harvard School of Public Health concluded regular anal cytology every two to three years for anal squamous epithelial lesions would not only provide life expectancy benefits for homosexual and bisexual men comparable to other accepted preventive health measures, but would also be cost effective (Goldie et al., 1999). See Chapter 6 for the technique for performing an anal Pap smear.

Sexual Health

Risk of Sexually Transmitted Diseases

Men who have unprotected sex with men are at an increased risk for contracting urethritis, proctitis, pharyngitis, hepatitis A and B (HAV and HBV), syphilis, gonorrhea, chlamydia, herpes, anal and genital warts, and HIV (Dean et al., 2000). HIV-positive, sexually active men may also suffer chronic or life-threatening complications from sexually transmitted diseases (STDs) that are harmless or manageable in HIV-negative men, such as cytomegalovirus, herpes, and HPV-related anal cancer (Dean et al., 2000). Because gay men are at an increased risk for contracting viral hepatitis, all men who engage in same-sex sexual activity should be vaccinated against the A and B strains (Centers for Disease Control and Prevention, 1996).

As many as one-third of men who have sex with men engage in unprotected anal sex at some point in their lives (Hickson et al., 1996). A recent (since 2000) increase in the incidence of STDs in gay men in some urban centers may indicate an increase in rates of unprotected anal sex. This hypothesis is supported by anecdotal reports that fewer men who have sex with men consistently practice safer sex. Gay men's sexual risk taking may be influenced by such psychosocial factors as self-esteem, mood prior to sexual encounter, optimism or fatalism, age, level of education, and substance use (Maurice, 1999).

HIV/AIDS
Of all the sexually transmitted diseases, HIV/AIDS has had the most devastating impact on men who have sex with men:

- Of the more than 702,000 Americans diagnosed with AIDS since 1981, 54% are men who reported same-sex sexual activity (Centers for Disease Control and Prevention, 1999).
- More than 10,000 new HIV infections continue to be recorded among U.S. gay and bisexual men every year (Vittinghoff & Douglas, 1999).
- Since 1998, African-American and Latino men who have sex with men constitute the majority of reported AIDS cases. They tend to become infected at a higher rate and at a younger age than white men (Centers for Disease Control and Prevention, 2000).
- Approximately 25% of active HIV-positive African-American men who have sex with men identify themselves as heterosexual (Centers for Disease Control and Prevention, 2000).

Understanding and Treating Sexual Health Problems

Patients involved in same-sex sexual activity are often reluctant to come out to their physicians or speak about specific sexual practices because of the fear of being patronized, ostracized, or rejected. At the same time, physicians often don't ask specific sexual questions because they fear offending the patient, they are unfamiliar with sexual practice, they are unfamiliar with treatment approaches, or they fear they may leave themselves open to charges of sexual misconduct. If the patient is older, the physician may be reluctant to ask about sexual practices (i.e., a generational obstacle) (Maurice, 1999). See 4.1 for the components of the health history that specifically address actual or potential health problems of gay and bisexual men.

4.1 Identifying Potential Health Problems of Gay and Bisexual Men: Health History

When taking a health history of a gay or bisexual patient, physicians should focus particularly on the following information, which can help identify any potential health problems.

Sexual Activities

1. Sex with men, women, or both
2. Preferred sexual activities (see 4.2)
3. Alternative sexual practices, such as sadomasochism or those

---

that involve the exchange of body fluids such as urine (i.e., 'watersports')
4. Engaging in sex with multiple partners (numbers of partners, gender of partners); settings of sexual activities (i.e., public/commercial sex venues); history of sex with sex trade workers
5. Knowledge of the use of condoms, including application, removal, use of lubricants, and difference in condom efficacy; discussion of contraception where indicated
6. Use of mood-affecting drugs before or during sexual activities
7. An HIV diagnosis in anyone with whom the client has had sex
8. Knowledge base of the risk involved with sexual practices and safer sex practices
9. Knowledge of the signs and symptoms of primary HIV infection
10. Needle exposure (in addition to parenteral drug use); other needle-exposure activities such as tattoos, body piercing

Occupational History

1. Current employment status
2. Client's occupation and responsibilities in relation to risk potential for HIV exposure (health care worker, police officer, commercial sex worker)
3. Any HIV exposures
4. The health care follow-up the client has pursued since exposure

Travel

(especially important in men who conceal their sexual preference and those who are in long-term relationships or married)

1. Sex-seeking behaviors when traveling alone
2. Sexual activities when traveling in areas where the number of AIDS cases is high, such as New York, California, New Jersey, Texas, and Florida, countries such as Haiti, India, Thailand, or sub-Saharan Africa

Medication History and Drug / Alcohol Use History

1. Current prescribed medications
2. Recreational drug use
3. Patterns of alcohol intake
4. Knowledge of drug interactions between the above (e.g., sildenafil citrate [Viagra] and nitroglycerin or inhalation nitrates); see Chapter 9

Medical History

1. Usual source and patterns of seeking health care
2. HIV testing in the past: has it ever been recommended, where was it done, what were the results, and does the client have documentation
3. Treatment for mental health problems, including affective disorders and substance use
4. Treatment for sexually transmitted diseases
5. Postexposure prophylaxis therapy for unprotected sex
6. Use of injection drugs/needle sharing for any reason (including steroids, piercing); client's partner's needle use
7. Any experience with being forced physically or emotionally to have sex or with victimization (e.g., physical violence, hate crimes)
8. Other information about sexual health past or present

Adapted from Ungvarski, P.J., & Grossman, A.H. (1999). Health problems of gay and bisexual men. *Nursing Clinics of North America, 34*(2), 313–31.

Providing Appropriate Sexual Health Care

Although the practice has not been corroborated by studies, it is common for physicians to see sexually active gay men or men having sex with men (in or outside a monogamous relationship) annually, and to see men who engage in high-risk sexual contacts every three to six months – or more frequently if patients need preventive counseling and education. The purpose of these regular visits is to provide screening for HIV and STDs and to review/redefine safer sex practices.

During these visits, for patients from the age of adolescence on, physicians should modify the routine physical examination to cover the following (Wolfe, 1999; Shalits, 1998; Penn, 1997):

- Counsel young men and men having sex with men about tobacco, drug, and alcohol use, how these substances can affect their safer sex practices, and harm-reduction strategies that they can use to manage their use and long-term effects.
- Discuss smoking cessation options and low-risk drinking guidelines with their clients. See Chapter 9 for diagnosis and treatment of substance-related disorders.
- Ask patients about sex with women, contraception options, and any plans for parenthood (see Chapter 3).
- Offer hepatitis A and B vaccination to all men who are sexually active with other men based on standard protocols.
- Discuss any lapses in safer sex practices openly and without judgment. See page 57 for some of the reasons men may engage in unprotected anal intercourse or other high-risk activities as well as strategies for modifying such behaviors.
- Revisit safer sex guidelines, ask specific questions designed to elicit any new information about high, medium, and low-risk activities, and review proper use of a condom. Some patients may ask about using the feminine condom for HIV protection, but its efficacy for anal sex is not yet known. (See patient guidelines in 4.2 for safer sex practices, 4.3 for condom use, and 4.4 for strategies for negotiating safer sex with sexual partners.)
- Discuss HIV testing; offer the test when warranted by risks associated with specific sexual practices or when requested by the patient. (See Chapter 7 for guidelines for HIV testing and counseling.)
- As part of preventive sexual education, explore the risks of specific sexual activities with the patient (see 4.9). In particular, men may be unaware that pathogens such as herpes, gonorrhea, and syphylis can be transmitted oro-anally. Note that the term 'gay bowel disease' used to describe oro-anally transmitted pathogens has been abandoned because it was stigmatizing and implied that heterosexuals do not engage in these practices (Scarce, 1999). This terminology should be avoided.
- Encourage patients to present promptly – either to the physician or to an anonymous STD clinic – for any STD because of associated risks of contracting HIV in the context of other untreated STDs. (See Chapter 7 for discussion about prophylaxsis for exposure to HIV.)

- Review the technique of a monthly testicular self-exam with all men, gay or straight.
- Explore the impact of travel on the health of gay men. Make sure they are up to date on vaccines, such as hepatitis A, B, diphtheria, tetanus, polio, flu, and regional specific pathogens. Review the risk of having sex in specific countries that have cultural, religious, or legal prohibitions, or where homophobic violence is high. Reinforce the need for safe sex practices even while on holiday.
- Provide opportunities for men who have penetrative anal sex to ask specific questions about anal health. In some cases, shame about anal sex or anal play or being labeled as 'gay' may prevent patients from asking for information. Given gay men's high risk of HPV, ensure that patients are aware that HPV can be transmitted through skin-to-skin contact, including digital touch.
- Explore the impact of homophobia in the client's work life, family, personal and couple life, including any past history of sexual harassment, physical and sexual abuse, violent attacks or 'gay bashing.' Review your patient's strategies for avoiding gay bashing and other violent crimes. See 4.5 for tips.
- Conduct basic screens for depression, anxiety, and substance abuse disorders with all gay men.

4.2 Guide to Safer Sex for Men

No Risk

- Dry kissing
- Body-to-body rubbing
- Massage
- Nipple stimulation
- Using unshared inserted sexual devices
- Being masturbated by partner without semen or vaginal fluids
- Erotic bathing and showering
- Contact with feces or urine on intact skin

Theoretical Risk

- Wet kissing
- Cunnilingus with barrier

- Analingus
- Digital-anal and digital-vaginal intercourse, with or without glove
- Using shared but disinfected inserted sexual devices

Low Risk

- Sharing nondisinfected personal hygiene items (razors, toothbrushes)
- Fellatio and ejaculation, with or without ingestion of semen
- Fellatio, with or without condom
- Penile-vaginal intercourse with condom
- Penile-anal intercourse with condom

High Risk

- Cunnilingus without barrier during menstruation
- Penile-vaginal intercourse without condom
- Penile-anal intercourse without condom
- Coitus interruptus (intercourse with withdrawal before ejaculation)

From Canadian Medical Association. (1995). *Counseling guidelines for HIV testing from the expert working group on HIV testing.* Ottawa: CMA.

4.3 How to Use a Condom – Sample Handout for Patients

- Put the condom on the end of your penis. A drop of lube on the head of your penis or in the tip of the condom will increase comfort.
- Hold on to the tip of the condom to squeeze out the air, to leave room for the semen when you ejaculate/'cum.'
- Unroll it all the way down to the base of the erect (hard) penis.
- Put the condom on before you enter your partner.
- You can use a water-based lubricant such as 'K-Y.' Do not use Vaseline or oily products like baby oil. Avoid irritants like nonoxonyl-9 contraceptive gels.

- After you ejaculate, hold on to the base of the condom and pull out while your penis is still hard.
- Use condoms to help prevent diseases.
- Always use a new condom every time you have sex.
- If being penetrated, watch that your partner has followed these suggestions and check that the condom remains on.
- Heat and friction damage condoms. Keep them in a case or in a shirt or jacket pocket.

Adapted from Ottawa–Carleton Health Department. (n.d.). *Protect yourself: Use a condom* (pamphlet).

4.4 Negotiating Safer Sex: Tips for Men Who Have Sex with Men – Sample Handout for Patients

- Consider delaying intercourse until you feel ready and safe. Stick to low-risk activities such as kissing, hugging, and touching (see 4.2).
- Discuss safer sex in a nonsexual setting before going home with somebody.
- Tell potential partners that you only have sex with condoms.
- Avoid alcohol and drug use in the context of sex, as they may cloud your judgment.
- Remember that some people lie about or are unaware of their HIV status or STD health status, so do not take any assurances at face value.
- 'No means no.' If you don't want to proceed with an activity, tell your partner.
- Hand your partner a condom, which sends a clear message that you intend to use one. Put a condom on yourself for the same reason, or put a condom on your partner as part of foreplay.
- Always keep condoms in visible places where you have sex (e.g., on the bed stand near the table, on the bed itself). Keep water-based lube at hand.
- If you are a teen, consider putting a safer sex poster above your bed.
- If you meet resistance about using protection, remember that

safer sex is about health protection and self-esteem. If your partner refuses to allow condoms, think twice about your partner's health status and respect for you.

- Don't rationalize that you can be unsafe 'just once': it takes only one error to contract HIV or another STD.
- If you find that you are putting yourself at risk repeatedly, talk to your doctor about strategies of harm reduction.
- Talk candidly to your doctor about the times you've not used a condom so that you can strategize for the future.

From Peterkin, Allan. (1998, April 20). Negotiating safer sex: Tips for men who have sex with men. *Toronto Star* (Toronto Star Lifeline).

4.5 Avoiding Homophobic Violence: Safety Tips – Sample Handout for Patients

Violence and harassment against the GLBT community is real. Not every attack can be prevented, and it is never your fault if you are attacked or harassed. There are things you can do to reduce your risk. Your primary consideration should be your personal survival.

- Stay alert. Awareness is your best self-defense; know what is happening around you. Be especially careful if you are alone or have been drinking. Watch where you are going and what is going on around you.
- Plan a safe walking route. Use well-lit, busy streets. Keep a safe distance between you and others, and always have an out (somewhere you can turn to run if you feel threatened).
- Walk with friends or a group. When you are out late at night, have a friend accompany you – don't go alone. If you feel uneasy, trust your instincts and go directly to a place where there are other people.
- Project confidence. Walk as if you know where you're going. Stand tall. Walk in a confident manner, and hold your head up.
- Carry a whistle. If you feel threatened, blow your whistle, bang garbage cans, honk your horn, or shout 'fire!' to attract attention. Noise may be your most effective defense.

- Take action if you feel threatened. Cross the street, change direction, run to a place where there are other people, or walk closer to traffic. Step out in the street on the other side of parked cars.
- If you are being followed in a car, turn around and walk quickly in the opposite direction. Get the license plate number and a description, if possible.
- If you are being followed on foot, turn around to let the person know that you have seen them. Immediately cross the street or run toward a place where a number of people will be.
- If you decide to bring someone home, introduce him or her to a friend, acquaintance, or bartender so that someone knows who you left with. Let your date know you spread the word about him or her.

Adapted from Public Health Seattle and King County GLBT website pages.

Safer Sex Practices: Some Questions and Answers

Physicians – particularly those who do not have a lot of experience working with gay or bisexual men – often have questions about safer sex practices and their implications. Here are answers to the most commonly asked questions.

1. *Why do men have unsafe or unprotected sex?*

As we near the end of the second decade of HIV/AIDS, many health care workers are puzzled or distressed by the increased incidence of unprotected sex or 'bare-backing' (intercourse without condoms) among gay or bisexual men. The reasons for the increase in unprotected sex are as many and varied as in the case for heterosexual couples (Barrie et al., 1998; Hospers & Kok, 1995; Elford et al., 1999; Kelly et al., 1998).

- Sex without condoms feels better and enhances feelings of closeness for both partners. Clinicians should acknowledge this fact in the context of discussing behavioral change.
- With the emergence of highly active antiretroviral therapy (HAART) and other successful treatment protocols, there is a growing perception among gay and bisexual men that the epidemic is under control,

that AIDS is treatable, or a 'morning after pill' is available. Since the advent of measuring viral load and use of the word 'undetectable' to describe quantities of virus in blood, many HIV-positive men have come to believe that they are noninfective, or that a partner with a low viral load is not infective. They mistakenly believe that a low viral load in the blood is the same as a low viral load in semen, or that a low or undetectable viral load means a complete absence of virus.

- Alcohol and drug use (including poppers) are often a factor in unsafe sex.
- Certain political organizations deny that HIV is the cause of AIDS. Some individuals who subscribe to this ideology interpret this as a reason to dispense with condoms.
- For some men, partaking in unsafe sex is a manifestation of survivor guilt or complicated bereavement related to multiple losses to AIDS among friends or lovers. An individual may have a fantasy of 'joining' a deceased friend or partner.
- Many men who have recently experienced a breakup of a relationship, a death in the family or of a friend or lover, or some other recent loss may act out complex unresolved conflicts or have periods of sexual de-repression.
- Fatalism about HIV infection is a growing trend among HIV-negative men in urban centers. Some believe that 'it's only a matter of time' before they seroconvert, whether they are careful or not, and this affects their motivation to practice safer sex.
- Some men make snap judgments about a particular or potential partner based on physical appearance (e.g., 'He looks healthy, so he must be safe') or on a partner's assurances that he is negative. Others believe that because they are 'tops only,' their risk of contracting HIV from being the penetrator is nonexistent.
- Partners who are both HIV-positive believe there is no reason to practice safer sex because they are already infected and may be unaware of the risk of cross-infection with other – possibly treatment-resistant – strains of the virus or the fact that cross-infection may nullify clinical gains they have made with new treatments.
- Some men may have been out of the casual sex scene for some time and may lack the skills they need to negotiate safer sex with a new partner.
- Lack of self-esteem and internalized homophobia play a key role in the decision to engage in unprotected sex.
- Men with a history of past sexual abuse may dissociate during sex,

use drugs to allow sexual activity, or accept an abusive element in relationships. This puts them at higher risk of engaging in unprotected sex.

- Certain men choose abstinence as a way to deal with their homosexuality, but may have periods of depression or alcohol/drug bingeing when away on holiday or in a foreign city, and may dispense with usual precautions.
- All human beings long for physical closeness, and this may include skin-to-skin contact and exchange of body fluids as a sign of love and connection. Intercourse without a condom feels more pleasurable, and many men who have practiced safer sex for many years are complaining of 'condom fatigue.'
- In the mid-1980s, the effects of the AIDS epidemic were visible on any street in any gay ghetto in the world. However, a new generation of young men may not have seen gay men sick with AIDS or experienced any losses yet. This may foster ongoing denial about the possibility of contracting HIV – 'it won't happen to me.'
- For some, 'bare-backing' is frequently an act of nihilistic rebellion. In some urban centers, there are reports of 'inoculation parties' where men intentionally choose to become infected. For others, the behavior may represent parasuicidal acting out.
- For some men, particularly those who are homeless or street involved, poverty may be a factor. They may be unable to afford condoms.

4.6 Strategies for Working with Patients Who Engage in Unsafe Sex

Faced with a patient who confesses that he has had lapses in safer sex practices, physicians should be aware that moralizing, scolding, and judgment are not usually effective. Instead, the physician should explore with the patient the reason(s) for the lapses and attempt to provide the information or support the patient needs to maintain safer sex practices. The most successful prevention strategies in North American AIDS service organizations have linked an individual's ability to protect himself with healthy self-esteem and empowerment.

It's important to acknowledge that a gay or bisexual man is unlikely to have completely safe sex every single time from the age of 16 to 80, and that tolerance for health-related risks will vary from person to person. Help the patient to describe a scenario where he is more likely to abandon condom use and how he determines risk in specific encounters. For example:

- Ask your patient about any doubts he might have about the role of HIV in the development of AIDS.
- Ask your patient about how he understands safe sex messages. This is particularly important with young men (including teens or individuals from rural areas) or men who are conflicted about their sexuality (including married men) who may have ignored safe sex messages or found them inaccessible.
- Ask your patient to speak openly about feelings associated with condom use. Acknowledge any sense of loss or frustration the patient may have about condomless sex as normal and universal.
- Ask about the relationship between being 'high' and having sex or, in particular, unsafe sex.
- Explore any history of physical or sexual abuse.
- Ask about his understanding of the impact that treatments have had on the risk of HIV transmission. He may, for instance, mistakenly assume that low viral load in blood means low viral levels in semen.
- Ask an HIV-positive patient to discuss how he would feel if he infected someone. This may allow him to reflect on the nature of his attachment to a partner and unacknowledge any feelings of ambivalence or rage.
- Ask an HIV-positive patient about his sense of belonging to the gay community, and his desire to protect others in the community. This can help encourage health altruistic attitudes that can reinforce safer sex practices.

When counseling patients:

- Explore any educational gaps. Challenge misperceptions and misinformation in a respectful fashion.
- Emphasize with both HIV-positive and HIV-negative men that HAART is not a cure and that it may be unsuccessful with treatment-resistant strains of the virus. Discuss the risk of

cross-infection, and encourage HIV-positive men to practice safer sex with all partners. Explain that the relationships between levels of the virus and infectiousness in blood and semen are still not fully understood. In particular, free-floating virus is not the only way that infection may occur. There may be other reservoirs of virus in the body that are still unmeasurable with current methodologies.

- Provide any loss counseling that may be required (see Chapter 7). Mention the risk of acting out or periods of sexual de-repression as part of grief counseling.
- Reinforce safer sex practices. Discuss strategies patients can use to help them practice safer sex (see 4.2, 4.3, and 4.4). Remind them that partners may be unaware of their STD/HIV status or may lie about it as part of the seduction process. Discuss strategies for eroticizing condom use and maximizing other forms of touch. Consider referring HIV-negative men who are experiencing lapses in safer sex practices to AIDS service organizations, which provide workshops on safer sex strategies as well as ongoing support groups.
- Conduct appropriate screening for depression, dysthymic disorder, anxiety, and suicidality.
- If required, provide counseling about the ongoing impact of sexual abuse (see Chapter 8).
- Consider having a free or donated supply of condoms in the waiting room.

4.7 When an HIV-Positive Patient Puts Others at Risk: The Physician's Role

Many physicians are concerned about how to respond when they know that an HIV-positive patient is putting others at risk. They try to balance their responsibility to their patient with their responsibility to protect public health. In some cases, reporting problem behaviors immediately to public health authorities may harm the physician's therapeutic relationship with the patient, and the patient may be too angry, fearful, or mistrustful to return for follow-up.

When working with an HIV-positive patient who engages in

unsafe sex practices, the physician may find it helpful to contact the local public health department to find out about his or her 'duty to warn' or report, and then share these guidelines and constraints openly with the patient. The physician may also inform the patient about the legal precedents now established in both the United States and Canada, which allow people to be found criminally liable for infecting uninformed partners with HIV.

When helping patients deal with problem behaviors or behaviors that put others at risk, it may be more useful and effective to explore risk and meaning with the patient on a case-by-case basis and encourage the patient to identify and pursue specific behavioral interventions. There is some evidence that criminal prosecution does not result in rehabilitation (Canadian HIV/AIDS Policy and Law Newsletter, 1996), and that support and counseling are more effective strategies in most cases. However, there may be certain individuals who cannot or will not change behaviors around unsafe sex (often because of complicating psychiatric conditions), and in such cases public health law allows public health authorities to issue restraining orders that forbid a person with a communicable disease to engage in conduct that could infect others, or lead to the infecting of others, and to detain anyone who contravenes such an order. Clinicians can call the local public health office for advice around specific cases and risk profiles.

From Health Canada. (1997). *CPA, HIV and psychiatry: A training and resource manual*. Ottawa: Health Canada.

2. How safe is oral sex?

Historically, most North American AIDS service organizations, including the AIDS Committee of Toronto and the Stop AIDS Project of San Francisco, have advised gay men that oral sex (fellatio) is much less risky than penetrative anal sex for transmitting HIV, and this is true. However, recent research (Nycum, 2000) indicates that oral sex – although less risky – is not risk free. Nycum summarizes the following findings:

- In 1992, a Dutch study reported that between 9 and 20 of 102 HIV-positive men may have been infected as a result of oral sex. However, this and other studies may have been flawed due to participants' fear of candidly reporting more risky behaviors, including unprotected anal sex.

- In 1996, the Gay Men's Health Crisis in New York City surveyed 54 studies done in North America and Europe between 1984 and 1995: most reported no significant risk from oral sex; a few identified some risk, but noted that it is significantly lower than from unprotected anal or vaginal sex.
- At the Conference on Retroviruses and Opportunistic Infections in February 2000, the Centers for Disease Control and Prevention reported that, of a group of newly infected individuals, nearly 8% reported oral sex as their only sexual practice/risk factor, and that 8 of 102, or 7.8%, were identified as infected through oral sex.
- At the same conference, researchers reported the results of extensive interviews with 122 people who had acquired HIV within the preceding year. Using very stringent criteria, they concluded that oral sex was responsible for 6.6% of the infections in the cohort and that those who were infected this way believed oral sex presented minimal or no risk of HIV transmission (Buchbinder et al., 1999).
- A San Francisco study determined a 2% risk of HIV infection through the mouth when a man fellated an HIV-positive man in the absence of a condom, and with the presence of ejaculate in the mouth.

Epidemiological studies that attempt to quantify the risk associated with oral sex must rely on the truthfulness of participants, who may find it difficult or embarrassing to admit that they have engaged in unsafe sexual practices. The actual number infected through oral sex may therefore be lower than some of the studies indicate. However, unprotected oral sex probably is riskier than was once thought, and patients should be aware of that fact.

When counseling patients, physicians should review the growing body of literature on seroconversion through oral sex and reinforce that oral sex is not 100% safe. The risk is greater in fellatio on an individual who has recently seroconverted and is, therefore, likely to have a higher viral load in blood and semen, and on individuals who are carrying more virulent or infectious strains of the virus. Despite these risks, oral sex is still considered a 'low risk' activity, particularly when patients follow certain guidelines designed to reduce risk (see 4.2, 4.8).

4.8 Guide to Safer Oral Sex – Sample Handout for Patients

- Avoid performing fellatio:
  - after tooth brushing or flossing;
  - when you have mouth sores, severely chapped lips, gum disease, or a sore throat (when you have a sore throat, there are more white cells in the area fighting the infection, which can be infected by HIV);
  - when you've recently had dental work;
  - if you wear braces (these may abrade penile tissue causing your partner to bleed in your mouth and increasing your risk of exposure);
  - if you have a co-infection or irritation due to another sexually transmitted disease, such as gonorrhea or chlamydia in the back of the throat, which can provide an entry point for the virus.
- Avoid contact with ejaculate or pre-ejaculate, as HIV has been noted to be present in pre-cum.
- Insist that your partner wash before you fellate him. (He may have recently ejaculated and have semen on his penis, even though it may not be visible.)
- Examine your partner's penis for evidence of discharge or sores (i.e., possible signs of other STDs) before sucking him.
- Consider licking the shaft but minimizing tongue contact with the glans or urethra.
- Consider using a condom for oral sex.
- Avoid deep throat penetration. It may irritate the tissue at the back of your throat, and any irritation can provide a more efficient route for HIV into the body.
- Keep dental health up to date to rule out the possibility of abscesses or severe gum disease.
- Be aware that the risk of being exposed to HIV in pre-ejaculate or ejaculate may increase with the length of time fellating, and the risk of developing mouth abrasions may increase with the number of partners.

From Nycum, B. (2000). *The XY survival guide.* San Diego: XY Publishing.

3. *Can a male monogamous couple abandon the use of condoms for anal intercourse?*

Gay couples who intend to be monogamous will often ask physicians this question. To help patients explore this issue:

- Try to have both members of the couple present during counseling.
- Ask both to be tested for HIV after six months with no sexual activity outside the couple.
- Review the couple's communication skills and levels of trust. How do they handle conflict? How likely are they to reveal problematic information to the partner? How willing is each partner to be responsible for the other partner's health or to allow the other to be responsible for his health? If one partner chooses to have a sexual relationship outside the couple, how will that information be revealed?

If the two partners choose to allow sexual activity outside the relationship, discuss steps they can take to reduce risk and protect themselves, including:

- limiting their 'outside' sexual activities to those that are low risk or specifically defined (i.e., no anal penetration, or double condom use for penetration; will receive but not give oral sex)
- being screened regularly for other STDs (see Chapter 6)
- promptly reporting to the partner any mishap or lapse in safe sex activities (e.g., condom breakage, ejaculate in mouth) so the partner can choose to abstain from sex or use condoms until HIV testing indicates that there is no risk.

4.9 Sexual Practices, Risks, and Risk Reduction

According to surveys, heterosexual physicians lack knowledge about specific male sexual practices and often feel uncomfortable discussing them. The following is a primer on specific sexual behaviors that will help physicians answer patients' questions in a matter-of-fact way.

Sexual activity	Risks/issues	Recommended practices
Oral Sex/Fellatio The most practiced activity in male-to-male sex.	Contracting STDs or acquiring HIV (see discussion above).	See 4.8 – Patient Guide to Safer Oral Sex. *Note*: Hygiene is extremely important. Penis should be washed before and after oral sex. If patient has deeper abrasions or bite marks, he should be encouraged to clean with soap and water, apply an antibiotic ointment, such as Polysporin, and consult a physician if redness or swelling occur, so oral antibiotics (like Cloxacillin) can be prescribed.
	The possibility of penile abrasions or bites.	
	Superficial phlebitis to superficial penile veins after rigorous sucking (rare).	
	Sensitive gag reflexes that may make some men uncomfortable performing fellatio.	Have the partner thrust toward the back of the tongue rather than hitting the palate or tonsils, which induces gagging. Suggest the individual: • take only part of the penis in the mouth, or lick the shaft until comfortable with receiving more • breathe through his nose • tilt the head back • vary the rhythm of sucking and keep the penis well lubricated with saliva • practice sucking on bananas, a toothbrush, or a dildo.
Kissing/Oral Contact (including deep kissing)	Risk of HIV/STD transmission is thought to be nonexistent.	Encourage patients to explore kissing as a satisfying, safe activity and a way to enhance physical intimacy.

Sexual activity	Risks/issues	Recommended practices
	Incidents of trauma to lips, tongue, or mouth mucosa are rare in the absence of biting.	

Oral/Anal Contact
(rimming)

Sexual activity	Risks/issues	Recommended practices
Few statistics exist on the popularity of this activity in either male-male, male-female, or female-female couples.	Many patients may be reluctant to tell a physician that they engage in rimming because of the general taboo related to the anus and exposure to fecal matter. Risk of contracting specific bowel pathogens (e.g., giardia, salmonella, shigella, and E. coli), hepatitis A and B, and other viral infections from rimming. Risk of HIV if exposed to blood.	Advise patients to: • be vaccinated for hepatitis A and B • consider using a dental dam over the anus as part of this practice • practice high levels of anal hygiene in themselves and in their partners (e.g., washing the anus with soap and water or using a disposable baby wipe) • inspect the receiving partner's anus for signs of discharge or sores (which may indicate herpetic or other STD lesions) or for the presence of blood from hemorrhoids • avoid douching as this changes the flora of the bowel and may lead to local trauma. Report any changes in bowel habits so physician can take stool cultures and provide treatment; notify sexual partners so they can be screened and treated. See Chapter 6 for protocols for treating bowel pathogens.

Sexual activity	Risks/issues	Recommended practices
Masturbation		
Penile masturbation	No risk of STDs or HIV during solo or mutual masturbation.	Avoid ingesting ejaculate.
		Prevent ejaculate from entering skin abrasions or splashing into eyes.
	Can be a source of guilt and shame for some patients (i.e., because of religious prohibitions or perception it is an 'immature' sexual activity).	Provide reassurance about the role of masturbation in normal healthy sexuality and reinforce its benefits as a tension release at all ages.
	Can become compulsive, particularly in combination with an addiction to pornography; may lead to avoiding human sexual contact; can be a form of AIDS-phobia.	Explore any fears openly and, where appropriate, refer for counseling.
Anal masturbation, digital play, or 'finger fucking'	Some risk of anal trauma; contact with anal pathogens.	Ensure fingers are free of abrasions and/or trauma.
		Keep nails short.
		Wash hands carefully before and after play.
		Avoid oral contact with fingers exposed to anus.
Anal Intercourse (sodomy)		
Villified historically and with emergence of HIV, but up to two-thirds of gay men report practicing anal sex.	High risk of STD and HIV transmission in unprotected anal sex.	When counseling patients about safe, comfortable anal sex, make sure patient wants to engage in receptive anal sex and is not being pressured by his partner.
	Risk of anal trauma. Sphincter tear can occur if a	

Sexual activity	Risks/issues	Recommended practices
	partner's penis is too large or if penetration is too fast, although transmural rectal perforation is rare.	Ensure good communication for both top and bottom.
	Incontinence related to repeated anal sex is thought to be rare, but there is an increased risk if the internal sphincter has been forced repeatedly through use of fists or large dildos.	Encourage recipient to be vocal in saying no or suggesting that his partner slow down when he feels discomfort.
	Perception that anus is dirty, unclean, or shameful.	Promote hygiene but discourage use of douching or invasive anal cleansing procedures. A baby wipe is sufficient to clean the external anus.
	Guilt about wanting to be penetrated (to be a bottom) because of cultural prejudice against passivity or taking on a 'feminine' role.	Suggest a high-fiber diet to keep the rectum clear of feces.
		Suggest erotisizing safer anal sex and using a sheathed penis during foreplay (a condomless penis rubbing against the anus can transmit herpes and HPV).
		Suggest ample water-based lubricant (such as K-Y gel) as any other forms of oil-based lubricant will dissolve condoms. Discourage the use of products containing the spermicide nonoxynol-9 as it irritates anal tissue, which could increase the risk of STD transmission.
		Advise patient to avoid rushing penetration.
		Encourage foreplay, including gentle digital

Sexual activity	Risks/issues	Recommended practices
		play of the recipient's anus prior to penetration. Remind patient not to force deeper penetration (the internal sphincter may take up to 30 seconds to relax).
		Suggest the recipient or bottom not play with his penis before his partner's penis is inserted as this causes external sphincter constriction.
		Encourage patients being penetrated to breathe deeply to encourage relaxation.
		Encourage partners to experiment with the positions they find most comfortable. Altering positions to where the bottom gradually sits on his partner's penis may allow better control of penetration.
		Encourage patients to avoid drugs when being penetrated, as these may obscure physical cues related to anal tearing and laceration or sphincter tears. Although drugs such as poppers are thought to dilate the anal sphincter, they may cloud judgment leading to unsafe sex activity.
		Instruct patients to stop anal penetration if bleeding occurs or if they experience pain.

Sexual activity	Risks/issues	Recommended practices
		Some feelings of rectal fullness, gas, or mucous discharge after penetration are normal short-term sequelae of anal sex.
		Review the risks of particular STDs through anal sex and review safer sex guidelines.
		Remind patients of the risk of HIV transmission from pre-ejaculate; reinforce that a condomless penis should not be inserted into the rectum even momentarily.
		Encourage the patient to have a strategy regarding condom breakage or failure (e.g., call a physician immediately for postexposure prophylaxis). Some couples use double condoms (i.e., 'double bagging') for protection.

Adapted from Goldstone, S. (1999). *The ins and outs of gay sex*. New York: Random House. Anal intercourse from Bell, R. (1999, February). ABC of sexual health: Homosexual men and women. Clinical Review. *British Medical Journal, 318*(13), 452–4.

4.10 Patient Guide to More Comfortable Anal Penetration

Anatomically, the anus is enervated by S4, the same nerve that supplies the genitals. The anal canal is externally sensitive to touch and temperature and internally sensitive to stretch sensation. The external sphincter is made of striated muscle and can be controlled voluntarily. The internal sphincter is made of smooth muscle with autonomic nervous system enervation, which responds primarily to stretch stimuli.

If you are experiencing pain when being penetrated, do the following exercises on a bed in private until you are confident you can accommodate a penis:

- Lie on a towel on a bed or on your back in a warm bath.
- Raise your knees toward your chest.
- Explore the perianal areas with a finger covered with a lubricant, such as petroleum jelly. (*Note*: before intercourse, substitute with a water-based lubricant because petroleum jelly damages condoms.)
- Apply gentle pressure by moving a finger in a circle round the anus – this will relax the sphincter enough to allow you to insert one digit.
- Once your anus can comfortably accommodate the finger, begin to stretch the sphincter with circling motions inside the anus. After several sessions, you will be able to insert a second finger and to continue.
- You can further dilate the anus by relaxation, not stretching, or by using an anal dilator of the St Mark's type or a self-retaining 'butt plug' left in situ on a regular basis. Soft rubber butt plugs can be purchased in most sex shops.

Adapted from Bell, R. (1999, February). ABC of sexual health: Homosexual men and women. Clinical Review. *British Medical Journal, 318*(13).

Sexual Dysfunction

Twenty to 30 million American men are affected by erectile dysfunction (Chan, 2001), and the incidence of sexual dysfunction in otherwise healthy gay men is thought to be no different than in heterosexual men. Surprisingly, little has been written about sexual dysfunction in gay men. This may be due to the fact that gay men are not being asked or they are reluctant to discuss sexual functioning and practices with their physicians.

In gay and bisexual men, high levels of internalized homophobia or unresolved issues about sexual identity can complicate their sexual functioning. This means that the definition of sexual dysfunction for gay and bisexual men must be broadened to include discomfort with any of the sexual practices that the patient wishes to engage in (e.g., difficulty performing fellatio or being penetrated anally).

Erectile Dysfuntion

Erectile dysfunction is defined as the consistent inability to achieve and maintain penile erection to permit satisfying vaginal or anal sexual intercourse, although anal sex is rarely mentioned in erectile dysfunction educational campaigns. Although the manifestations of erectile dysfunction are the same in both gay and straight men, anal penetration requires a more rigid erection than vaginal penetration. Given the variability of sexual practice and sexual roles among men who have sex with men, it's also conceivable that a 'bottom,' who does not have a full erection during sex, may complain less vociferously to his doctor than a man who customarily acts as a 'top.' The incidence of erectile dysfunction in gay and bisexual HIV-positive men is reportedly high. Up to 30% of HIV-positive men experience erectile dysfunction, due to the underlying disease with peripheral neuropathies, low testosterone, and also the side effects of HAART drugs, specifically DDI and its analogs (Leiblum & Rosen, 2000).

For all patients, effective management of erectile dysfunction or discomfort with certain sexual practices begins with counseling and sexual education. Counseling may help the patient to identify issues such as relationship conflict, alcohol, or drug and tobacco use, and outline strategies to decrease performance anxiety and increase communication around sex. If the cause of erectile dysfunction appears to be psychogenic and performance anxiety is high, consider couple counseling, individual counseling, referral to support groups, or a trial of sildenafil (Viagra) to restore confidence. Referral to a gay-affirmative sexologist, urologist, or sex therapist may be advised.

It is important to acknowledge that some gay men may not be in regular or exclusive relationships, and some counseling strategies may not be suitable with new or anonymous partners. Physicians should be aware that some HIV-positive men have been denied medical help for erectile dysfunction 'because they shouldn't be having sex anyway,' so clinicians should always ask about previous treatment attempts and encounters with medical personnel.

Sadomasochism

Men involved in sadomasochistic activities face health risks, such as:

- secondary STD infections, spread via shared or poorly cleaned toys, props, or surfaces, especially when engaging in activities that draw blood
- exposure to blood and possible HIV transmission, particularly during anal play (including anal fisting) – due to the delicacy of rectal mucosae and the concentration of blood vessels in the rectum
- physical injury and damage to internal organs from whipping or flagellation
- infection of the urinary tract and injury to the urethra during urethral catheterization
- exposure to blood-borne diseases from piercing activities.

To reduce the health risks associated with these activities, patients should be advised of the following:

- Ensure all dildos, gloves, whips, and other toys are cleaned thoroughly. Cover dildos with condoms. Toy insertion should be gradual and never forced. If blood is drawn, any toy or surface that may be contaminated must be sterilized or disposed of.
- Ensure the tips of whips are cleaned with peroxide, particularly if blood is drawn (HIV and hepatitis transmission are possible).
- Never deliver blows to the kidneys, head, or genitals. Wear gloves if wielding the whip, and avoid contact with droplets of blood propelled from broken skin.
- Dispose of any needles and piercing implements safely after use. Never share needles.
- Do not consume drugs and alcohol during play as they impair judgment and heighten the tendency to overextend comfort and safety levels. Tops may become overly vigorous, while bottoms may submit to more extreme treatment than their bodies are reasonably able to handle.
- Avoid direct contact with fluids, orifices, cuts, or fresh piercings. Use surgical or latex gloves when manually contacting body fluids. Gloves reduce the risk of fluids entering the body through open cuts or nicks and minimize the danger of scratching or scraping delicate tissue with one's fingernails (i.e., when fisting) or contract-

ing STDs. Use rubber calving gloves for fisting. For more information, consult (www.safeguards.org/tips/sandm.htm) on the safety of fisting.

- Use lubricant on gloved hands if they are entering a partner's anus or vagina to prevent friction and the associated tearing of delicate tissues.
- When engaging in piercing activities, observe the same precautions as professional body piercing services (see Chapter 10); sterilize all implements and services before and after piercing; the person doing the piercing should wear gloves.
- When engaging in watersports, advise only those who have the knowledge and expertise to use catheterization equipment. Only sterile equipment should be used. Avoid getting urine in the rectum, vagina, eyes, or mouth.
- When engaging in scenes that incorporate bondage or suspension, conduct regular checks to ensure circulation to extremities is not restricted and body weight is correctly supported to prevent compression damage to nerves.

4.11 Glossary of S/M and Other Terms

The following is a glossary to sexual terms and activities, including sadomasochism.

BD: Bondage (restraining a person) and discipline (erotic punishment).

Bottom: Submissive participant.

D/S: Dominance (in charge of another/others) and submission (submitting to the dominant figure).

Edge play: Activities considered more radical than other S/M activities, which may involve a heightened level of danger. Includes knife play (used for cutting, scratching, intimidation), blood play (piercing, shallow cutting activities that draw blood), electricity (inflicting electric shocks), and breath play (controlled strangulation or asphyxiation).

EPE: Erotic power exchange; wherein S/M roles are engaged only during sexual interaction.

Fetish: Erotic attraction to an inanimate object, material, mode of dress, or scenario.

Fisting: Insertion of a fist and potentially a portion of one's arm into the rectum or vagina of a partner.

Piercing: Play piercing involves the temporary, shallow insertion of sterile needles for erotic stimulation. Similar precautions as with permanent body piercing should be observed, including the sterilization of piercing sites, equipment, and hands. Permanent piercing may also be practiced and should only be performed by those who are knowledgeable regarding correct placement, insertion, and possible complications.

Safe word: A term agreed upon in advance that stops a scene, used to distinguish between a desirable 'no' and a legitimate command to end the scene. As 'no' and 'stop' may be part of the erotic power exchange, it is best to select an unrelated word to be used in case of emergency, or if a person becomes uncomfortable with the scene and no longer wishes to continue.

Scat: Involves playing with feces, either one's own or that of a partner.

Scene: The performance of or engaging in S/M activities. May range from a nonsexual exchange of words to an intense round of bondage and flagellation. It is a situation agreed upon and staged by participants, incorporating any variety of activities.

S/M: Sadomasochism. Sadism is deriving pleasure from giving extreme stimulation; masochism is the derivation of pleasure from receiving extreme stimulation.

SSC: Stands for 'safe, sane, consensual,' the three encouraged regulations within the S/M community. All activities are to be enjoyed in a safe manner in spite of inevitable risk, using appropriate precautions, not impaired by intoxicants that may cloud judgment, and between consenting parties only.

Switch: A person who may be either dominant or submissive; one who derives equal pleasure from assuming the role of top or bottom.

Top: Dominant participant.

Toys: Props used during play (e.g., whips, restraints, dildos).

TPE: Total power exchange; wherein partners live out an S/M relationship in all aspects of their interaction with one another, at all times observing set rights and obligations established by each party involved.

Vanilla: Refers to non-S/M erotic practices and those who engage in them.

Watersports: Activities involving urination.

Whipping: Use of implements to administer blows, usually but not exclusively to the back or buttocks.

From Jacques, T., et al. (1999). *The safe edge: SM 101*. Toronto: AIDS Committee of Toronto.

Anal and Genitourinary Health

Testicles

The incidence of conditions of the testicles, such as epididymitis, torsion, varicocoele, mass, and hydrocoele, is no different in gay men than in straight men. Physicians should review the testicular self-exam with all gay patients, regardless of age. A quick review of men's genitourinary health management can be found online (www.emedicine.com).

Anus and Rectum

The incidence of hemorrhoids, both internal and external, is no higher in gay men than in heterosexual men, and treatments are the same.

Anal fissures are usually the result of a traumatic event, such as the passing of a large stool, and are commonly indicated by pain or bleeding on defecation or after anal sex. Compared to constipation and straining, which lead to spasm of the sphincters and an increased risk of tears, anal sex is thought to be an infrequent cause of anal fissures. Management tends to be conservative: the use of stool softeners, sitz baths, and glycerine suppositories. A paste of .25–.5% nitroglycerine may also be applied twice daily until symptoms subside. If an internal sphincter tear leads to sphincter spasm, this often causes decreased blood supply and delays healing of the sphincter. Surgical interventions such as internal anal sphincterectomy, anal dilatation, or local injection of botulism toxin by a surgeon may be required.

Proctitis occurs more frequently in men who have sex with men who contract anal STDs. Symptoms are usually rectal bleeding and mucous discharge. If the infection is due to herpes simplex, pain can be significant. Diagnosis is usually made by proctoscopy or sigmoidoscopy. Culture swab and sensitivity for evidence of gonorrhea, syphilis, chlamydia, shigella, salmonella, and herpes should be performed. Antibiotic treatment is offered to the patient, often in combinations with other agents, such as Flagyl (see Chapter 6).

Prostate

The comparative incidence of prostate cancer in gay men is unknown, as is the impact of prostatic cancer on enjoyment of passive penetrative anal sex. Screening for prostate cancer and the treatment for benign prostatic hypertrophy (BPH) involve the same procedures for both gay men and straight men. However, it is important to advise gay male patients not to engage in penetrative anal sex before PSA screening as this will lead to false elevations of PSA and possibly unnecessary interventions. Clinicians are also advised to not make presumptive comments or jokes about 'enduring' rectal prostatic exams; these are offensive to gay men. To review treatment and screening protocols, including use of the PSA diagnostic test, see standard urological texts. Treatment of prostatitis is outlined in Chapter 6. Gay men who have been treated for prostatic cancer or had surgery for BPH or prostatic cancer may have difficulty accessing support to help them deal with the impact on their lives. A useful website can be found at (www.mindspring.com/ujerrysh/prosstop.html).

Penis

Physicians should review the risks of priapism and resulting vascular injury with patients who engage in recreational use of Viagra or wear 'cock rings' (i.e., restrictive bands worn at the base of the penis to prolong erection). Any patient who has an erection that won't subside within half an hour of nonstimulation should be advised to present to the emergency room. Needle evacuation or injection of epinephrine into the corposa may be necessary to avoid secondary scarring of erectile tissue.

Trauma to the penis can occur in a number of ways, including sexual bites, piercing of the glans, or a tearing off of the frenulum during sex. The insertion of a urethral catheter or other object as part of S/M play can also lead to urethral trauma and strictures. Superficial phlebitis of the dorsal veins of the penis, secondary to rigorous oral sex, usually responds to aspirin, warm compresses, and rest. Inflammation of the glans, penis, or foreskin, secondary to superficial, candidal infections, is not uncommon in gay men, and it usually responds to standard topical anticandidal treatment, such as Nystatin or clotrimazole. Patients may report erythema after use of latex condoms or spermicide, although this is rare. Erythema suggests an allergy and can be managed by avoiding latex products or wearing a lambskin condom with a superimposed external latex condom (lambskin condoms alone are not effective in preventing HIV exposure). For treatment of specific STDs, such as gonorrhea, syphilis, and HPV, see Chapter 6.

CHAPTER FIVE

Gay, Lesbian, and Bisexual Adolescent Physical and Mental Health

Loren is a 19-year-old straight-A student from an Orthodox Jewish family. After watching an Oprah program on gay teens, she mentions to her parents that she has had crushes on girls and doesn't see anything wrong with that. Her father responds that if he had a child who was gay, he would sit Shiva as if she had died and have no further contact with her. Loren experiences her father's comment as a threat. She becomes more obsessed about getting high grades and begins to experiment with controlling her food intake. Her family physician notices her weight loss and explores family stressors, but because he is aware of her religion's position he does not ask about issues of sexuality. Loren's eating disorder becomes worse.

Zak, a good-looking, athletic, affable 16-year-old, has been having physical fights with his father. Because he fears that he may be gay, Zak is thinking of committing suicide. He goes alone to the community emergency department where the intake worker comments, 'I bet you can't keep the ladies away.' Zak contemplates leaving.

 The male staff doctor overhears the remark. When taking Zak's history the doctor says, 'I'm sorry the secretary made some assumptions about you. Can we start over?'

 The doctor then conducts a sensitive sexual history and gives Zak an opportunity to talk about his sexual concerns. He also arranges a sensitivity workshop on gay and lesbian teens for the ER staff.

Adolescence is a vulnerable time for all youth, regardless of sexual orientation. All teens experience body changes, a growing desire for autonomy, an increasing interest in sex and sexuality, disenchantment with adults, changing relationships with parents and siblings, pressure from peers to use alcohol and drugs, and concerns about school, career, and relationships. In terms of health care, adolescents are an underserved population: since 1950, they are the only population group that has not experienced an improvement in their overall health. Much of the morbidity and mortality that occurs in this age group is related to risk behaviors (such as unsafe sex, using drugs or alcohol, or driving while impaired) or mood disorders (depression and suicide). Effective interventions to reduce or prevent disease and illness in this age group can have a profound impact on how adolescents will experience the rest of their lives.

While all youth have health needs, the growing body of literature on gay, lesbian, and bisexual (GLB) teens confirms that they have health care problems and needs distinct from heterosexual youth (Lock & Steiner, 1999). This has led an increasing number of adolescent caregivers to consider the care of gay, lesbian, and bisexual youth a subspecialty of adolescent medicine. Yet, because of their invisibility and stigmatization, the needs of young lesbians and gay men are often ignored (Durby, 1994). The standard reference for physicians interested in gay adolescent health is *Lesbian and Gay Youth: Care and Counseling* (Ryan & Futterman, 1998).

The Physical and Mental Health Needs of Gay and Lesbian Youth

The most prevalent health and social problems gay and lesbian youth experience are depression, family rejection, suicide, substance abuse, running away, homelessness, prostitution, truancy, victimization, violence, STDs, high-risk sexual behavior, and poor health maintenance (Brotman et al., 2000). As the following facts illustrate, the stresses on homosexual youth and their health needs differ significantly from those on straight youth. Lesbian, gay, and bisexual youth are particularly vulnerable to family issues, violence and hate crimes, substance use, suicide, and HIV and other STDs.

Family Issues

- 19% of gay men and 25% of lesbians suffer physical abuse by family members as a result of their sexual orientation (Philadelphia Lesbian and Gay Task Force, 1992).

- Conflict over their sexual orientation forces approximately 25% of adolescent gay males to leave home (Remafedi, 1987).
- Almost half of homeless and runaway youth self-identify as gay or lesbian (Traveler's Aid: Victim Services, 1991; Kruks, 1991).

Violence and Hate Crimes

- Gay and lesbian youth are particularly vulnerable to antigay hate crimes (Dean et al., 1992).
- Hate crimes against lesbian and gay youth are often perpetrated by family members and community authorities (Herek, 1989).
- Gay and lesbian youth are often forced to leave home and/or school as a result of homophobic victimization and abuse (American Academy of Pediatrics, 1993).

Substance Use

- Approximately 30% of adolescent lesbians and gay men report excessive alcohol use, while nearly 25% of study respondents report using illicit drugs (D'Augelli & Hershberger, 1993).
- The adolescent lesbian and gay male cohort accounts for a significant percentage of reported substance use in the gay community (Stall et al., 1986).
- Use of substances other than alcohol is more prevalent among gay youth than older gay men (Addictions Research Foundation, personal communication).
- Substance use makes gay and lesbian youth even more vulnerable to health risks, such as HIV infection and suicide (Futterman et al., 1993). Alcohol and drug use are linked with an increase in high-risk behavior, including condom noncompliance (Chitwood & Comerford, 1990).

Suicide

- Suicide is the second most frequent cause of death among youth between the ages of 15 and 24 (Fisher & Shaffer, 1990). Gay and lesbian youth account for 30% of all teen suicides, but only 10% of the teen population (Gibson, 1989).
- Gay and lesbian adolescents are two to three times more likely to attempt suicide than their heterosexual peers (Jalbert, 1999).

- 42% of gay and lesbian youth make at least one suicide attempt. The methods used, in order of frequency, include overdose, alcohol abuse, use of firearm, use of razor blade, knife, car, and fire (Hershberger et al., 1996).
- 53% of gay street youth report attempting suicide at least once; 47% report multiple attempts (Kruks, 1991).
- As a group, gay male youth and adults account for the largest percentage of suicide attempts. Risk factors include coming out at a young age, gender atypical appearance, low self-esteem, substance abuse, running away, prostitution, sexual abuse, and arrest for misconduct (Remafedi et al., 1991).
- Researchers note a significant positive correlation between attempting suicide and rejection, recognition of being gay, early first sexual experience, stress arising from coming out at a young age, and substance abuse (Kruks, 1991).
- Gay and lesbian youth who attempt suicide tend to have lost more friends as a result of their homosexuality, have low self-esteem, be more open about their sexual orientation, experience more victimization, and have more mental health problems than other gay and lesbian adolescents (Hershberger et al., 1996).

HIV and Other STDs

- Worldwide, half of all people with HIV became infected between the ages of 15 and 24 (Goldsmith, 1993). The median age of people with HIV has dropped from over 30 during the 1980s to 25 by 1991, with 25% of newly infected persons aged 22 or younger (Rosenberg et al., 1994).
- Studies estimate 30% of all young gay males are infected with HIV; young gay men have a one in five chance of being infected before age 25 (Coates et al., 1995).

Factors that Put GLB Youth at Risk

Many of the health and social problems gay teens experience are due to the fact that they internalize hostile messages from society about homosexuality (see 5.1). Lack of ease with sexual orientation is associated with high risks to overall health (Lock & Steiner, 1999), and homophobia may impede the natural development of sexual identity during adolescence (Gochros & Bidwell, 1996).

Many gay teens who hide or deny same-sex attraction develop a false self: a pretending self who complies with social assumptions that gays and lesbians are deviant or unhappy. This kind of dissimulation damages an emerging self-esteem and hampers the normal development of trusting, intimate, open relationships within which secrets and feelings can be explored. Because of their fear of ostracism, ridicule, violence, and rejection (including expulsion from their families or support networks), gay teens must often explore the feelings and behaviors of their same-sex attraction in isolation. In fact, 80% of gay and lesbian youth experience severe social isolation (Hetrick et al., 1987). One of the main sources of stress for many gay teens is the school environment (see 5.2), and this may partly explain the high rates of truancy among gay and lesbian youth.

The stress on gay teens leads some to over-function or become perfectionists. They become star athletes or students, often at the expense of developing an authentic sexual self or intimate relationships. Their struggles often go undetected because they have chosen socially acceptable defenses against psychosexual conflicts. Other gay teens react differently. For some, the stress of developing their sexual identity may interfere with school socialization and success and with the learning process. Some youth develop significant emotional and mental health problems.

Lesbian, gay, and bisexual adolescents' unease with sexual orientation and their sense of isolation is compounded by a lack of 'out' role models, age-appropriate information and materials, or places for gay teens to meet (i.e., non-bar or nonsexualized venues). Gay groups, clubs, and media publications seldom address the developmental concerns of gay teens. Social isolation from their peers, and lack of appropriate outlets for adolescent socialization, leads many young lesbians and gay men to seek out peers in more adult, high-risk environments where they are more likely to be exploited. Gay and lesbian teens may also suffer immuno-suppressing stress, depression, and low self-esteem due to stigmatization and invisibility, and this may lead to high-risk behaviors as negative coping mechanisms.

5.1 General Stresses on Gay and Lesbian Teens

- Invisibility
- Family assumption that homosexuality is a defect

- Stigmatization
- Stereotypes imposed by others
- Emphasis of homophobia and heterosexist attitudes in teen culture
- Absence of visible, positive role models
- Managing identity day to day in terms of disclosure (i.e., some people know, some don't)
- Disruption in peer relations when homosexuality is suspected or disclosed
- Interpersonal conflict related to disclosure
- The keeping of secrets in close relationships, precluding further intimacy
- Isolation from gay community supports
- Discrimination, harassment, violence
- Health-related anxieties, including HIV

Adapted from Gochros, H., & Bidwell, R. (1996). Lesbian and gay youth in a straight world: Implications for health care workers. In K.J. Paterson (Ed.), *Health care for lesbians and gay men: Confronting homophobia and heterosexism* (pp. 1–17). New York: Harrington Park Press.

5.2 School Stresses on Gay and Lesbian Teens

- 97% of high school students report regularly hearing homophobic comments from their peers; 53% report hearing such remarks from school staff (Massachusetts Governor's Commission on Gay and Lesbian Youth, 1993).
- In general, the public school system is unwilling to protect gay and lesbian students against harassment and discrimination (Fontaine, 1997). Gay and lesbian victims of harassment in school often do not disclose the incidents out of fear of further victimization and negative consequences (Sears, 1992).
- Schools fail to create a safe environment for gay and lesbian youth. Information about homosexuality is rarely taught, and gay and lesbian students do not have role models or support within the school (Fontaine, 1997). Homophobia, heterosexism, exclusion of homosexuality from school curricula, and absence of resources contribute to the invisibility of gay and lesbian youth in secondary schools (Herr, 1997).

- More than half of prospective teachers admit they would not be comfortable working with openly homosexual colleagues (Sears, 1992), while 85% oppose integrating homosexual subject matter into existing curricula and 77% would discourage classroom discussion of gay and lesbian issues (Sears, 1992).
- Approximately 25% of guidance counselors rate themselves highly competent in meeting the needs of gay and lesbian youth; however, less than 20% have received formal training on serving this student population (Price & Telljohan, 1991).

Barriers to Care

Gay and lesbian teens, in both Canada and the United States, are hesitant to access health care because of fear of judgment and humiliation (Dempsey, 1994). When they do seek out care, they encounter many barriers, including practitioners' heterosexist language; inadequate social/sexual history taking; the absence of any representation of lesbian or gay youth in health care settings; lack of educational materials for gay, lesbian, or bisexual youth; practitioners who do not have the knowledge or skills to provide complete, satisfactory answers to their questions; and concerns about confidentiality (Nelson, 1997).

Preventive Care

To provide effective primary care for this population, practitioners need the skills to take a sensitive patient history, identify risks, and identify interventions that will reduce risk. The Canadian Task Force on Preventive Health Care (CTFPHC) has identified several specific, evidence-based interventions that should be included in the adolescent periodic health exam. The guidelines are available online (www.ctfphc.org/) and are summarized in 5.3.

5.3 Best Practices for Periodic Health Exam in Adolescents

- Clinical tobacco cessation interventions
- Counseling to promote regular physical activity
- Counseling to prevent motor vehicle injuries (seat belt use, avoidance of driving while impaired)

- Counseling to encourage the use of bicycle helmets
- Counseling to avoid HIV infection: abstinence, monogamy, and/or condom use
- Counseling to avoid sharing needles for injection drug use
- Counseling to avoid unintended pregnancy: sexual abstinence or regular contraceptive use
- Counseling to lower risk of cervical cancer: use of barrier contraceptive or sexual abstinence
- Ensuring up-to-date primary series of immunizations; after their primary series in infancy and early childhood, adolescents should be considered for hepatitis B vaccine and varicella vaccine (if no documented infection in childhood)
- Consider MMR booster
- Td booster – age 14 to 16 and every ten years thereafter
- Pap smears for sexually active women

Adolescent Pregnancy

- Folic acid supplementation in women considering pregnancy
- HIV testing for high-risk youth and pregnant women (see Chapter 7)
- Routine urine culture in pregnant women at 12 to 16 weeks of pregnancy

History taking is key to providing high-quality preventive primary care. In the nonsexually active adolescent, a physical examination is unlikely to contribute significantly to overall preventive care. The adolescent's height, weight, and blood pressure should be documented, and other exam maneuvers may help build rapport and confidence between patient and practitioner.

Adolescent Sexual Health

Adolescents carry a disproportionate share of morbidity from sexually transmitted infections. Prevalence rates for most STDs peak in young people between the ages of 16 and 24, and the relatively high rate of HIV infections in the 20 to 25 age group indicates a failure of HIV prevention efforts with teens. While all adolescents are at risk of STDs, gay youth – who face the additional developmental challenge of negotiating a minority sexual identity – are the most vulnerable. Physicians can play a vital role in helping adolescents who are sexually active to reduce the risk of STDs, including HIV, improve their health, and enhance their ability to survive the difficult developmental transition from adolescence to adulthood. The goal of adolescent sexual health is to screen all adolescents and identify those at risk, educate youth about STD/HIV transmission, and counsel them about strategies to reduce their risk.

Sexual History and STD Screening

An adolescent's need for STD screening is based on the level of risk identified in the sexual history. For items that should be discussed when taking an adolescent's sexual history, see 5.4. In general:

- Adolescent males who are sexually active with other males should be routinely screened for STDs, including gonorrhea, syphilis, chlamydia, and enteric pathogens. (See Chapter 6 for a more thorough review of STD screening.)
- Lesbian adolescents who have sex only with other women are at low risk for STDs and HIV. However, a lesbian identity does not preclude sexual activity with men. All adolescent women should be offered relevant, realistic contraceptive and STD prevention advice.

5.4 Sexual History Taking

Behavior

- Same-sex and opposite-sex partners
- Age of coitarche and ages of partners
- Consensual vs. nonconsensual sex
- Past history of sexual abuse
- Types of sexual experience:
  'Outercourse': kissing, petting, masturbation
  'Intercourse': vaginal-penile, oral-genital, oral-anal, anal-genital
- Condom use
- Concurrent substance abuse
- Sex for food or money

Identity / Sexual Orientation Disclosure

- To family
- To friends, partners/roommates
- To classmates/coworkers
- To teachers/supervisors/counselors

Adapted from Hoffman, N., & Ocepek, D. (1994). *Protocol for primary care of lesbian and gay adolescents.* Conference on the Primary Care Needs of Lesbian and Gay Adolescents. Washington, DC: Health Resource and Services Administration, December 5–6.

Counseling and Education

A recent survey (Crosby et al., 2000) of young adults seen in an STD clinic underscores the misperceptions that youth have about STDs and the importance of education:

- Nearly half the group believed douching protected against STDs.
- Almost 40% thought urinating after sex fought off STDs.
- One in five believed birth control pills protected against STDs.
- 16% percent thought washing their genitals after sex was effective protection.

Because adolescents tend to be infrequent visitors to primary services, it is essential for physicians to provide anticipatory care even during visits for episodic illness (see 5.5).

5.5 Physicians' Guide to Anticipatory Adolescent Sexual Health Care

- Anticipatory care starts at the door to your office. Display posters, brochures, and books about sexuality prominently. This will tell teenage patients that you recognize that sexuality is an important health issue.
- Before asking screening questions, explain that any information the youth gives you will be kept confidential. Reassure all

adolescents that questions about sexuality are a routine part of any health visit for that age group.

- Normalize different types of sexual activity and set an open, nonjudgmental tone: 'Some of my patients your age date boys, some girls, some both.' This can be a very powerful tool with most people, but especially with youth. Begin with the assumption that many adolescents have experimented with same-sex activity and that questions about identity are normal.
- Use inclusive questions to set the tone: 'There are many ways of having sex with another person, such as kissing, hugging, and caressing different parts of the body as well as having sexual intercourse. Have you had any kinds of sexual experience? Were they with boys or girls or both? Have you ever been attracted to any boys or girls? Are you now? Do you have any concerns about your sexual feelings or the sexual things you have been doing?'

Adolescent Mental Health

To understand and treat the mental health needs of gay, lesbian, and bisexual youth, physicians should recognize the stressors and health risks discussed above. In addition, they should know something about the developmental process involved in sexual identity.

The Development of Sexual Identity

The development of sexual orientation is a complex interplay of biological, psychological, social, cultural, religious, and familial factors (D'Augelli, 1996). Most gay teens report a sense of sexual attraction or fascination with members of the same sex well before puberty but do not come to identify these feelings as homoerotic until later. Sexual encounters are commonly the means through which gay and lesbian adolescents gain knowledge of homosexuality (Paroski, 1987). Although both boys and girls are having their first same-sex experiences and are identifying themselves as gay or lesbian earlier than previous generations, the consolidation of sexual identity may not occur during adolescence.

Troiden (1989) summarizes the developmental phases of gay teen identity as follows:

- **Sensitization.** Sensitization usually occurs in prepuberty. The child feels different but does not attach the difference to sexuality. He or she may have same-sex crushes or fascinations, but they are not sexually derived. The child may also exhibit some gender atypical behaviors that are noted by others (e.g., tomboy characteristics for girls or effeminate traits in boys), but such differences are not universal.
- **Identity confusion.** Identity confusion usually occurs during the teenage years. The teenager starts to wonder about certain feelings or considers that certain preoccupations could be considered gay or lesbian. This frequently causes anxiety because these thoughts are often inconsistent with the teen's emerging sense of self. The teen also begins to wonder if he or she is now a member of a stigmatized group. He or she may weigh negative cultural stereotypes of gays and lesbians and assess the physical and emotional risks of being gay or lesbian in the culture, often concluding 'I'm not like that.' As a result, the teen may deny his or her feelings and avoid sexual behavior altogether or modify gay typical behaviors and engage in heterosexual dating and sexual relationships. Some teens engage in verbal or physical harassment of other vulnerable gay teens, or express antigay sentiments as a way of denying their own attractions. Others may use drugs or alcohol either to subdue or express their sexual urges.
- **Identity assumption.** The teen may come to accept same-sex romantic and physical attractions. This allows the youth to emerge into the next phase of identity development where the teen sees herself or himself as lesbian, gay, or 'queer' (a term often used by youth). The youth's realization of sexual identity continues to be complicated by internalized homophobia and discomfort. Positive interaction with other gay people allows socialization and acquisition of new coping skills.
- **Commitment.** The youth accepts her or his lesbian, bisexual, gay, or queer identity and allows herself or himself to live as a gay person, pursuing same-sex emotional and physical attachments.
- **Coming out.** The final stage of coming out to friends, family, peers, and colleagues usually follows the commitment phase.

Although Troiden's phases were based primarily on the developmental experience of gay males, Young (1995) developed a similar developmental model for lesbian teens, which consists of the emergence of emotional relationships; processing the implications of these relationships for identity and sexuality; searching; labeling; fitting in; noticing differences; and – finally – integrating into the community. Other models of identity formation are described in Chapter 8. When working with gay and lesbian youth, clinicians are encouraged to keep developmental models in mind when formulating treatment plans – recognizing their theoretical limitations when applied to different ethnocultural groups.

5.6 Counseling Interventions for Stages of Identity Development

Identity stage	Possible feelings / behaviors	Counseling interventions
1. Confusion	Feeling 'different.' Same-sex attractions, dreams, fantasies.	Provide support. Provide readings. Explore strengths in 'differentness.' Discourage premature self-labeling.
2. Comparison	Continued sense of difference from peers. Strong same-sex attractions, preoccupations. Anxiety about fitting in. Social isolation, alienation, shame.	All of above, plus: Explore fears, anxieties, shame. Identify positive role models. Locate age-appropriate peer support resources.
3. Tolerance	Actively seeking out bi/ homosexual peers or adults. Living 'double life' with secret bi/gay self. Denial of sexuality.	All of above, plus: Maintain safe, supportive relationship with adult. Discourage inappropriate sexuality with adults. Encourage gay/lesbian/bi peer social activities. Address fears of exposure.

Identity stage	Possible feelings / behaviors	Counseling interventions
4. Acceptance	Increased contact with GLB peers. Severe loneliness/alienation if peers not available. May be scapegoated at home/school.	All of above, plus: Encourage 'safer sex' if sexually active. Explore coming-out issues. Affirm basic self-worth. Explore and build self-esteem.
5. Pride	Us/them attitude about heterosexuality. Belief in superiority of GLB lifestyle. Aggressively 'out' stance. Sexual activity to bolster identity. Anger at prejudice, discrimination.	All of above, plus: Support self-acceptance and pride. Encourage bridging with supportive heterosexuals. Caution about 'crashing out.'
6. Synthesis	Rejoining supportive heterosexuals. Increased empathy. Renewed emphasis on work, school, family roles.	Support efforts to bridge gay/lesbian/bisexual self with aspects of identity.

From Fontaine, D.H., & Hammond, N.L. (1996). Counseling issues with gay and lesbian adolescents. *Adolescence*, *31*(124), Table 1, 824–5.

Assessing Adolescent Mental Health Needs

Given what we know about normal gay and lesbian development, and how homophobia and heterosexism can influence this development, physicians, counselors, and other health care workers working with gay and lesbian teens should anticipate counseling issues that may emerge (e.g., self-acceptance, coming out safely, substance use). They should also encourage the youth to talk about any concerns regarding stress at home or school, discrimination, physical violence, sexual abuse or exploitation, depression, anxiety, and plans and goals for the future.

To identify the presence of mental health problems, the clinician must perform a thorough psychiatric assessment. The issues involved in a more detailed psychosocial assessment relevant to lesbian, gay, and bisexual youth are outlined in 5.7.

5.7 Mental Health Assessment

Background / Family History

1. Family
   a. Relationships
2. Living situation
3. Work
4. School
   a. Academic
   b. Activities and interests
5. Social relationships
   a. Adults and peers
   b. Social networks
6. Disclosure
7. Self-concept/self-image
8. Conscience/values
   a. Capacity for judgment and decision making
   b. Personal values: What is important/worthwhile?
9. Emotional states
   a. General feelings – What makes you happy/sad?
   b. Anxiety (duration, severity, frequency)
   c. Depression (duration, severity, frequency)
   d. Anger
   e. Other
10. Reality testing
    a. Judgment and insight
    b. Impulsivity
11. Fantasy – imagination
12. Future time orientation/expectations
    a. Goals

Past Psychiatric / Mental Health History

1. Mental health treatment/counseling history
   a. Inpatient
   b. Outpatient
   c. Medications
   d. Experience with mental health professionals/counselors

2. Family history
   a. History of severe and persistent mental illness
   b. Family use of mental health services – inpatient, outpatient
   c. Youth's perception of these experiences

Substance Use (see Chapter 9)

1. Drug
   a. Cigarettes
   b. Alcohol
   c. Marijuana
   d. Cocaine
   e. Amphetamines
   f. Nonprescribed narcotics
   g. Inhalants
   h. Tranquilizers
   i. Hallucinogens
2. Mode of administration
   a. Oral
   b. Nasal
   c. Intravenous/intramuscular
3. Age at initiation
4. Duration/frequency of use

Sexuality

1. Sexual orientation/sexual identity
   a. Sexual desires/attractions
   b. Sexual behavior and experience
      – Sexual readiness

      – Types and number of partners
      – Frequency and range of sexual behavior
      – Knowledge and use of safer sex practices
  c. Sexual fantasies
  d. Sexual identity/labeling (heterosexual, gay/lesbian, bi-
      sexual, homosexual, queer)
  e. Psychological conflicts
2. Sexual development
  a. Awareness of desires – age, context
  b. First sexual experience(s) – gender, age, age of partner
  c. Sexual abuse
  d. Disclosure or suspicion of sexual identity (consequences
     and response)
      – Parents/family/guardians
      – Peers
      – School environment
      – Workplace
      – Adults
  e. Decision making about disclosure
      – Is it safe?
      – Consequences
      – Who to tell and when

Gender Identity

1. Core gender identity
  a. Sense of masculinity and femininity
2. Cross gender behavior
  a. History and personal significance
3. Gender dysphoria
  a. History
  b. Current status
  c. Goals/desires (i.e., hormonal/surgical treatments)
4. Emotional response/psychological responses to sexuality issues
  a. Changes in sociability
      – Social engagement or withdrawal
      – Changes in peer group (loss of close friends?)
  b. Emotional responses
      – Emotional changes (temporary or long-lasting?)

- Knowledge of help seeking and response
- Substance use related to sexual experience
- Nature of responses
- Temporary or significant duration?
5. Social relationships/supports
- Adults
- Peers
- Networks
- Disclosure to others
- Self-concept/image

Evaluation of Suicide Risk

1. Current/past suicidal actions/feelings/fantasies
   a. Methods
2. Concepts/intentions of outcome
3. Life circumstances/situation at time of attempt
4. Past experience/history of suicidality
5. Motivations for suicidal behavior
6. Experiences/concepts of death
7. Depression and other predominant emotional states/affects
8. Family and environmental circumstances
9. Assessment of impulsivity
10. Assessment of suicide within the peer network

Victimization/Abuse/Exposure to Violence

1. Victimization and harassment related to sexual orientation
   a. Verbal (insults, harassment including gossip/slander)
   b. Physical (threats, assault)
   c. Sexual (sexual harassment, abuse/rape)
   d. Nonverbal/nonphysical experiences with stigma
2. Victimization based on ethnicity, gender, or other characteristics
   a. Verbal
   b. Physical
   c. Sexual abuse
3. Childhood abuse history
   a. Corporal punishment, physical abuse

b. Sexual abuse
- Family members
- Others
c. Emotional/verbal abuse
4. Exposure to crime/violence
a. Relationship to violence
- Family
- Intimate relationship(s)
- Peers – in school/out of school/community
- Gang participation
5. Traumatic events
a. Accidents
b. Major illnesses
c. Family dissolution
d. Other

From Ryan, C., & Futterman, D. (1998). Appendix F in *Lesbian and gay youth: Care and counseling*. New York: Columbia University Press.

Treating Depression

It is important for clinicians to realize that any depressed teen may require a psycho-educational approach (i.e., What is depression? What are the options for care?). She or he may already feel stigmatized about being gay and may have concluded that depression is a consequence of homosexuality. It's important to help the youth make the distinction between depression or another Axis I diagnosis and the struggles involved in accepting sexual orientation. Keep in mind that new awareness of same-sex attraction or recent disclosure may have precipitated a crisis. Ideally, a depressed teen should be offered a combination of medication and individual or group gay-affirmative psychotherapy, as well as – if indicated – family education and family therapy. (For more detailed treatment of guidelines for depression, anxiety, and substance abuse, see Chapters 8 and 9 or a standard adolescent psychiatry text.)

The clinician should follow the teen's adherence to treatment, keeping in mind that all adolescents have a tendency to reject authoritarianism in matters of care. Ensure that information about the youth's sexual identity and specific diagnoses is kept confidential. Respect the teen's wish to not come out to other providers or family members.

Exploring Suicidality

Clinicians are familiar with specific risks and behaviors associated with suicidality in teenagers. When working with teens, be direct and matter-of-fact in exploring thoughts of death and suicidal ideation. Clinicians may mistakenly believe that raising these issues might heighten suicidality, but in fact most teens find comfort in discussing these issues directly. When exploring suicidality:

• Make the distinction between fleeting suicidal thoughts of a passive nature and imminent suicidal ideation, including a plan.
• Explore the risk factors listed above to assess current risk.
• Determine whether thoughts of death and self-harm are linked to internalized homophobia, and identify whether this is something that can be worked on over time.

If, based on the assessment, a teenager is at high risk of attempting suicide, the clinician should offer the teen the option of voluntary hospital admission as the first step in a treatment plan and reiterate that information about the youth's behavior and sexual identity will be kept confidential. If the teen is not cooperative, the clinician should complete the forms required for closed treatment and notify the teen's parents about the safety issue. Whenever possible, teens should be admitted to an adolescent unit where clinicians are familiar with issues related to gay teens. At no time should the teen be forced to come out if he or she is not ready.

If, based on the assessment, a teenager is at low risk of attempting suicide, the clinician should discuss danger signs with the teen and develop a 'safety contract' that sets out how the teen will deal with these signs (e.g., talking to a friend or family member, booking an appointment, or using one of the gay teen hotlines). In the United States, teens can call the Trevor Talk Line (1-800-850-8078) to talk about mental health and suicidality. In Canada, teens can call the Lesbian, Gay, Bisexual Youthline (1-800-268-9688).

Counseling a Teenager about Coming Out

Once a teenager develops a trusting relationship with a practitioner, he or she may begin to ask questions about sexual identity and coming out. See 5.8 for a list of common questions, and visit the Parents and

Friends of Lesbians and Gays (PFLAG) website (www.pflag.com) for thoughtful answers.

5.8 Common Questions about Sexual Identity / Coming Out

- How do I know for sure I'm gay?
- Can I have a family of my own?
- Will I lose my straight friends?
- How will I meet gay friends?
- How do I tell my parents?
- Whom should I tell?
- Should I come out at all?
- I feel alone; who can I talk to?
- Will I be accepted?
- Will I get HIV or AIDS if I come out?
- I don't fit the stereotype; can I still be gay?
- Is it normal to be gay?
- Am I the only one?
- Am I your only gay patient?
- Can gays and lesbians be healthy?
- I played around with another girl/guy. Does that make me gay?

From Parents and Friends of Lesbians and Gays (PFLAG), available online (www.pflag.com).

When faced with teenagers' concerns about coming out, it is important for the clinician to dispel any sense of urgency that young people may feel. Emphasize that they must work on their own level of self-acceptance and self-esteem and ignore any pressure, political or otherwise, to come out to others until comfortable with their own identity. Clinicians should also be aware that teens with acute psychosis or suicidality may not have the ego strengths to explore sexuality. This work should be deferred until appropriate.

Premature coming out or untimely coming out can have serious consequences for an adolescent, including physical violence and ejection from school or family. It can also damage self-esteem. See 5.9 for a series of questions that practitioners should discuss with adolescent patients before they 'come out' to their parents. These questions can be explored in one meeting or over a series of meetings as part of ongoing counseling about sexual orientation, self-acceptance, and telling others. See 5.10 for a Survival Guide that may help gay and lesbian teens manage the process of coming out and telling others.

5.9 Coming Out? Some Questions

1. Are you sure about your sexual orientation?
2. Are you comfortable with your gay and lesbian sexuality?
3. Do you have supports should your family react badly?
4. Are you knowledgeable about homosexuality should you be asked questions about it?
5. What is the emotional climate at home? Is this the right time? Is the family stressed? Will they be more accepting at another time?
6. Can you be patient if this is not the best moment to reveal your sexuality to your family?
7. What is your motive for coming out now?
8. Do you have available resources?
9. Are you financially dependent on your parents? What would you do if they cut off your financial support on learning of your homosexuality?
10. What is your general relationship with your parents? Do you speak about intimate details or generally not? If not, how will any discussion of sexuality go over?
11. What is your parents moral, societal, and religious view on homosexuality?
12. Is this your decision or are you under pressure from elsewhere to reveal your sexuality?

5.10 Who and When to Tell? A Survival Guide

- Don't come out if you risk violence or cutting off financial or educational resources.
- Don't come out if you are angry, in the midst of an argument, or to punish someone.

- Come out to one person at a time so you can deal with reactions individually.
- When coming out to parents, it may be useful to come out to both parents together rather than individually.
- Sound out parental reactions regarding homosexuality before you come out by bringing up an article, television show, or documentary that deals with homosexuality.
- Do not come out if your family is in crisis. Wait until things have settled down.
- Come out in a private place where feelings can be expressed.
- Come out when you feel good about yourself, not when you're feeling depressed or anxious.
- Come out when sober, not high on alcohol or drugs.
- Be prepared for parents or others to deny your sexuality or ignore your revelation until they are ready to cope with it.
- Be ready for questions and for stereotypical or ignorant comments.
- Be prepared for emotional upset from the person you're telling.
- Have information and books/pamphlets ready for the individual to learn more about gay life.
- Maximize your supports with friends or a supportive adult to help counter negative reactions from the person you tell.
- Explore the materials provided by some of the gay-affirmative church groups in each of the religious denominations so that you can help counter or educate the person about negative attitudes toward homosexuality based on religion.
- Don't bring up difficult issues such as specific sexual practices, risks of AIDS, or grandchildren until later. However, keep the lines of communication open by suggesting that these issues be discussed later.
- Remember that once you've come out, you can never take it back, and that information may be spread. This lends more weight to the notion that you should come out gradually, person by person, to individuals you trust.

From Nycum, B. (2000). Coming out, you're what? *The XY survival guide*. San Diego: XY Publishing.

Helping Families Deal with Their Reactions to
Their Child's Homosexuality

Clinicians should never reveal a teen's sexuality to his or her parents – that would be a breach of trust or confidentiality. However, when a child does come out, parents will often turn to the family physician to explore their sense of confusion and feelings of loss, anger, or shame. A clinician who has counseled the child should agree to see the parents only with the teen's approval and after reassuring the teenager and explaining to the parents that any information the child has discussed with the physician will be kept confidential. To safeguard a trusting relationship with the teen, the clinician may decide to refer the parents to another colleague.

How are parents likely to react? In a survey of parental reactions to a child coming out, 43% had strongly negative reactions and 41% faced negative reactions from friends (Remafedi et al., 1991). According to a PFLAG survey (www.pflag.com) 74% of parents reported sadness, 58% regret, 49% depression, and 74% fear for the well-being of their child. Families reported considerable disruptions, and only 11% initially responded supportively to the child's revelation. According to teens, parents' reactions can be very difficult: between 19% and 41% of gay and lesbian teens reported an increase in family verbal abuse, and between 4% and 7% reported a new onset or increase in physical abuse.

According to an article published in the *Journal of Pediatric Health* (Kreiss & Patterson, 1997), family acceptance usually lags behind the youth's own development and acceptance of sexual identity. The researchers have proposed a model of family adaptation that consists of the following:

- **Initial rejection** – often because the information may be in conflict with the family's cultural or religious beliefs.
- **Denial, guilt, anger, grief, fear, confusion, and withdrawal from the youth** – which can last from months to years, with considerable disruption in all communication.
- **Identity acceptance** – where the family gradually comes to accept the reality of the youth's sexual orientation, even if they don't approve, and communication begins to improve.
- **Commitment** – where parents are able to disclose their daughter's or son's homosexual identity to others without intense feelings of shame.

The rate at which each family negotiates these phases will vary and is often complicated by cultural and religious factors. Some families move to commitment quickly, others never move past rejection.

Parents will likely have a number of questions (see 5.11). They may also wonder why they never suspected it before and feel they failed in their ability to be close to their child. When considering how to answer these questions, it's essential for clinicians to realize that parents need information and support. They also need the opportunity to verbalize stereotyped myths, to vent fears, and to have their fears patiently explored. For some parents, the primary experience is grief for the loss of their 'old' child and the loss of possibilities, such as being a grandparent. They may also want to talk about their fears for the child's health, happiness, future well-being, and how he or she will fit in a homophobic society. The clinician's role is to:

- Help parents understand how their attitudes have been shaped by prevailing homophobic and heterosexist assumptions in the culture.
- Reassure them that it takes time to work through these issues.
- Provide resources, including pamphlets and books, and refer parents to the local chapter of Parents and Friends of Lesbians and Gays (PFLAG).

5.11 My Child Is Gay: Parents' Questions

- Now that I know, what should I do?
- Is my child different now?
- Why did he or she have to tell us?
- Why didn't our child tell us before?
- Why is my child gay?
- What have I done wrong?
- Why am I uncomfortable with his or her sexuality?
- Should we consult a psychiatrist or psychologist to change this?
- Will my child be ostracized, have trouble finding or keeping a job, or even be physically attacked?
- How do I consolidate this news with my religious views?
- What about HIV and AIDS?
- We have accepted the situation, but why must my child flaunt it?

- Will my child have a family of his or her own?
- How do we tell family and friends?
- How can I support my child?

Helping Parents Help Their Children

Once parents have worked through some of their issues of anger, grief, loss, betrayal, and discordance, they usually ask how they can help their child. They may also ask for guidance on setting age-specific limits, such as curfew, dating, and sleepovers. The following suggestions come from an article 'Coming Out, You're What?' in the *XY Survival Guide* (Nycum, 2000):

- Parents are advised to listen, but to ask questions when the child has finished speaking, to avoid saying it's a phase, to thank the child for being honest and open, to congratulate the child for knowing himself or herself so well, and to acknowledge love regardless of choices, behaviors, and identities.
- Parents are encouraged to say that the news is unsettling or uncomfortable, but that they are willing to work on their attitudes.
- Parents should realize that they have no effect or influence on changing the child's orientation – that their only choice is to accept it.
- Parents are encouraged to ask the child if they can help with any stresses at work or school, and that they are open to hearing about these problems.
- Parents should promise support, locate resources, and encourage their child to bring friends home for visits, and also to come out to his or her doctor.
- As a sign of solidarity with their child, parents may wish to become politically active by putting rainbow stickers on their car, lobbying for rights within the schools, or confronting homophobic comments in their workplace or social milieu.

Helping Teens Feel Safer at School

As teenagers develop trust in their practitioner, they may talk about particular experiences of violence or verbal abuse at school. If this happens, it's important for the clinician to reiterate that the teenager has a right to feel safe and respected by classmates and teachers, and that the problem rests with a homophobic system, not with the teen. Teens should be told that harassment is wrong and criminal, whether or not they are gay, and that they should explore their legal options.

To help teens feel safer at school, clinicians should:

- Explore issues of safety with the child and the impact they have on emotional and physical health.
- Advise the child to transfer schools if the situation has reached destructive or dangerous proportions. Otherwise, with the teen's permission, contact the school's administration or guidance counselor to discuss the bullying or harassment.
- Give the teen resources on youth groups and information about a new phenomenon in North American schools, called Gay and Straight Alliances (GSAs). GSAs are political groups that seek to promote the rights of gay and lesbian teens and confront homophobic attitudes within schools. Gay and Straight Alliances insist that school should be a safe place for students, regardless of orientation or gender, and they seek to end discrimination, harassment, and violence related to sexuality. Information on GSAs and an information kit for setting up a GSA can be obtained from the Gay, Lesbian, and Straight Education Network at 212-727-0135.
- Emphasize to teenagers that they are not the only gay student in their school, and that they may be able to find support at the grass-roots level, which can be empowering and may help counter feelings of helplessness and isolation.
- Educate teachers, administrators, and students about gay and lesbian teen issues, STD prevention, and safe school environments. An interested physician may offer to help with the school's health and sexuality curriculum, provide an in-service for teachers, speak on gay and lesbian health issues, provide up-to-date resources for guidance counselors, write or edit a health article for the school newspaper, or donate lesbigay-themed books to the school library.

5.12 A Quick Guide to Counseling Gay, Lesbian, and Bisexual Adolescents

Here are some suggestions for clinicians and mental health professionals working with gay and lesbian teens.

Attitude and Environment

- Have up-to-date pamphlets and lists of resources and books in the waiting room that would be of interest to gay, lesbian, bisexual, and questioning teens.
- Be aware of your own homophobic/heterosexist attitudes (see Chapter 2) and how these might manifest when working with young people. Where appropriate, consult with informed colleagues or refer adolescent patients to gay and lesbian affirmative care.
- Choose your language carefully, avoid labels, and try to find out about the teen's comfort level with certain language and incorporate that into your discussions.
- Always reinforce that you're there to give facts and not to judge. Be aware of your educational role.
- Convey a nonjudgmental attitude to the teen. Affirm gay and lesbian identity as a healthy alternative form of sexual expression (Shapiro, 1991).
- Provide unconditional acceptance and model respect for the teen.
- Safeguard confidentiality so that the teen feels safe revealing information to you. Explain to the teen – before starting therapy – any exceptions to patient–provider confidentiality (e.g., a situation where the youth posed imminent harm to self or others, and the physician has a duty to inform family or other support group members).
- Invite the teen to have a third person in the room, if you think it would make him or her feel more comfortable.

Skills and Strategies

- Normalize the fact that some teens experience uncertainty or confusion about their sexual orientation. Explain that teens often explore romance and sex with both boys and girls. This will make it easier for the teen to talk about any same-sex activity. However, do not implicitly favor heterosexuality by identifying homosexual experimentation as a phase that will pass.
- Keep in mind that the teenager may come for assessment for reasons other than sexuality, so respect the agenda within a given appointment.

- When exploring issues of self-esteem and academic perform-ance, including over-functioning, be sure to ask teens about sexuality issues and how they may affect their behavior.
- Keep in mind that the teenager may present as homophobic initially, and may insist on not discussing sexuality at all. Listen for hints in the teen's communications that would allow you to ask empathetically about issues related to sexual confu-sion, exploration, or orientation.
- Ask the teen what his or her day-to-day life is like and the stresses and pressures it presents. Be sure to ask about issues of harassment, ridicule, and verbal, physical, and sexual abuse.
- Be prepared to counter the teen's negative stereotypes and myths patiently but rigorously, keeping in mind that these attitudes are prevalent in teen culture as well as society at large. Be prepared to explore the teen's resistance to a gay identity on religious grounds, and provide resources prepared by specific religious denominations that are gay affirmative.
- Keep in mind that a teen may identify as gay before same-sex activity has taken place, or may deny being gay although same-sex activity is currently taking place. One same-sex en-counter does not define orientation, although a teen may fear that it does.
- Don't rush teenagers into sexual labels or declarations about their orientation. Allow them to explore these issues gradually, and offer ongoing appointments where they can discuss sexu-ality issues in a supportive environment.
- Always emphasize that homophobia/discrimination is the teen's primary difficulty, not sexual orientation.
- When teenagers are ready, and if safe and appropriate, encour-age them to politicize their sexual orientation and to respond to it as a form of discrimination.
- Remember that teenagers may minimize their difficulties, and do not take their interpretation at face value.

Safer Sex and Support Strategies

- Be ready to answer frank questions about sex and to repeat-edly explain the use of condoms and barrier methods.
- Provide information on STDs and contraception and explore issues of safer sex in the context of emerging sexual explora-tion and relationships.

- Help the teen to identify key stresses at work, home, and school, and to problem-solve by developing short-term and long-term solutions.
- Help the teen identify the most supportive adult and peer in his or her social environment who can be an ally and added source of support and information.
- When appropriate, role play to give the teen practice being assertive, contradicting homophobic comments, or negotiating safer sex.

Referrals

- Always ask about depression, psychosis, suicide, and drug use. Arrange timely treatment, when appropriate, in lesbigay affirmative settings – if you are not able to provide this care yourself.
- When appropriate, refer the teen to a youth group.

Family-Based Strategies

- Offer to liaise with parents, but only when initiated and accepted by the teen.
- Reiterate that conversion and reparative therapies are never appropriate and have been condemned by the American Psychological, Psychiatric, and Social Work Associations (see Chapter 8).

CHAPTER SIX

Diagnosing and Treating Sexually Transmitted Diseases

Helen saw her family doctor for recurrent yeast infections. During the initial part of the exam, Helen told her doctor about her new relationship and her excitement about the upcoming gay pride weekend. From her stories and appearance, the provider assumed Helen was a lesbian and did not ask about risk factors for HIV.

Several months later, Helen returned and saw the physician covering for her original doctor. The symptoms had not resolved. The new provider looked beyond Helen's pink triangle T-shirt to ask about the number and gender of Helen's previous sexual partners. He discovered that although she identified herself as lesbian, Helen had been in a two-year relationship with an IV-drug-using man. He suggested HIV testing for both Helen and her current partner as well as some strategies to incorporate safer sex into their relationship.

Terry, a 26-year-old gay man, presents to his family doctor with symptoms of extreme fatigue and nausea. The doctor orders routine blood work, including liver function tests. Four days later, Terry returns for follow-up – obviously jaundiced.

Glancing at the results of Terry's liver enzymes, the physician announces: 'You have hepatitis A. A lot of homosexuals get it.' He does not take any other history information – although he does send Terry back to the lab for hepatitis B and C serology.

Concerned about his diagnosis, Terry does some reading about hepatitis. He has never had any risky sexual encounters or shared needles. He soon realizes his illness is more likely due to the mussels he ate several weeks ago while visiting the East Coast. His hepatitis A resolves in six weeks. He never returns to his family physician.

Effective diagnosis and treatment of sexually transmitted diseases (STDs) is vital to patient health, regardless of sexual identity or orientation. STDs, uncomfortable diseases in and of themselves, can also have long-term negative effects on fertility and make people more vulnerable to infections such as HIV. Those STDS, such as herpes or syphilis, that lead to ulceration or inflammation of the genitourinary tract increase the risk of HIV transmission in men and women. Timely and effective STD care has the potential to improve physical and reproductive health and to reduce the spread of communicable diseases, including HIV. In fact, in Tanzania, communities with improved STD treatment demonstrated a 42% decrease in new, heterosexually transmitted HIV infections (Grosskurth et al., 1995).

A sexually transmitted disease occurs when at least two separate sets of mucous membranes have somehow been in contact with each other and an unwanted pathogen has made its way from one person to another. The pathogen doesn't care whether those membranes self-identify as gay, lesbian, straight, bisexual, or celibate, and neither should diagnosis or treatment. When diagnosing or treating an STD, clinicians should focus on specific behaviors (e.g., which mucous membranes? how?), rather than on sexual identity or sexual orientation.

With the exception of HIV, discussed in Chapter 7, rates of sexually transmitted infection in men who have sex with men have fallen to levels equal to or lower than that of the general sexually active population. However, young gay males continue to engage in risk behaviors that put them at significant risk (Health Canada, 1998). This chapter provides advice on taking a sexual history as well as exploring STD issues of particular relevance to the lesbian and gay populations. For up-to-date information regarding specific STD pathogens and their treatment, readers are referred to treatment guidelines published by the Centers for Disease Control (www.cdc.org) or Health Canada (www.hc-sc.gc.ca).

Taking a Sexual History

Excellent STD care depends on taking an excellent sexual history. A sexual history allows the clinician to:

- assess both risks and symptoms
- determine the most appropriate screening tools or diagnostic tests

- set the stage to discuss risk reduction
- provide specific health instruction (e.g., 'You've mentioned that you have had four partners in the last six months, yet you don't like to use condoms ... Can you tell me more about your thinking on that?' Based on the response, the clinician can give tailored advice on risk reduction).

Most physicians do not find it easy to take effective sexual histories. According to one study of HIV pretest counseling, in 73% of the encounters physicians did not elicit enough information to characterize patients' HIV risk status (Epstein et al., 1998).

To achieve the accuracy required for effective STD diagnosis and treatment, most practitioners need to improve their history-taking technique (preferably with some practice and feedback). Developing an ease with sexual history taking requires preparation and practice. One strategy to improve sexual history taking is to combine it with anticipatory care of other things (a must when caring for adolescents). Clinicians should also develop an opening line that they feel comfortable with, such as: 'Your sexual health is an important part of your overall health. I need to ask you some specific questions to understand how best to address all your health needs and make sure we lower your risk of sexually transmitted infections. Are you okay with that?' See 6.1 for a Sexual History Checklist and 6.2 for a list of questions to use when taking a sexual history.

6.1 Sexual History Checklist

Preparation

- Be aware of your own biases – don't let them intrude.
- Assure the patient all information will be kept confidential.
- Explain why this information is important.
- Make no assumptions about sexual identity or orientation.
- Avoid technical terms and jargon.
- Start with the least threatening questions and work up to the most sensitive questions.
- Remember – most people will talk freely about personal matters if the environment is nonthreatening and their caregiver

seems to genuinely care about them. If your patients seem uncomfortable, they may be mirroring your own discomfort.

Screening for Risk

- Numbers of partners (male and female)
- Types of sexual activity: specific behaviors
- Condom usage
- Context of risk taking: drugs, alcohol, known or anonymous partner, sex for money
- History of previous STD in self or partner
- Abuse or rape

Symptom Review

- Genital sores/lesions
- Dysuria
- Discharge: rectal, vaginal, penile, urethral
- Genital itching/burning
- Abdominal/pelvic pain
- Abnormal bleeding: vaginal, rectal, urethral
- Skin rash
- Testicular pain/swelling
- Lymphadenopathy
- Last menstrual period/most recent Pap smear results

6.2 Sexual History: Some Questions

- Have you begun to have sex yet?
- When I use the word 'sex,' I generally mean intercourse or penetration as well as oral sex. Is that what you are thinking too?
- When was the last time you had sex with anyone? Was it someone you knew well? About how many sexual partners do you think you have had in the past month? Year?
- Do you have sex with men? Women? Both? (Always ask for all three – never rely on your personal prediction of the answer!)

- How many days since you last had sex with your regular partner? A casual partner?
- Did you use a condom or other protection the last time you had sex with your regular partner? Your casual partner?
- How many times in the past week/month/year did you have sex without using a condom or other protection?
- What methods do you use to prevent unwanted pregnancy?
- Have you ever used injection drugs? Have you ever had sex with someone that you know used injection drugs?
- I need to understand your specific sexual practices. Do you use your mouth on your partner's penis/vagina/anus?
- Do you put your penis in your partner's mouth/vagina/anus?
- Does your partner put his penis in your mouth/anus/vagina?
- Do you use any sex toys or dildos during sex? Do you share those with your partner? Do you clean them before sharing them? How?
- Do you use any bondage or domination during sex? Is there ever any blood involved? Do you feel comfortable and knowledgeable about how to stay safe during your scenes?
- Do you ever use drugs such as amyl nitrate (poppers) or ecstasy (E) to enhance your sexual experience?
- Do you ever use enemas or douches as part of your sexual activity?

Risk Assessment and Screening

Proper STD care also involves screening asymptomatic individuals based on risk. See 6.3 for a general approach to screening symptomatic and asymptomatic individuals and 6.4 for tips on collecting specimens.

6.3 Tips for STD Screening

Who to Screen?

Anyone who:
- is sexually active <25 years of age
- is a known contact of any STD

- has had a new or >2 partners in the past six months (male); or has had a new partner in the past two months or >2 partners in the past year (female)
- is street involved and/or uses substances (particularly injection drugs)
- has unprotected sex
- has a history of previous STDs
- has symptoms of dysuria, urethral discharge or itch, meatal erythema, lesions, or rash (male); or vaginal discharge, lower abdominal pain, abnormal bleeding, deep dyspareunia, dysuria (when urinary tract infection is ruled out), lesions, or rash (female)
- is male and has sex with men
- is pregnant (test for HIV with consent)

Why?

- 50% of males can be asymptomatic. Left untreated, complications may include prostatitis, epididymitis, and sterility.
- 70% of females can by asymptomatic. Left untreated, complications may include pelvic inflammatory disease (PID), and sterility may result.

Which STDs?

- gonorrhea
- HIV
- HPV
- HSV (herpes simplex virus)
- syphilis
- chlamydia
- hepatitis B (if unvaccinated)
- hepatitis C (if IV drug user, snorts cocaine, or is a contact of hepatitis C)

When?

In asymptomatic patients, screening is most effective when:
- relevant postexposure incubation period is respected
- patient has not taken antibiotics for at least 48 hours

Incubation Periods

- gonorrhea – 2 weeks
- chlamydia – 2 weeks
- HIV – 12 weeks
- syphilis – 6 weeks
- hepatitis B* – 6–26 weeks
- hepatitis C* – 2–24 weeks

*Symptomatic clients who initially tested hepatitis-negative should be retested in three months.

6.4 Tips for Specimen Collection

Males

- Evaluate entire genital area carefully. Using gloves, retract the foreskin if uncircumcised in order to inspect the glans. Examine extragenital area to detect other manifestations of STDs (i.e., pharynx, conjunctiva, lymph nodes, skin rashes, and/or lesions).
- Observe and palpate scrotum to detect any lesions, tenderness, or swelling, with special attention to the epididymis.
- Examine the meatus for urethral discharge, stripping the urethra by milking the penis from the base to the glans three or four times to detect small amounts of urethral discharge. Note amount and color of any discharge detected.
- Examine the perianal region.
- *Note*: voiding reduces the amount of exudate in the urethra and may decrease the ability to detect organisms. To get the best gonococcal specimen possible, it is preferable for the patient not to void for at least four hours. In reality, a last void of one to two hours is acceptable.
- Swabs — collect urethral specimens for N. gonorrhea prior to those for chlamydia. This is because N. gonorrhea is harbored in the urethra, whereas chlamydia is an obligate intracellular parasite situated in the epithelial cells.

Females

- Evaluate entire genital area carefully. Using gloves, examine

extragenital area to detect other manifestations of STDs (i.e., pharynx, conjunctiva, lymph nodes, skin rashes, and/or lesions).
- Observe and palpate the external genitalia, including the labia, to detect lesions, swelling, erythema, discharge, or odor. Be sure to separate labia so as to adequately visualize the vaginal orifice.
- Conduct speculum examination, noting vaginal walls' color, lesions, and amount of discharge.
- Swabs — Collect N. gonorrhea swabs prior to chlamydia. Cervical mucus need not be removed prior to taking N. gonorrhea swabs, but it is advisable to remove vaginal secretions and endocervical mucus by swabbing before chlamydia screening.
- Conduct bimanual examination — carefully palpate vaginal walls, cervix, uterus, and adnexa for enlargement or masses. Move cervix laterally to determine its mobility and any cervical motion tenderness.

Reprinted with permission from the Ottawa–Carleton Health Department. (n.d.). *Specific considerations in approaching STD care in lesbians and gay men.*

Hepatitis A

Hepatitis A is generally caused by fecal-oral transmission due to contaminated food or water. The virus can be transmitted during heterosexual or same-sex oro-genital contact.

Presence of IgG anti-HAV antibody confirms lifelong immunity. Demonstrated immunity or hepatitis A vaccine is especially important for those also infected with hepatitis B or C. Acute hepatitis A in the presence of active hepatitis B or C can lead to fatal hepatitis. Hepatitis A vaccine is also recommended for travelers to endemic areas, men who have sex with men, injection drug users, and persons with chronic liver disease.

Hepatitis B

Hepatitis B is considerably more infectious than HIV. The virus is transmitted through breaks in mucosal surfaces during insertive/receptive penile, vaginal, oral, and anal intercourse. Any sexual activity involving mucous membranes can potentially transmit hepatitis B.

Persons with existing HIV infection who acquire hepatitis B are at higher risk of becoming chronically infected. Hepatitis B immunization should be offered to all sexually active adults with more than one partner in the preceding six months, those who have a history of a sexually transmitted infection, men who have sex with men, injection drug users, sex trade workers, and lesbians who have sex with men. The vaccine is also used in occupational settings with risks of exposure to blood (i.e., hemodialysis units and certain long-term-care facilities).

Chlamydia

Chlamydia is spread by contact with infected body fluids and can live in the vagina, cervix, rectum, urethra, pharynx, and eyes. Heterosexual and male-to-male transmission is well documented. Female-to-female transmission is theoretically possible but not well studied.

Because the pathogen can be asymptomatic in men and women, screening is recommended for those with a high pretest probability of infection (see 6.3). Specimens must contain epithelial cells – pus contains few such cells. Nucleic acid tests are the most sensitive and specific and can be obtained from a urine sample. Consult your local lab for specific collection instructions.

Genital Warts

More than twenty subtypes of the human papillomavirus (HPV) can infect the genital tract. Warts are caused by skin or mucous membrane contact with an infected person or inoculation via hands or shared sex toys. Heterosexual and same-sex spread is possible.

Intra-anal warts indicate receptive anal intercourse. Perianal warts commonly occur without anal penetration. Certain serotypes of HPV are associated with cervical and anal dysplasia. Clinically apparent warts of the anus or cervix should be referred for colposcopic examination. Cervical Pap smears are recommended for all women according to current clinical practice guidelines. Anal Paps are also recommended but less widely used in clinical practice. Consult the cytology experts in your area for up-to-date advice regarding anal Paps.

Gonorrhea (GC)

Transmission of gonorrhea has been well documented in male-female and male-male sexual contact. Female-female transmission is theoretically possible but not well studied. The pathogen can infect the penis, vagina, anus, mouth, and throat. Long-term, asymptomatic carriage is possible in both men and women.

Syphilis

Syphilis is transmitted in blood and semen and through contact with an open sore (chancre) of an infected person. Heterosexual and male-male transmission is well documented; female-female transmission is theoretically possible but not well researched.

Fifty percent of new syphilis cases diagnosed in 1999 were in men who have sex with men (Centers for Disease Control, 2001). Primary infection can present in atypical ways. Primary syphilis can present similar to anal fissures, with pain and bleeding on defecation. Unlike fissures, the atypical chancre will be indurated and associated with bilateral inguinal adenopathy.

Co-infection with syphilis and HIV needs aggressive screening and treatment. All newly diagnosed HIV patients should be screened with a VDRL. Request a confirmatory test as the first line for those who are significantly immunocompromised.

Bacterial Vaginosis (BV)

BV indicates a change in the microbial ecosystem of the vagina, including an overgrowth of anaerobic bacteria, loss of normally acidic pH, and a relative absence of lactobacilli. BV is more frequently found in women who have sex with women than in heterosexually matched controls (Marrazzo et al., 2000). Monogamous lesbian couples tend to be concordant for the presence or absence of BV. There is evidence that BV may be associated with a higher risk of genitally acquired HIV (Taha et al., 1998). Treat BV in those who are symptomatic and in anyone considering pregnancy (Ralph et al., 1999). Female partners of symptomatic women should also be tested and offered treatment.

Trichomoniasis

Trichomoniasis can be transmitted sexually and via fomite. Transmission heterosexually and between women is well documented. In men, the protozoa live only in the urethra, so male-male transmission is unlikely. Long-standing asymptomatic infection is possible. Female partners of infected women should be tested and treated.

Diagnoses and Treatment of Specific Clinical Syndromes

Proctitis

Proctitis (also known as colitis) refers to inflammation of the rectal mucosa and the tissues surrounding the anus. Clinical symptoms include rectal pain, rectal bleeding, mucousy rectal discharge, tenesmus, and left lower quadrant abdominal pain. If the cause of proctitis is due to gonorrhea, cytomegalovirus (CMV), or herpes simplex, the rectal pain may be intense.

For men and women who practice receptive anal intercourse, proctitis is most often due to sexually transmitted infections. The most common pathogens are herpes simplex, gonorrhea, chlamydia, and cytomegalovirus.

People infected with HIV are at higher risk of severe herpes and CMV proctitis, which may require IV antibiotics. Even in cases with an apparent clinical diagnosis (i.e., herpes simplex), cultures should be ordered to rule out co-infection. Be sure to obtain samples for viral culture, chlamydia, and GC. If there is a change in bowel habits, order stool cultures. If symptoms do not resolve with antibiotics, request imaging of the rectum and sigmoid colon (proctoscopy, sigmoidoscopy).

6.5 Collecting Rectal Specimens for Culture

Collect blindly or through an anoscope. An anoscope is preferred for symptomatic individuals – use of an anoscope minimizes fecal contamination. With the blind method, insert a swab 2 to 3 cm into the rectal canal. Use lateral pressure to avoid fecal material (this will also aid collection of columnar cells for C. trachomatis). If there is visible fecal contamination, discard swab and obtain another.

Treatment for proctitis is directed at the specific pathogen. In some settings (i.e., anonymous clinics where follow-up is difficult), give empiric treatment for chlamydia and GC at the time of cultures. Consider HIV testing, syphilis screening, and hepatitis A and B immunization in all cases of sexually acquired proctitis. Manage pain with topical anesthetics (i.e., xylocaine viscous 2% applied QID and before defecation), sitz baths, and measures to avoid constipation or straining (e.g., high-fiber diet, high-fluid intake).

Pelvic Inflammatory Disease (PID)

PID is a syndrome that involves infectious inflammation of the endometrium, fallopian tubes, and pelvic peritoneum. PID is often polymicrobial: sexually transmitted pathogens (gonorrhea and chlamydia) interact with nonsexually transmitted pathogens including bacteroides, hemophilus, E. coli, and streptococci.

Symptoms include lower abdominal pain, dyspareunia, vaginal discharge, fever, and increased menstrual flow. Signs may include cervicitis (30%), cervical motion tenderness, and adnexal mass. Diagnostic measures include cervical swabs for C. trachomatis and GC, a vaginal swab/wet prep, and a bimanual exam. Ultrasound may be required when a tubo-ovarian abscess is suspected.

PID cannot be ruled out when results of laboratory investigations are normal. When the diagnosis is equivocal, consider treatment. Referral and hospitalization is required for severe illness, tubo-ovarian abscess, inability to tolerate oral therapy, HIV-positive patients, pregnancy, or when there is a possibility of a surgical emergency (i.e., ectopic pregnancy).

Therapy should provide excellent coverage for GC and chlamydia. Re-evaluate all women treated for PID 48 to 72 hours after initiation of therapy. Women with a previous episode of PID are ten times more likely to experience a recurrence.

Prostatitis

Strictly speaking, prostatitis is not a sexually transmitted disease. However, men with symptoms of prostatitis often present to STD treatment clinics, so the clinical approach to prostatitis is included here. Evidence-based practice guidelines can be found online (www.agum.org.uk/CEG/s46_prostatitis.html). Acute prostatitis is caused by organisms generally found in the urinary tract, including gram negatives, enterococci, and staph aureus. There is no evidence that the incidence of prostatitis is higher in men who have sex with men than in the general population.

Prostatitis generally presents as an acute systemic illness with lower urinary tract symptoms (dysuria, frequency, urgency), prostate symptoms (low back pain, perianal, penile, and occasionally rectal pain), and symptoms of bacteremia (fever, chills, rigors). On exam, the prostate is exquisitely tender, swollen, and tense. Investigations include mid-stream urine for culture and microscopy, and blood cultures. Because many of the symptoms of prostatitis are also present in sexually transmitted infections, a screening genitourinary history/physical and cultures should be completed during the initial workup of all male patients presenting with genito-urinary symptoms – regardless of sexual orientation or risk behavior.

Because of the severity of the illness, start empiric therapy against urinary tract pathogens immediately after cultures have been drawn. IV therapy may be required. Quinolones, which are active against gram negatives and achieve good penetration into prostatic tissue, are the standard oral therapy. Because prostatitis is due to uropathogens, sexual partners do not require treatment.

Chronic prostatitis is a subacute condition characterized by a variety of symptoms involving genital pain: perianal pain, lower abdominal pain, penile pain (especially the tip), testicular pain, ejaculatory discomfort, rectal and lower back pain, and dysuria. The classification, diagnosis, and treatment of chronic prostatitis is multilayered and evolving. For more information, see the online practice guidelines cited above.

Anal Intercourse

Anal intercourse is a high-risk activity for STDs, and it is not only gay men who are at risk. Although the majority of men who have sex with men practice anal intercourse, so do many heterosexuals. In a 1995 study of California households, 8% of males and 6% of females reported having anal sex at least once a month during the last year and most of them one to five times a month. In that same study, 60% of the people who practiced anal intercourse did so without ever using a condom (Erickson et al., 1995). Halperin (1999), an expert in heterosexual risk, has calculated that women practice unprotected anal intercourse seven times more often than men who have sex with men. These findings highlight for clinicians the importance of taking an accurate sexual history for all patients and of counseling patients about the proper use of condoms.

Anal sex is the most significant risk factor for HPV-related anal cancer. Cytological screening at three-year intervals for patients who practice anal sex is recommended. Annual screening for patients who are HIV-positive has been suggested but is not available in all settings. See Chapter 7 for specific sampling techniques.

CHAPTER SEVEN

HIV Issues

Bill is a 40-year-old nurse working in internal medicine at a Toronto hospital. He and his HIV-positive partner, Joe, are traveling to Philadelphia for a nursing convention. When they reveal at Customs that they are traveling together, their luggage is searched and Joe's HIV medications are discovered. They are refused permission to enter the United States because of Joe's HIV-positive status, even in the context of a professional visit. They cancel the trip.

Kim is a 27-year-old woman whose parents came to Canada from Korea twenty-five years ago. When she was 16, they discovered a love letter she had written to her girlfriend and told her she had to leave the house immediately. During several years on the street, Kim exchanged sex with both men and women in return for housing and food. On several occasions she used IV drugs, although she never developed an ongoing addiction.

Kim left the street when she was 20 and is now training to be a carpenter. She has been with her partner, Lana, for the past five years. They are considering trying to become pregnant using alternative insemination from a private fertility clinic. During a 'preconception' exam the doctor mentions HIV testing but describes Kim as 'low risk' based on her current relationship.

HIV raises a number of complex issues and creates challenges for the people infected, clinicians, and other caregivers. This chapter discusses testing issues, counseling, and the role of primary care practitioners in treatment. Because of the rapidly evolving nature of HIV care, specific treatment protocols will not be covered. For up-to-date approaches to treatment, consult the following websites: AEGIS (www.aegis.com); AIDS Knowledge Base (www.hivinsite.ucsf.edu/Insite); The Body (www.thebody.com); CATIE (www.catie.ca).

Testing Issues

Testing is a significant part of HIV care and prevention. It is the means by which people with HIV are diagnosed and are then able to receive the care they need. It is also an opportunity to counsel and educate everyone who is at risk about how to protect themselves and prevent the spread of HIV.

Until recently, HIV testing required a venous sample that was submitted to a laboratory for an ELISA screen. Positive screening tests are then confirmed with a Western Blot, which checks for specific proteins on the HIV particle. The most significant issues about HIV testing have been confidentiality and the time between when the blood is drawn and when test results are received (sometimes two to three weeks). In most jurisdictions, patients can choose between nominal, non-nominal, and anonymous testing:

- Nominal testing follows the same routine as any blood test: a patient's name, health card number, and identifying information accompanies the sample to the lab.
- Non-nominal testing uses a code (name or number) known only by the patient and the clinician ordering the test. The result can be traced back to the patient, but the process helps protect the patient's identity and confidentiality.
- Anonymous testing collects no identifying information. Patients are given a number to collect their test results, but the results cannot be traced back to them.

Now another testing option has become widely available: the rapid HIV test (see 7.1). It uses the same HIV enzyme immunoassay technique as the ELISA screen and, if positive, requires a confirmatory testing. However, the rapid HIV test does not require the services of a laboratory. It can be done at the point of care in a physician's office.

7.1 Potential Advantages / Disadvantages of Rapid Point-of-Care HIV Testing

Pros

- Rapid HIV testing allows patients to receive their test results within 30 minutes, rather than waiting two to three weeks (or longer in remote communities) for standard testing results.

- The technique uses blood obtained from a finger-prick, which is less painful for patients and lowers the chance of occupational exposure via needle-stick injuries (Quinn et al., 2000).
- On-the-spot testing eliminates the 'failure to return' phenomenon seen when results take two to three weeks to process.
- No advanced laboratory equipment is required, making it easier for remote, hard-to-reach, and high-risk populations to access testing services.
- Although a positive result from rapid testing must be confirmed by more extensive analysis, patients who receive a positive preliminary result can take immediate steps to reduce the risk of transmission.
- Rapid testing can be administered to pregnant women who have had no prenatal care or whose HIV serostatus is unknown at the onset of labor. When a pregnant woman tests positive, clinicians can take steps to reduce the risk of transmission from mother to child during delivery and begin antiretroviral therapy to HIV-positive mothers and their infants (if desired).
- For people who have had a possible exposure to HIV (occupational or nonoccupational), the rapid HIV test allows them to make a more informed decision about whether to start or continue postexposure prophylaxis (PEP). The decision to start PEP must be made within 72 (and preferably within 36) hours of exposure. The rapid test can also be used to test the possible source of infection (if the person gives consent). If the person tests negative, then PEP can be avoided or discontinued.
- Because of its high sensitivity, rapid testing provides a reliable negative result – the risks of a false negative are extremely low.
- Patients who test negative can be tested and counseled in a single visit.
- The rapid HIV test gives patients another testing option.

Cons

- The rapid point-of-care test is hypersensitive and produces a substantial proportion of false-positive results. Although it provides test results quickly, approximately two-thirds of the positive results generated will be false. This is likely to create high levels of anxiety in patients tested, who now have to await confirmed results.

- Rapid tests may be administered by health care practitioners who are inexperienced in dealing with HIV testing and counseling and who are unprepared to meet clients' care and counseling needs.
- Because the results are available so quickly, the clinician does not have the same time or opportunity to prepare clients for results (e.g., counseling, support, psychological preparation) as with standard testing.
- Patients who receive a negative result no longer have to return for a second visit. This compresses pretest and posttest counseling into a single appointment, potentially reducing the clinician's ability to promote HIV risk-reduction techniques.
- The compression of counseling and testing into a single session, coupled with the ease of testing and the ability to obtain immediate results, may lead to testing without voluntary, specific, informed consent – particularly with certain clients, such as women in labor whose HIV status is unknown, people who must make decisions about postexposure prophylaxis, people under pressure to submit to testing in order to receive medical attention, prison inmates, health care workers, and members of high-risk populations.
- Proliferation of rapid HIV testing may lead to breaches of confidentiality; supervision of testing, training of test providers, and protection of records may be inadequate.
- For many individuals, willingness to undergo HIV testing is contingent upon privacy and confidentiality; therefore, public perception of rapid screening as insecure may lead to fewer people being tested. Unlike laboratory facilities, where quality assurance controls are firmly established, proper testing protocols for point-of-care testing are impossible to enforce.

Adapted from Elliott, Richard, & Jürgens, Ralf. (2000). *Rapid HIV screening at the point of care: Legal and ethical questions.* Canadian HIV/AIDS Legal Network.

HIV Test Counseling

Regardless of the testing method used, all HIV testing requires skilled pretest and posttest counseling, informed consent, and access to follow-up resources. See 7.2 for test counseling guidelines.

7.2 HIV Counseling Checklist for Physicians

Pretest Counseling

- A person's request for HIV testing should be honored.
- Explore risk history and discuss reasons for the test.
- Assess the person's risk of having been exposed to or of being infected with HIV.
- Provide information about HIV infection and testing, including the meaning of positive, negative, and indeterminate test results and the impact of the window period.
- Discuss risk reduction and explore specific ways in which the person can avoid or reduce risk-producing behavior.
- Identify testing options available in the region, specifically nominal, non-nominal, and anonymous testing.
- Discuss the potential benefits and harms of being tested and of being found HIV-positive.
- Discuss the confidentiality of test results in relation to office or clinical procedures, communicating results to other health care officials, provincial reporting requirements, and partner notification.
- Discuss the stress related to waiting for test results and possible reactions to learning the results.
- Assess the window period by identifying the most recent risk event and plan an appropriate time for testing.
- Obtain and record informed consent, whether provided in writing or verbally, before testing is conducted.
- Arrange a return appointment after a predetermined interval for a face-to-face visit to inform the patient of his or her test results.
- A person has the right to decline testing.

Posttest Counseling

- HIV test results are given only in person.
- Assess the patient's understanding of the test result.
- Encourage the patient to express feelings and reactions.

Negative or Indeterminate Result

- Discuss any need for repeat testing.
- Review the ways in which HIV is transmitted.
- Review risk-producing behavior and assess the patient's commitment to risk-reducing strategies.

Positive Result

- Assess the psychological response to being HIV-positive.
- Plan how the patient can overcome adverse psychological reactions to being found HIV-positive.
- Arrange additional psychological and social support services as needed.
- Provide reassurance about the person's immediate safety.
- Arrange for medical follow-up.
- If possible, review transmission modes and risk-reduction strategies.
- Arrange for partner notification, if necessary.

Other Important Issues (emphasize early if poor follow-up is likely)

- Discuss health, reproductive, and treatment issues.
- Review importance of partner testing and notification and offer assistance if the person needs it.
- Reiterate the patient's right to privacy and confidentiality with respect to medical information.

From Canadian Medical Association. (1995). *Counseling guidelines for HIV testing from the expert working group on HIV testing.* Ottawa: CMA. Reprinted with permission.

Preventing Sexual Transmission of HIV

Sexual transmission accounts for 75% of worldwide HIV infection (Royce et al., 1997). Sexual transmission is related to two factors: the infectivity of the positive partner and the susceptibility of the exposed partner.

There is a strong correlation between infectivity and the amount of virus found in the genital tract, which is directly related to serum viral load (Quinn et al., 2000). The most significant factor in susceptibility is the presence of inflammation or trauma in genital mucosa. This means that STDs – particularly those that cause ulceration, such as herpes and chancroid – can play a significant role as cofactors in HIV infection (Fleming & Wasserheit, 1999; Quinn et al., 2000).

Safer Sex

Depending on their sexual practices, men who have sex with men can be at high risk of acquiring HIV and other STDs. When counseling about risk reduction, it's useful for clinicians to recognize that sexual activities fall on a continuum of risk. All patients have the right and responsibility to choose the level of risk they feel comfortable with when they have sex. The role of the health care practitioner is to offer information and support to patients to help them achieve their health goals. The continuum of risk in 7.3 outlines sexual practices, starting from the most risky sexual activity for HIV transmission to activities considered no risk (Safer Sex Institute, 2000). The safest activities are those that avoid any way in which HIV-infected blood, semen, or vaginal fluid can get from one person's body to another person's mucous membranes or bloodstream. Clinicians may wish to use this list during sexual history taking to help patients identify where their sexual activity places them on the continuum and to help them generate strategies for change, if desired.

7.3 Safer Sex: A Continuum of Risk

Higher Risk

- Unprotected anal intercourse
- Unprotected vaginal intercourse
- Sharing needles (for drugs, piercing)
- Sharing implements that draw blood (whips, knives)
- Unprotected oral sex on a menstruating woman
- Unprotected oral sex on a man with ejaculation
- Unprotected oral-anal contact
- Getting urine or feces in mouth, vagina, rectum (for receptive partner)

- Unprotected fisting or finger fucking
- Unprotected oral sex on a man without ejaculation
- Unprotected oral sex on a nonmenstruating woman
- Sharing uncovered sex toys

Low Risk

- Anal intercourse with a condom
- Vaginal intercourse with a condom
- Oral sex on a man using a condom
- Oral sex on a woman using a latex barrier
- Oral-anal contact using a latex barrier
- Fisting or finger fucking using a glove
- Petting, manual-genital contact
- Deep (French) kissing
- Spanking, whipping that does not break the skin
- Bondage and discipline play

No Risk (Safer Sex Institute, 2000)

- Masturbation (alone or with partner)
- Hugging, touching
- Massage
- Talking dirty, phone or Internet sex, fantasy

Treating HIV Infection

With continued advances in the treatment and management of HIV disease, people living with HIV have the potential to live much longer and enjoy a better quality of life than could have been imagined five or ten years ago. However, the continuing complexity and controversies in HIV treatment – When should we begin treatment? Which drugs should we use first line? Second, third, fourth line? When should we switch? – make it a challenge for any practitioner to maintain competence in HIV care.

What Is the Role of the Primary Care Provider?

There is increasing evidence that greater experience and specialization in HIV care leads to better patient outcomes (Hecht et al., 1999). The experience of the provider is particularly important when it comes to making medication decisions and treating complications of HIV disease. In settings where family doctors are the point of initial care and contact for patients with HIV, those family physicians must have access to specialized consultation services. A model of 'shared care' between a family doctor and an HIV consultant can be very effective in ensuring a balance between a high standard of HIV-related care and an ongoing physician/patient relationship that provides accessible, continuous, and coordinated care.

What Skills Should Family Doctors Have to Provide HIV Care?

1. *Competence in screening for HIV/STD risk and providing information about HIV testing and risk reduction.*
Family doctors and other primary care providers are in a unique position to assess patients' risk behavior for HIV and other STDs and to help them reduce their risk. Primary prevention of HIV involves both education and counseling about safer sex practices and screening/treatment for any STD infections that may make patients more vulnerable to HIV infection. To be competent in screening and educating patients, clinicians must:

- be knowledgeable about risk, transmissibility, and pathogenesis
- have strong sexual history taking skills
- be able to provide a safe, confidential atmosphere where patients can explore issues relating to sexuality and risk
- have an open, nonjudgmental attitude and a willingness to meet people wherever they are to provide information and support about potentially difficult behavior changes.

General inquiries about risk for STDs and HIV should be a part of routine primary care, especially during the annual health exam. Individuals who are uncertain of their risk, have had more than one sexual partner, or have ever engaged in risk behaviors should be offered HIV pretest counseling and screening.

2. *Familiarity with the signs and symptoms associated with seroconversion, HIV infection, or opportunistic infections secondary to HIV.*
The symptoms of HIV infection vary according to the stage of infection (see 7.4). Clinicians should be familiar with these symptoms. It is par-

ticularly important to recognize and diagnose acute seroconversion illness. Diagnosing HIV early provides the opportunity to prevent further transmission and to provide treatment that can slow or prevent long-term disease progression. To diagnose patients as early as possible, clinicians should maintain a high index of suspicion when encountering patients with acute, nonspecific febrile illnesses.

Clinicians should also be familiar with some presentations of symptomatic HIV disease, including chronic yeast infections in women, oral hairy leukoplakia or thrush, skin changes associated with Kaposi's sarcoma, and unexplained weight loss and night sweats. Pneumocystis carinii pneumonia (PCP) is one of the most common presentations of advanced, previously undetected HIV disease. When clinicians encounter a syndrome of nonproductive cough, progressive dyspnea, and fevers, they should investigate, because early detection of PCP could be lifesaving.

7.4 Symptoms of HIV Infection and AIDS

Stages	Common symptoms
Seroconversion illnesses	Fever, rash, swollen lymph nodes, headaches, loss of appetite, sweating, sore throat, and other flu-like symptoms
Asymptomatic stage	No signs or symptoms
AIDS-related complex	Flu-like symptoms, weight loss, diarrhea, fever, fatigue, memory loss, dry cough and shortness of breath, depression, swollen lymph glands, thrush, shingles, herpes simplex, oral hairy leukoplakia, idiopathic thrombocytopenic purpora, pneumococcal pneumonia
AIDS	Pneumocystis pneumonia (PCP), Kaposi's sarcoma, tuberculosis, mycobacterium avium complex (MAC), HIV-related lymphoma, toxoplasmosis encephalitis, cytomegalovirus infection (CMV), cryptococcus, cryptosporidium, candidiasis, wasting, encephalopathy, herpes, progressive multifocal leukoencephalopathy, histoplasmosis, cardiomyopathy, coccidiodomycosis, Hodgkin's disease, isospora, salmonella, varicella, lymphoid interstial pneumonia

3. *Basic knowledge of the workup for a newly diagnosed patient, prophylaxis for opportunistic infections, and general principles to support treatment decisions and adherence.*

Care of the newly diagnosed HIV patient involves a variety of tasks, including:

- staging the HIV infection using a detailed history, physical exam, and selected laboratory investigations
- initiating, where appropriate, specific treatments for opportunistic infections and co-infections and ensuring appropriate preventive care, including immunizations
- providing and monitoring treatment for HIV disease
- counseling to address psychosocial and environmental issues, such as safer sex and contact tracing.

1. Staging the Infection

History

To stage the infection, the clinician should obtain an HIV-related history, including date of positive test, reason for test, the client's estimate of when seroconversion may have occurred, previous trials of medications, and the dates and results of any previous tests including genotyping. Ideally, unless other markers confirm the diagnosis, the clinician should have documented proof of a positive HIV test before initiating any HIV care.

If the patient has already been receiving HIV care in another setting, the clinician should obtain the following patient information:

- most recent CD4 count and viral load (if known)
- lowest previous CD4 count
- current medications
- previous medications, including their sequence, duration, and any adverse effects
- medication adherence history
- history of opportunistic infections.

Review of Symptoms and Physical Exam

The clinician's initial physical exam of a newly diagnosed HIV patient must be thorough enough to provide an adequate baseline for future assessment and to detect any HIV-related conditions that require immediate treatment (e.g., thrush). See 7.5 for a summary of the review of symptoms and physical examination.

7.5 Guide to Review of Symptoms for HIV Staging

Head, eyes, ears, nose, throat (HEENT)	Change in vision, floaters, change in hearing, tinnitus, sore throat, oral discomfort, gingivitis, sinusitis symptoms
Respiratory	Cough, shortness of breath, hemoptysis
Cardiovascular (CVS)	Chest pain, palpitations
Gastrointestinal (GI)	Nausea and vomiting, diarrhea, anorexia, melena, hematochezia, perianal lesions
Genitourinary (GU)	Urethral discharge, penile lesions, testicular pain, frequency of urination, nocturia, dysuria
Pelvic	Menstrual history (cycle, irregularities), obstetric history, vaginal discharge, dyspareunia
Musculoskeletal (MSK)	Arthralgias and arthritis
Dermatologic	Rashes, infections, shingles
Central nervous system (CNS)	Headaches, paresthesias, neuralgias, memory loss
Psychiatric	Mood, concentration, emotional liability, sleep, libido
General	Unintended weight change, unexplained fevers, night sweats

Physical Examination

General	Weight, height, blood pressure, pulse, respiration rate, temperature
HEENT	Fundoscopic, extraocular movements, visual fields, tympanic membrane, canals, teeth, gums for gingivitis, oral ulcers, thrush, oral hairy leukoplakia, pigmented lesions (Kaposi's), warts, thyroid
Nodes	Cervical, occipital, axillary, inguinal

Chest and CVS	Detailed routine examination
Breasts	Routine breast examination
GI	Surgical scars, tenderness, masses, hepato-megaly, splenomegaly, perianal lesions
GU	Testicular masses, urethral discharge, lesions, rashes
Pelvic	Rashes, lesions, vaginal discharge, cervical discharge, adnexal tenderness or masses

Laboratory Investigations

Routine laboratory investigations in newly diagnosed patients may be used as a screen for other occult disease or to provide a baseline for functions that may be affected by HIV medications in the future. The suggested routine laboratory tests are: CBC, differential, smear, glucose, electrolytes, BUN, creatinine, AST, ALT, ALP albumin, cholesterol, triglycerides, and urinalysis. Because of the likelihood of exposure to sulfonamides or dapsone during the course of HIV infection, consider G6PD deficiency testing for patients of Mediterranean, African, and Southeast and South Asian origin.

HIV-specific investigations provide essential information about the patient's immune status and level of viral activity. The CD4 counts and viral load can be used together to estimate the stage of HIV disease as well as the patient's prognosis and risk of progression to opportunistic infections and AIDS. Because of their importance in treatment decisions and prognosis, order two separate sets of viral loads and CD4 counts, done about four to eight weeks apart, as baseline. Patients who are stable require repeat CD4 and viral loads every three to six months.

Clinicians should be aware that both viral load and CD4 counts are subject to variation. In fact, infections and vaccinations can cause an artificial elevation in viral load that can persist for up to one month, and this should be taken into account when ordering viral load tests and interpreting results. To reduce the variation in CD4 counts, take the samples at approximately the same time of day and send them to the same laboratory.

2. Initiating Treatment and Providing Preventive Care

Screening and Treatment for Other Infections

People living with HIV can enjoy optimal health when the risks of other co-infections are eliminated or reduced. When treating a newly diagnosed patient, consider screening for a range of illnesses that could have an adverse impact on his or her health (see 7.6).

7.6 Guide to Screening for Newly Infected Patients

Disease	Test	Reason / action
Syphilis	VDRL Confirmatory, if VDRL is positive	Screening, high rate of HIV and syphilis co-infection. Possible biological false positive VDRL. Treat if positive.
Hepatitis A	Anti-HAV	Screening for immune status, especially if from endemic areas, high-risk activities. Vaccinate if not immune.
Hepatitis B	Anti-HBs (HepBsAb)	Immune status, especially if from endemic areas or IDU: vaccinate if not immune. (IDU = intravenous drug user.)
Hepatitis C	Anti-HCV	Carrier status, especially if IDU, dialysis, blood transfusion: vaccinate for Hep A and B if positive.
Toxoplasmosis	Toxoplasma IgG	Screening, prophylaxis if positive and prevention of infection if negative. Repeat if negative and when CD4 < 100.
Cytomegalovirus	CMV IgG	If negative and needs transfusion, should get CMV negative blood or leukocyte depleted blood.

Clinicians need to pay particular attention to the genital tract and reproductive system in women and to the anal canal in men, as both are adversely affected by this disease. For example, HIV can prolong and intensify pelvic inflammatory disease, cervical HPV infection, and vaginal candidiasis. Order cervical screening for women with HIV, including testing for chlamydia and gonorrhea and cytology for HPV. Because of the virulence of HIV/HPV co-infection, order cervical cytology more frequently for HIV-infected women than for non-HIV-infected women. Pap smears should be done six months apart and then yearly unless an abnormality appears. Refer high and low-grade squamous intraepithelial lesions (LSIL, HSIL) for immediate colposcopy. If the cytology identifies ASCUS (atypical squamous cells of undetermined significance), repeat the test every four to six months until normal. If the patient receives two successive reports of ASCUS, refer for colposcopy.

The carcinogenic impact of HPV on the cervix is similar to its impact on the anal canal. In fact, the rates of anal cancer in gay men who practice receptive anal intercourse are higher than the rates of cervical cancer in women who don't receive Pap smears. One study reported that 95% of gay men with HIV and 65% of HIV-negative men had HPV DNA in their anal canals and surrounding skin (Palefsky et al., 1998). Another study reported a high incidence of anal high-grade squamous intraepithelial lesions among HIV-positive and HIV-negative homosexual and bisexual men (Goldie et al., 1999). Although research is underway to determine proper screening intervals, current data suggest that all HIV-positive men and women who have had anal intercourse should be screened annually for anal HPV. Men and women who practice anal intercourse but are HIV-negative should have an anal Pap smear every three years (Goldie et al., 1999). The clinical effectiveness and cost-effectiveness of screening for anal squamous intraepithelial lesions in homosexual and bisexual HIV-positive men is in line with other accepted clinical preventive interventions (Goldie et al., 1999). See 7.7 for a guide to obtaining and interpreting the anal Pap smear.

It should be noted that in many North American health care settings, protocols for collecting, interpreting, and registering the results of anal Pap smears are less developed than corresponding systems for cervical smears. Practitioners are advised to consult their local cytologists for specific advice regarding the clinical use of the anal Pap.

7.7 Guide to Obtaining and Interpreting an Anal Pap Smear

- Ask the patient to lie on his/her side in a knees-to-chest position.
- Do the Pap smear before the digital exam (avoids contamination by lubricant).
- Place one hand as close to anus as possible and spread buttocks. You want to be able to see anoderm once buttocks are spread.
- The other hand is holding a dacron swab or cytobrush. (Dacron is less irritating. Don't use cotton-tipped swabs.)
- Insert the swab or brush an inch or two into patient's anus. (The swab must be above the squamo/columnar junction, usually at the dentate line.)
- Once successfully in, twirl the brush or swab while moving it in and out several times.
- Remove it and immediately roll it across a microscope slide. Finish by spraying cytology fixative across the slide, as with any routine Pap smear.
- The cytologist can read through small amounts of feces or blood.
- Send requisition to lab as a request for anal cytology.
- Results are graded using the same criteria as cervical Pap smears.
- Investigate any abnormals (i.e., ASCUS, LSIL, HSIL) with anoscopy using magnification and acetic acid. High-grade lesions need ablation.

Preventive Care and Treatment

Vaccinate HIV-positive patients to prevent illness. Clinicians should be aware that, as HIV infection progresses, the immune system loses its ability to develop antibodies in response to immunization, so protective vaccines should be administered as early as possible in the course of infection. Killed, inactivated, or recombinant vaccines are considered safe; live viral or bacterial vaccines (including oral polio vaccine, BCG, and varicella-zoster) are contraindicated. Controversy exists over the role of MMR, Hib, and Lyme disease vaccine. Before administering these vaccines, consult with an HIV specialist or an infectious disease specialist. See 7.8 for recommended vaccines.

7.8 Guide to Vaccines for People with HIV

Vaccine	Adult dose	Notes
Pneumococcal vaccine	0.5 mL IM single dose repeated every 5–6 years	High rates of bacterial pneumonia in HIV-infected people with low CD4+ counts.
Influenza vaccine	0.5 mL IM in deltoid, annually	
Tetanus – diphtheria vaccine	0.5 mL IM repeated every 10 years	Should have had a primary series and recommended as a booster.
Polio (inactivated poliomyelitis vaccine)	0.5 mL SC once	Use as booster if patient has received a primary series.
Hepatitis B vaccine	1 mL IM in deloid × 3 doses given at 0, 1, and 6 months	Increased risk of becoming chronic hepatitis B carrier if HIV-positive patient contracts acute hepatitis B.
Hepatitis A vaccine	1 mL IM × 2 doses given at 0 and 6–12 months	Indicated if hepatitis B or C positive, travel to endemic countries, men who have sex with men, intravenous drug users, or community outbreak.

Managing Tuberculosis (TB)

In the care and treatment of people with HIV, TB deserves special mention. HIV is a significant risk factor for TB reactivation, and active

TB, in turn, can hasten the progression of HIV disease. It is essential that clinicians screen all patients with HIV for TB.

If the patient has no history of a previous positive TB test, use a two-step Mantoux (5TU PPD) three weeks apart for the initial screening. If both tests show less than 5 mm induration, consider it a negative test. Then screen the patient annually using a one-step routine Mantoux.

If the patient tests positive (i.e., >5 mm), use a chest X ray, induced sputums, and TB urine to rule out active TB. If the TB is active, refer the patient promptly to a specialist. If there is no evidence of active infection, initiate INH prophylaxis (regardless of age) for nine to twelve months. (The risk of reactivation outweighs the risks of INH-induced hepatitis.) Give pyroxidine to reduce risk of neuropathy. Because of the magnitude of risk from HIV and TB co-infection, consider prophylaxis for any patient with a past history of a positive Mantoux or a history of exposure to active TB. Anergy testing for those with a negative Mantoux is no longer recommended.

3. Treating HIV Disease

The specifics of HIV treatment change rapidly. The emergence of new classes of drugs, like fusion inhibitors, and alterations in combination protocols require an active approach to continuing medical education. Family physicians may need to consult with specialists who know about recent treatment trials, unusual medication interactions, or strategies for treatment failures. Since clinicians may have only one opportunity to make a medication decision that could have a dramatic impact on outcome, it is essential to involve experienced and knowledgeable practitioners in some of the specifics of HIV treatment (e.g., which medications, when).

The bulk of HIV care, however, will fall on the shoulders of the primary care team. The lifelong management of a chronic disease as complex as HIV depends on primary care for patient education and counseling, disease monitoring, adherence issues, service coordination, family support, and care of other diseases (e.g., hypertension, diabetes) that will occur over the course of a lifetime.

Antiretroviral Medication: When Should It Begin?

When making the decision to initiate antiretroviral therapy, consider:

• the patient's viral load, CD4 count, and overall clinical status

- potential short-term and long-term side effects
- results of viral genotyping testing, where available
- the patient's ability to adhere to a complex medication regime
- potential drug interactions.

Adherence is likely the most significant predictor of successful antiretroviral therapy. When patients fail to achieve at least 90% adherence to their medication regimen, drug-resistant strains of the virus replicate. Consider antiretroviral therapy only for a highly motivated patient who feels ready to make the commitment to the regime and assume the risk of side effects.

Medication Side Effects

Medication side effects and drug interactions can pose a significant threat to treatment adherence and the patient's health and quality of life. A complete discussion of medication side effects is beyond the scope of this book. For more detailed information on all aspects of antiretroviral therapy, contact the Canadian AIDS Treatment and Information Exchange (CATIE) online (www.catie.ca) or the AIDS Knowledge Base (www.hivinsite.ucsf.edu/Insite).

Monitoring Therapeutic Response

Once medication has been initated or changed, patients should be seen two and four weeks after the change to check for side effects, verify adherence, and monitor biochemical parameters such as CBC, liver enzymes, and renal function. The plasma viral load should be checked at week eight to ensure a response to therapy. It must have decreased by at least 1.0 log HIV-1 RNA copies/mL to be considered effective. Note that reduction of the virus to undetectable levels may not occur until weeks 16 to 24. Once suppression is achieved, measure viral load every three to four months to ensure continued suppression.

When should medication be changed? The decision to change a patient's antiretroviral should be based on the patient's immune response, his or her personal experience of the medication, and/or clinical signs that the regimen is not effective. A change should be considered when the clinician observes:

- an inadequate drop in plasma viral load (defined as a decrease of less

than 1.0 log after either eight weeks or the lack of full suppression by four to six months)
- a detectable level of viral load after months of successful suppression
- a drop in the CD4 count that occurs while on medication
- clinical progression of HIV while on medication
- inability to tolerate side effects
- inability to adhere to the treatment regimen.

Treating Opportunistic Infections

Despite treatment advances, HIV still causes significant damage to the immune system, making it difficult for patients to fight off other opportunistic infections. To help patients maintain optimal health, it is essential that clinicians provide proper prophylaxis against opportunistic infections associated with HIV. See 7.9 for current U.S. Public Health Service guidelines for prevention of opportunistic infections.

7.9 Prophylaxis for Opportunistic Infections

Pathogen	Indication	Preferred regimen	Alternatives
Pneumocystis carinii	CD4+ cell count <200/ul or <14%. Oropharyngeal candidiasis or an AIDS-defining illness.	TMP-SMX 1 DS tablet three times/week or daily.	Dapsone 50–100 mg/day + pyrimethamine 50 mg/week or atovaquone 1500 mg/day or aerosolized pentamidine.
Toxoplasma gondii	IgG antibody to toxoplasma and CD4+ cell count <100/ul.	TMP-SMX 1 DS tablet daily.	Dapsone 50–100 mg/day + pyrimethamine 50 mg/week or atovaquone 1500 mg/day.
M. tuberculosis	5 TU Mantoux skin test >5 mm or contact with active tuberculosis.	INH 300 mg daily + pyridoxine 25 mg daily for 9 months.	Consult public health.
M. avium complex	CD4+ cell count <50/ul.	Azithromycin 1200 mg weekly.	Clarithromycin 500 bid, or rifabutin 150 mg bid, daily.

Psychiatric Manifestations of HIV

The clinician will already be familiar with diagnosing DSMIV-Axis I conditions in the context of medical illness. Keeping a high index of suspicion regarding the role HIV disease plays, including the specific psychiatric presentation, is vital. When prescribing psychoactive drugs, the physician should aim for medications with a low side effect profile and 'start low and go slow' regarding dosing. Cross-checking drug-to-drug interactions between HIV and psychiatric medications is *essential*.

An excellent review, 'Practice Guidelines for the Treatment of Patients with HIV/AIDS' (*American Journal of Psychiatry, 157*(11), November 2000), can be obtained from 1-800-668-5111, order #2318. The guidelines are also available online (www.psych.org). The Canadian Psychiatric Association has also prepared a videotape called 'Learning to Care: An Introduction to HIV Psychiatry' and a training module, which can be obtained at 613-234-2815, ext. 38. See also *Therapists on the Front Line: Psychotherapy with Gay Men in the Age of AIDS* (Caldwell et al., 1994).

4. Counseling

HIV infection is a disease of progressive and multiple losses. Although hopeful and effective treatment protocols have emerged over the past five years, people living with HIV experience devastating changes related to the loss of health, drop in economic status, loss of employment, disfigurement, discrimination, and bereavement. Clinicians must be aware of and responsive to their patients' psychosocial needs. When dealing with these important issues, physicians may seek the assistance and support of other health care professionals and community groups (Peterkin, 1993).

The Doctor–Patient Relationship: Comanagement

Because there is no definitive cure for HIV disease and treatment benefits vary, it is important to establish an effective, trusting doctor–patient relationship and an environment where the clinician and patient can share information and make decisions jointly. If a patient decides to refuse drugs or treatment, the physician has a responsibility to explain the risks but should respect the patient's decision.

Many people living with HIV use complementary therapies such as nutritional, vitamin, and naturopathic supplements, massage, hypnosis, and imaging. Provided that there is nothing intrinsically harmful in these therapies and they do not interact adversely with combination antiretroviral therapies, there is no reason for the clinician to discourage their use. However, it is important for the clinician to know about any products or substances the patient is taking in case there is potential for adverse interactions.

Treatment and Adherence Issues

When the path of HIV infection was a predictable progression to death, the task of the family doctor or psychiatrist was to help a person deal with the losses and grief caused by HIV and assist the person to die. With advances in diagnosis and treatment, HIV has been reconceptualized from a terminal illness to a chronic (though still life-threatening) illness. Now, patients living with HIV face a greater and less defined challenge: how to incorporate HIV into a longer life with more uncertainty.

The antiretroviral treatments for HIV (discussed above) create issues for patients and clinicians. Clinicians are being asked by patients to help weigh the pros and cons of the antiretroviral 'cocktail': When should it begin? Given the incapacitating side effects, do they have to take it when asymptomatic? Why should they take something that makes them sick even when they don't feel ill? Because HIV chemotherapy can have a substantial impact on patients' physical and emotional well-being, difficult underlying questions are raised concerning the patient's feelings about his or her life:

- Do I want to live and get better? (I had made my peace with dying ...)
- How do I define a future? Do I have an identity beyond being HIV-infected?
- I've been on disability for the past six years – how can I think of finding a job again? What if I lose my benefits?
- I never thought I would ever be in another relationship after my partner died and I got sick ... I'm terrified.
- My family expected I would be dead by now – I don't know how to face them.
- What if my treatment fails or I can't tolerate the side effects?

Mental health practitioners can play a crucial role in helping patients make decisions about beginning or adhering to complicated medication regimes with significant side effects. They may also be able to help patients identify personal issues that may affect their ability to adhere to a treatment regimen, such as an addiction problem, serious mental illness, or low levels of self-esteem. If patients appear to have any of these issues, they should be referred for drug treatment, counseling, or psychotherapy before starting antiretroviral therapy. These services may help them prepare for treatment and adhere to treatment regimens. See 7.10 for a summary of factors associated with poor adherence and 7.11 for inventions that can help improve adherence.

7.10 Factors Associated with Poor Adherence

- Increasing length of time since starting therapy
- Psychological distress (particularly depression)
- Alcohol abuse
- Lack of confidence in therapy efficacy
- Little effect on biologic markers
- Number of pills to take
- Dosing frequency
- Lack of HIV symptoms
- Presence of side effects
- Changes in daily routine (e.g., holidays, sickness of partner or children, new job)

7.11 Factors Likely to Facilitate Drug Adherence

Teaching on:
    HIV infection dynamics
    Development of resistance
    Goals of therapy
    Names of drugs
    Reason for dosages and modes of administration
    Side effects
    Choice of drug combination

Drug administration:
    Establishment of a daily drug administration schedule
    Utilization of alarms and pill boxes

Reinforcement for successful adherence:
  Improvement of biologic markers
  Reduction in the number of office visits

Social support:
  Involvement of close contacts
  Treatment of other conditions that patients may suffer from,
  such as drug addiction
  Telephone follow-up or home visit by nurse

Adapted from Williams, A., & Friedland, G. (1997). Adherence, compliance and HAART: Patient-focused strategies to increase medication adherence. *AIDS Clinical Care, 9*(7), Table 1, 53.

Legal and Financial Issues

To help patients maintain an appropriate sense of control over their lives, explore legal and financial concerns early, including:

- medical and extended health benefits, including drug coverage
- patient's assets, debts, and disability and life insurance policies
- a living will or advanced directives
- power of attorney
- other issues such as discrimination, housing concerns, wrongful dismissal, child custody, income maintenance, survivor benefits
- the impact of return to work on drug coverage.

Refer the client to appropriate legal, social service, and/or AIDS service organizations to address these concerns.

Spiritual Issues

Patients' spiritual needs, which are different from their psychosocial needs, may go unrecognized by the physician if the patient does not express them in traditional religious terms. Like all patients with potentially life-threatening conditions, people living with HIV question the meaning of life, suffering, death, and existence after death. Throughout the process of spiritual questioning and exploration, patients need an ongoing sense of purpose, creativity, and love. Every ill patient wishes to find peace with his or her life. Emotional and spiritual reactions to HIV disease will vary. Some patients may feel anger at a God who allowed them to become ill, or experience a sense of moral guilt about their past choices. Others experience a resurgence of religious faith and find great comfort in prayer, meditation, and traditional ritual.

Sexuality

HIV has a major impact on a person's sexuality. The impact may be psychological. For example, patients may experience guilt, loss of body image and self-esteem, and fear of infecting others, which can lead to changes in sexual behaviors (e.g., hypersexuality, decreased libido, impaired performance). The impact can also be physical. HIV drug protocols are known to produce erectile dysfunction (see Chapter 4). When working with HIV-positive patients, clinicians should reinforce the following points:

- People with HIV are not required to be abstinent as long as their sexual activity does not infringe on the health or rights of others. Discuss safer sex practices openly. Explore strategies for dealing with lapses in safe sex practices (see Chapter 4).
- It's important for people with HIV to inform current, past, and future sexual partners so that they can make informed decisions and choices about their health. Discuss the rejection the patient may experience when he or she discloses. Talk about the potential for breach of confidentiality.
- Most AIDS resource centers offer individual, couple, and group sessions that explore couple and dating issues and ways of eroticizing safer sex.

If a patient chooses to stay in a dysfunctional or abusive relationship out of fear of loneliness, consider referral for counseling (Peterkin, 1993).

Women's Issues

HIV-positive women face some unique issues related to pregnancy, childbirth, disclosure, and their traditional role as family caregiver. Women who are contemplating pregnancy or who have young children may have a number of concerns that clinicians can address through counseling, including:

- I want to get pregnant and have a child, but I don't know if it's okay to do that if I'll die before my kids grow up.
- I'm taking medications to help protect me during this pregnancy. What if they harm the baby?
- The doctor is too far away. I can't take my kids to that appointment – the whole community will know about my HIV.

Women will also have concerns about their sexuality and the stigma associated with HIV, which may affect their treatment decisions or ability to adhere to their medications:

- It's bad enough being a single parent, but if anyone knew I was HIV-positive I would never find a good relationship. It's easier staying off the medications.
- I've met a wonderful man – but I know he'll dump me if he knows I have HIV. He says he hates using condoms ...

HIV-positive women also face special demands in their traditional role as caregivers. They may feel guilty about being 'bad mothers,' or may fear losing custody of their children. Those who are caring for ill partners or children may be extremely anxious about the welfare of their family. All these issues should be identified and explored early in the course of the illness (Citron, 1999).

Gay Men's Issues

Gay men, the first population group affected by HIV in North America and the group hardest hit, have suffered stigmatization because of HIV. HIV creates complex personal and social challenges for gay men, who already may be misunderstood and stigmatized for their sexual orientation. When working with gay clients, clinicians should be sensitive to the following issues:

- Some gay patients may be hostile to or distrustful of physicians because of previous homophobic and 'AIDS-phobic' encounters.
- Many gay men who are infected have already lost partners and friends and have not fully grieved these losses. Provide an opportunity for the grieving to occur.
- Gay men need to have their partnerships and chosen families acknowledged by their health care providers. Discuss power of attorney for medical care with your patient. Whose wishes does he want

you to follow – his family of origin or his life partner? Put the information in his chart. Encourage him to take the legal steps that will ensure his wishes are followed.

- Some gay men experience a resurgence of guilt about their sexual identity or past behaviors when they discover that they are HIV-positive. Identify and explore internalized homophobia in counseling.
- Despite an overall low new infection rate in the gay community, some men may be inconsistent about practicing safer sex. Discuss the reasons for these lapses frankly and frequently (see Chapter 4). The counselor's goal should be to help the patient link his healthy identity as a gay man with safer sex practices.
- Family members vary dramatically in their support for an ill gay member. Some may be very involved; others are aware but cannot discuss the illness; others completely 'excommunicate' the gay man. Do not assume the family will be supportive. Discuss the situation with the patient.

Death and Dying

Many people with HIV have seen friends die from the disease in circumstances of pain, isolation, and dementia and are afraid that they will face the same fate. Others have seen friends or partners fail on new treatment regimens and worry about the distant long-term effects/risks of their own HAART treatment. When a patient raises the subject of dying, the clinician should be prepared to discuss realistic options for palliative care at home or in other settings with the patient and his or her partner, spouse, or family. Patients needs to be reassured that:

- They will be free from pain.
- Their wishes about legal matters or medical interventions will be respected.
- Surviving children will be cared for.
- They will have support from the family of origin and/or choice.
- They will not die alone, and their dignity will be preserved.

Care for the Family Caregiver / Care Team Member

Families who care for people with end-stage HIV or AIDS need support, education, and opportunities to vent any frustrations. The family physician can help provide support for family members and friends dealing with emotional issues, such as:

- feelings of anger, guilt, helplessness, and isolation
- fears of contagion, loss of sexual intimacy, and anxiety about their own HIV status
- anxiety concerning impending death
- guilt about survival or treatment success when a family member is ill.

Family members should be kept informed of the disease process as it affects their loved one. Children in the family should be given age-appropriate information. In addition, family caregivers may need to be given permission to take care of their own health and to take some respite from caregiving.

Care for the Physician and Other Professional Caregivers

Although most doctors working in HIV primary care derive satisfaction and challenge from their work with HIV and AIDS patients, they also express concerns about burnout, which is often characterized by stress and unresolved grief. Key stresses include:

- lack of supervision, training, or support
- overidentification with young, ill, or dying patients
- conflicts with their personal beliefs (such as homophobia)
- stigmatization associated with caring for people with HIV or AIDS
- coping with patients' struggles with adherence to and ambivalence about emerging treatment protocols or treatment failures
- fear of contagion
- administrative conflicts and lack of team support
- caring for persons with a history of multiple losses, physical disfigurement, and dementia or other psychiatric pathology
- difficulty learning and mastering new treatment protocols
- public perception that HIV is now a 'manageable' disease and thus less worthy of community resources.

It is essential that professional caregivers have realistic expectations of their own abilities to manage their patient's disease process. They also need support as well as opportunities to vent and to be a part of a team that shares responsibilities. The team should meet regularly for educational updates, clinical problem solving, conflict resolution, and grief work. Given the demanding nature of their work, all professional HIV/AIDS caregivers need to find a balance between their professional and personal lives.

Postexposure Prophylaxis

Postexposure prophylaxis (PEP) is short-term antiretroviral therapy offered to people who have had a possible high-risk exposure to HIV immediately after the exposure occurs.

Occupational PEP

The rate of HIV transmission from a known HIV-positive patient to a health care worker via a sharp injury is 0.3%. Rates are somewhat higher when exposure occurs through a hollow-bore needle, the injury was deeply penetrating, or if blood was injected during the injury. Risks are also greater when the source patient has a high viral load and/or a lower CD4 count (Robert & Bell, 1994).

PEP is routinely offered to health care, emergency, and other workers who have a high-risk occupational exposure. See 7.12 for a commonly used protocol for occupational PEP. Readers are encouraged to contact their local facility for updates in approaches to occupational PEP or to consult online www.cdc.gov.

7.12 Recommendations for HIV Postexposure Prophylaxis in Occupational Settings

Type of exposure	Action
Massive percutaneous exposure (e.g., deep injury with large-bore needle previously in source patient's vein or artery) or exposure to a lesser amount of blood with a high HIV titre	Recommend: AZT (200 mg tid) and 3TC (150 mg bid) with or without IDV*
Massive percutaneous exposure (as above) to blood with a high HIV titre	Recommend: AZT (200 mg tid) and 3TC (150 mg bid) and IDV (800 mg tid)

Type of exposure	Action
Percutaneous exposure to a lesser amount of blood with a low titre, to fluid containing visible blood, or to other potentially infectious fluid (semen; vaginal, cerebrospinal, synovial, pleural, peritoneal, pericardial, or amniotic fluid) or tissue	Offer: AZT (200 mg tid) and 3TC (150 mg bid)
Mucous membrane or high-risk skin exposure to blood	Offer: AZT (200 mg tid) and 3TC (150 mg bid) with or without IDVH
Mucous membrane or high-risk skin exposure to fluid containing visible blood or other potentially infectious fluid or tissue	Offer: AZT (200 mg tid) with or without 3TC
Percutaneous, mucous membrane, or skin exposure to other body fluid (e.g., urine)	Do not offer prophylaxis

*AZT – zidovudine; 3TC – lamivudine; IDV – indinavir.

Possible toxicity of the other drug might outweigh benefit.

If IDV is not available, saquinavir (600 mg tid) can be substituted.

High-risk skin exposure – high HIV titre in source patient; prolonged contact; extensive area involved; skin integrity compromised.

From Canadian Medical Association. (1997). HIV postexposure prophylaxis: New recommendations. *Canadian Medical Association Journal, 156*(2), 233. Reprinted with permission.

http://www.cma.ca/dmaj/vol-156/issure-2/0233.htm

Nonoccupational PEP

Although evidence about the efficacy of nonoccupational PEP is lacking, clinicians may consider offering PEP for possible high-risk exposures, such as sexual assault, receptive anal intercourse, or sharing needles with someone who is known to be HIV-positive or is at high risk of acquiring HIV.

Nonoccupational PEP generally follows the same protocol recommended for high-risk occupational exposure (i.e., AZT, 3TC, and a protease inhibitor). The Centers for Disease Control (1998) guidelines for nonoccupational exposure to HIV recommend the following:

- Evaluate all persons requesting PEP for their risk and counsel them about risk reduction and primary prevention of HIV. The role of hepatitis C testing should also be explored.
- Offer HIV testing (especially in the setting of sexual assault) to determine HIV status at time of exposure.
- Evaluate medically at time of presentation and at regular intervals for the following six months (i.e., 4 weeks, 12 weeks, and 6 months). HIV antibody testing should be offered during those evaluations.
- Provide medical care and follow-up for all those who are found to be HIV-positive at time of presentation for PEP.

In general, clinicians may consider prescribing PEP for a nonoccupational sexual or needle-using exposure under the following conditions:

- The person presenting has had a high-risk exposure to HIV. This includes anal intercourse (unknown partner) or any penetrative sex with a person either confirmed HIV-positive or known to be at high risk for HIV (e.g., an injection drug user).
- The person has a high likelihood of complying with medications.
- There are no contraindications to the medications.
- Treatment is offered as soon as possible after the exposure: within one to two hours is the preferred window of time. The benefits of beginning treatment more than 36 hours after exposure are not known. PEP should not be offered beyond 72 hours.

Because nonoccupational PEP has not been studied extensively, it is difficult to comment on its efficacy. When prescribing PEP for a nonoccupational exposure, clinicians should obtain the patient's informed consent and document in the chart that they have discussed and the patient understands the following:

- the need to initiate or resume relevant risk reduction behaviors (i.e., condom use, drug treatment)
- the lack of information on the efficacy and/or toxicity of antiretrovirals in this setting
- the known side effects of the prescribed medications
- arrangements for follow-up medical care
- the timing and frequency of follow-up HIV testing
- signs and symptoms associated with acute HIV seroconversion

- the need for adherence to maximize effectiveness of PEP and reduce the risk of developing drug-resistant strains of the virus.

Women who have been exposed and are pregnant or who could become pregnant as a result of their exposure – and who intend to continue their pregnancy – may require expert obstetrical advice about the PEP regime that is least harmful to the developing fetus.

If patients choose to take PEP, monitor for toxicity, including a CBC and liver and renal function at initiation and two weeks into therapy. If the patient develops any signs or symptoms of HIV seroconversion during PEP therapy, refer to HIV specialty services.

CHAPTER EIGHT

The Mental Health of Gays, Lesbians, and Bisexuals

Michael is a 59-year-old former seminarian who has struggled with his sexual orientation over the years, particularly because of prohibition suggested by his religious beliefs. He has had sexual explorations with other men in the past, but usually in the context of heavy drinking, which he says allowed him 'to get over my hang-ups for the night.' He requests psychotherapy with someone who welcomes looking at the roles of spirituality in mental health. In his first session of psychotherapy, he reveals that his religious order had previously sent him to a psychiatrist to help him diminish feelings of same-sex attraction.

Eleanor is a 50-year-old woman who has been married for twelve years and has two children ages 10 and 8. Although she and her husband have had marital difficulties for some time, she has decided to leave him after falling in love with a 30-year-old female neighbor whom she met at the local community center, where both of them were playing with their children. Eleanor has had no previous history of same-sex exploration and has never considered herself a lesbian. She consults her family physician, wondering if she is having a 'nervous breakdown.'

History

Throughout the twentieth century, the attitudes of mental health professionals toward gay and lesbian sexuality generally followed the prevailing mores of the times, informed by dominant religious and judicial doctrine. The notion of bisexuality was largely ignored. Psychotherapists working within a homophobic and heterosexist culture, intellectual tradition, or institution have traditionally considered homosexuality to be an illness to be cured or sublimated. In fact, it was only in 1973 that the American Psychiatric Association removed homosexuality from its list of mental disorders. In 1975 the American Psychological Association adopted a resolution which stated that 'homosexuality per se implies no impairment in judgment, stability, reliability or general social or vocational capabilities.'

Before that time, psychoanalytic thought was largely informed by the illness model of homosexuality and invariably categorized male same-sex attraction as a neurotic structure, arrested development, mental disease, moral flaw, hormonal imbalance, personality disorder including narcissism, defense against heterosexuality, or a variant of masochism. Female homosexuality has been less discussed and debated in the psychoanalytic literature. This gap likely reflects the tendency to ignore or neglect women's issues rather than tolerance for same-sex female relationships (Hopcke, 1989). Until ten years ago, most psychoanalytic training institutes throughout North America would not accept gay or lesbian trainees.

Because an illness model seeks cause, psychoanalysis tended to look for developmental contributors to same-sex attraction, such as the overprotective mother, the absent father, early abuse, family trauma, or mis- or nonidentification with the same-sex parent. Psychological distress in gay and lesbian patients was linked to the intrinsic flaw or vulnerability manifested in their homosexuality, which might explain why the individual might be unable to cope in society or sustain intimate relationships. As a result of this view of same-sex attraction, mental health professionals tended to recommend conversion therapy: the use of psychoanalytic and behaviorist principles to cure or eradicate homosexual impulses and behavior. However, over the last three decades conversion therapy has been condemned by all the major medical and psychological organizations (see 8.1).

8.1 The Current View of Conversion Therapy

All the major medical and psychological organizations have condemned conversion therapy and actively oppose its practice:

'Clinical experience suggests that any person who seeks conversion therapy may be doing so because of social bias that has

resulted in internalized homophobia, and that gay men and lesbians who have accepted their sexual orientation positively are better adjusted than those who have not done so.'
— American Psychiatric Association

'For nearly three decades, it has been known that homosexuality is not a mental illness. Medical and mental health professionals also now know that sexual orientation is not a choice and cannot be altered. Groups who try to change the sexual orientation of people through so-called conversion therapy are misguided and run the risk of causing a great deal of psychological harm to those they say they are trying to help.'
— American Psychological Association

'Confusion about sexual orientation is not unusual during adolescence. Therapy directed at specifically changing sexual orientation is contraindicated, since it can provoke guilt and anxiety while having little or no potential for achieving changes in orientation.'
— American Academy of Pediatrics

'Most of the emotional disturbance experienced by gay men and lesbians around their sexual identity is not based on physiological causes but rather is due more to a sense of alienation in an unaccepting environment. For this reason, aversion therapy is no longer recommended for gay men and lesbians. Through psychotherapy, gay men and lesbians can become comfortable with their sexual orientation and understand the societal response to it.'
— American Medical Association

From 'Reparative Therapy' and related web links (www.aglp.org).

Based on the evolution of knowledge and thinking in the mental health profession, it is now possible to conclude:

1. The search for a cause of homosexuality itself proved to be heterosexist in that a cause for heterosexual orientation was never posited.
2. Mental health vulnerabilities are now increasingly linked to the im-

pact of social, familial, and institutional homophobia on normal psychological development and self-esteem and are no longer linked to same-sex attraction itself. Therefore, homophobia is a significant psychosocial stressor and chronic health risk (Shaffer et al., 1995).

What Are the Mental Health Needs of Gays and Lesbians?

According to the mental health literature across professional disciplines published over the last thirty years, both gay men and women have a increased incidence of alcohol and drug abuse, depression, suicidality, low self-esteem, and eating disorders. Such findings are important to all mental health clinicians, including social workers, nurses, doctors, psychologists, family physicians, psychiatrists, and counselors.

8.2 Mental Health Disorders: Summary of Key Research Findings

- Lesbians and gay men tend to experience major depression disorder, generalized anxiety disorder, and conduct disorders at higher rates than heterosexuals (Sorenson & Roberts, 1997).
- Among gay men there is an elevated prevalence for current major depressive disorder (Sorenson & Roberts, 1997) and bi-polar disorder (Atkinson et al., 1998).
- There appears to be a high lifetime prevalence of affective disorders among both lesbians and gay men (Williams et al., 1991).
- Methodological limitations prevent researchers from collecting reliable data on the incidence of suicide ideation and attempts and completed suicides among gay men and lesbians (Herek et al., 1997). Studies indicate that gay men and lesbians experience an elevated lifetime prevalence of suicide ideation and attempts (D'Augelli & Hershberger, 1993). The incidence of suicidal ideation and attempts are three to seven times higher among gay and lesbian youth compared with heterosexual youth (Ferguson et al., 1999). However, there is no evidence to support elevated rates of *completed* suicides among homosexual populations (Shaffer et al., 1995).
- Lesbians and gays account for approximately 30% of youth suicides (Remafedi, 1999).

However, most of the studies seldom define lesbian or gay identity in a systematic way, use rigorous sampling methods, include men and women of different races, cultures, or classes, or establish control groups with gays and lesbians who were not consulting mental health professionals. Those that have taken a more rigorous approach (see Shaffer et al., 1995) have demonstrated that gay men and women have specific vulnerabilities linked to internalized homophobia, including anxiety and affective disorders (Williams et al., 1991) and alcohol and substance abuse. More significantly, gay men and lesbians are more likely to have experienced a hate crime, violence, or sexual abuse than straight men and women (Finn & McNeil, 1987). According to the research:

• The primary issues for which lesbians and gay men have specific counseling needs are depression, suicidal ideation, alcohol abuse, sexual orientation, domestic violence, sexual abuse and assault, and hate crimes (Trippet & Bain, 1990).
• Societal antigay attitudes and the associated stressors – prejudice, stigmatization, and antigay violence – place lesbian and gay populations at an increased risk for mental distress, mental disorders, substance use, and suicide (Rosario et al., 1996).
• Although they may not experience certain health problems found in heterosexuals, lesbians and gay men may confront other problems related to the stigmatization of homosexuality (Rothblum, 1994).
• Internalized homophobia is linked with adjustment difficulties, including intimacy and sexual problems (Meyer & Dean, 1998).

While lesbians and gay men may have specific, treatable mental health needs, they may not be receiving the care they need. The research indicates the following points:

• Gay men and lesbians seeking mental health services often face negative attitudes toward homosexuality or find their sexual orientation receives more attention than the central problem for which they sought therapy (Garnets et al., 1991).
• Gay men and lesbians in need of counseling turn to friends as often as to professional therapists due to the latter's inexperience with or insensitivity to gay and lesbian issues (Trippet & Bain, 1990).

Fine-Tuning the Comprehensive Mental Health History for Gay and Lesbian Clients

Mental health professionals working with a gay or lesbian patient must perform a sensitive, comprehensive history – as they would with any patient. History taking is the basis for developing a diagnosis and treatment plan that reflects the patient's current problem, developmental stage, and social reality. Clinicians are familiar with the fundamental components of this history. However, the history-taking process should be adapted somewhat to meet the needs of gay and lesbian patients. For example, clinicians should include the following:

- Background information, age, occupation, housing arrangements, presence or absence of primary relationship and gender of partner, makeup of family as defined by the client
- Current complaint, including current symptoms, stressors, losses. HPI: context and history of current complaint. Potential role of sexuality or revelation of sexuality in current crisis
- Standardized diagnostic interview tools to rule out presence of Axis I DSM-IV diagnosis, such as anxiety, affective disorder, psychosis, and substance abuse (see below for risks for lesbigay clients)
- Past psychiatric history: diagnosis, treatment, past experience of psychotherapy, counseling, and satisfaction with psychotherapeutic method/approach (individual versus group, short-term versus long-term)
- Past history of treatment, including medications, alcohol, street/party drugs, tobacco, caffeine
- Past medical history, impact of chronic illness, relevant medical history through review of systems, and in particular to rule out organic causes of psychological presentation
- Discussion of quality of medical care received in the past, history of homophobic/heterosexist interactions in the context of medical care
- Family history regarding family of origin, history of psychiatric illness, treatments, substance abuse in the family
- Background: birth history, history of neonatal illness, developmental history, political/religious/racial/class descriptors of family, early childhood memories, description of relationship to mother, father, siblings; presence of gender atypicality as a child, history of physical, sexual, or emotional abuse, including history of teasing, violence due to gender atypicality (i.e., tomboy girl, sissy boy)

- General family attitudes about sexuality and homosexuality
- Quality of parents' relationship
- School experiences: behavioral, learning, social difficulties, ostracism by peers for difference, including gender atypicality
- History of trauma, loss, geographic moves
- Quality of friendships with males/females. History of avoiding intimacy due to fear of revelation of sexual orientation
- Emergence of same-sex crushes, attraction
- Personal response to adolescent body developmental changes
- Early sexual experimentation: same-sex, opposite sex, both; quality: shameful, coercive, pleasurable, loving?
- Experience of adolescence, including rebellion, forensic history, running away, school leaving, experimentation with drugs, street involvement (including prostitution)
- History of emergence of sexual orientation and identity; distinction between fantasy versus behavior versus self-identification
- If relevant, history of coming out: when, to whom, response, to whom is the individual out now versus not. Why? Previous strategies used to hide sexual orientation, current experiences of homophobia/ heterosexism in family of origin, workplace, or religious community; knowledge/experience of gay community; levels of support
- Relationships: history of relationships with men, women, or both, including past history of marriage, duration and quality of relationships; identification of current significant relationships, stressors on these relationships; parenting concerns; history of loss of relationships to AIDS; history of rape or domestic violence
- Sexual concerns: libido, sexual performance, physical self-esteem, body image, safer sex practices, including context of alcohol/drug use during sex; risk of past or recent exposure to STDs, including HIV (if appropriate), history of testing for HIV. Why? Why not? Educational level/fears around testing in STDs
- Occupational history, history of education, principal jobs held, current job satisfaction; colleagues'/superiors' knowledge of/attitudes to sexuality; fears of violence, exposure, nonpromotion, or sexual exploitation in workplace
- Personal history, methods of relaxation, self-soothing, socializing, hobbies, interests, creative pursuits, goals, expectations, spiritual focus, relationship to religion of origin, involvement with church, temple, synagogue, struggles with homophobic messages within specific religious tradition, other existential concerns.

Once the clinician has obtained a comprehensive history, he or she will posit a formulation of the biological, psychological, developmental, and social components of the person's case, including a DSM-IV 5-axial diagnosis. To formulate the psychosocial difficulties of a lesbigay patient, pay particular attention to the client's experience of being different and how that difference has been tolerated or exploited by others.

Treating Mood and Anxiety Disorders

Clinicians are already familiar with diagnosing specific depressive syndromes, including major depression, psychotic depression, dysthymia, bereavement, bipolar depression, and anxiety disorders such as generalized anxiety disorder, panic disorder, obsessive-compulsive disorder, and posttraumatic stress disorder (Sorenson & Roberts, 1997; Atkinson et al., 1998). When treating mood/anxiety disorders in gay and lesbian patients, clinicians should consider the following (Cabaj & Stein, 1996):

- Gay and lesbian patients have often had discriminatory encounters with mental health care workers, so they may need time and reassurance to develop trust. In some patients, lack of trust may lead to missed appointments and lack of adherence to prescribed medications. Aim for a collaborative model of care with appropriate levels of psycho-education and presentation of therapeutic options.
- Older gay and lesbian patients may have had a past history of restorative or conversion therapies and may refuse psychotropic medications out of fear of brainwashing and mind control.
- Gay and lesbian clients are prominent consumers of alternative natural products and will often ask for opinions on an alternative to prescription medications or for information on interactions with prescribed drugs. (For more information on natural products, see Chapter 10.)
- In some patients, the use of alcohol/drugs must be closely monitored as they may increase side effects, drug interactions, and complicate clinical nonresponse in the treatment of mood/anxiety disorders (see Chapter 9).
- Many psychotropic drugs, including antidepressants, anxiolytics, and mood stabilizers, impair sexual functioning. Gay and lesbian patients may be reluctant to discuss these side effects (perhaps because

they have not discussed their sexuality with their caregiver), or they may be particularly vocal about them. The preferred antidepressants in terms of minimal sexual side effects are Nefazadone, Moclobemide, Buproprion, or Mirtazapine.

- Avoid overemphasizing STDs/HIV in your psychiatric history, but where risk exists, always include acute or chronic HIV infection in your differential diagnosis of psychiatric illness. There have been documented cases of mania and depression being the first indication of new or ongoing HIV infection. Unsafe sexual practices may also indicate parasuicidal behaviors and may be manifestations of depression/dysthymia, mania/hypomania, or substance misuse.
- When conducting a psychosocial history (particularly with gay men) be sure to explore the presence of bereavement, grief, multiple and/or complicated losses related to AIDS. Explain to the patient the difference between bereavement and depression as well as treatment distinctions for both problems.
- Inquire about and monitor suicidal ideation closely in all gay and lesbian patients. As reported above, the incidence of attempted suicide is higher in gays and lesbians, particularly when they are young (D'Augelli & Hershberger, 1993; Remafedi et al., 1991).
- When prescribing a new psychotropic drug for patients being treated for HIV infection/AIDS, ask the pharmacist to run a medication interaction profile with the patient's other medications. Start with a minimal dose of the psychotropic and increase slowly, monitoring for side effects, including toxicity, drug interactions, as well as clinical response.

Treating Patients Who Have Experienced Violence or Abuse

It is not uncommon for clinicians working with gays and lesbians to be asked to treat or refer someone dealing with issues of sexual, physical, or emotional abuse (see 8.3 and 8.4). In fact, many lesbians and gays have experienced violence or sexual abuse, and clinicians should ask all gay and lesbian patients – regardless of age and social class – about any past history of sexual, physical, or verbal assaults.

8.3 Antigay Violence and Mental Health

- The most visible, violent, and legitimized form of hate crime in the United States is homophobia and heterosexism-motivated violence (Herek et al., 1997). Gays and lesbians are among the most frequent victims of hate-motivated crimes in the United States (Finn & McNeil, 1987).

- According to a 1997 study, one in five respondents had been the victim of homophobic crime in the previous year. More than half reported having been victims of homophobic crime at least once during their lifetime (Herek et al., 1997).
- Male aggressors perpetrate the majority of homophobic violence (Herek et al., 1997).
- Qualitative differences between antigay violence and generic violence include a greater degree of violence in homicides; a high likelihood of the assailant being unknown to the victim; and a high ratio of the number of assailants to victims in antigay violence (Comstock, 1991).
- Law enforcement data typically underreport antigay violence (Dean et al., 2000).
- Victims of antigay violence often choose not to report the crime out of fear that discussion of their sexuality will subject them to further victimization, in particular by the police (Berrill, 1992).
- Lesbians are more likely to be assaulted by someone they know, while gay men are typically assaulted by one or more strangers (Herek et al., 1997).
- The majority of assaults against lesbians occur in their homes, while gay men are most often assaulted in a public place (Herek et al., 1997).
- Sexual assault may be a component of gay-bashing incidents (Knisley, 1992).

When treating patients for abuse, clinicians should keep in mind that 'lesbian and gay hate-crime survivors may perceive that their sexual orientation places them at heightened risk for all kinds of negative experiences in a dangerous world over which they have little control ... Survivors of bias victimization may tend to interpret all of the negative events in their lives as resulting from sexual prejudice. One important goal for interventions with victims, therefore, may be to assist them in regaining a balanced view that allows them to recognize the objective dangers posed by society's prejudice, while not being overwhelmed by a sense of personal vulnerability and powerlessness' (Herek et al., 1999).

8.4 Sexual Abuse and Mental Health

- Research indicates that sexual abuse and assault may affect victims' mental health and increase the tendency to use substances and engage in HIV risk behavior (Dean et al., 2000).
- Childhood and adolescent sexual abuse is associated with substance abuse, depression, suicide ideation, and a need for mental health services (Remafedi et al., 1991).
- Male-male assaults account for 5% to 10% of reported rape cases (Bureau of Justice Statistics, 1994).
- Adolescent and adult gay men are more often victims of male-male rape than their heterosexual counterparts (Scarce, 1997).
- Most rape crisis centers and medical personnel are unequipped to meet the psychological and physical examination needs of male assault victims (King, 1990).
- Men who were sexually abused as children typically demonstrate higher levels of internalized homophobia and become sexually active at a younger age than other gay men (Knisley, 1992).
- Gay men who have a history of sexual abuse have a higher rate of HIV risk taking than men who have no such history (Bartholow et al., 1994).
- Studies indicate that male-male rape almost always involves unprotected anal intercourse, which adds anxiety about HIV transmission to the trauma of sexual assault (Kalichman & Rompa, 1995).
- More than one-third of young gay men have sexual encounters with older or stronger partners, involving force that qualifies as sexual abuse (Doll et al., 1992).
- The rate of childhood sexual abuse and adult sexual assault for lesbians is comparable to rates for the general female population, which refutes the assertion that lesbians choose their sexual orientation in reaction to assaultive sexual experiences with men (Herman & Hirschman, 1981).

After a Violent Physical Assault

- Refer for urgent physical care, emergency room rape protocols, and documentation and photographing of injuries (when indicated).

If there is a risk of stalking or retaliation, ensure the patient's immediate safety by recruiting supportive friends or family members, or by involving the police. Explore alternative housing options when indicated.

- Encourage the patient to maximize supports after a trauma and to report the incident to the police. Keep a list of gay and lesbian community contacts who deal with issues of gay bashing and violence. Encourage the patient to document carefully what has happened, the time, place, and any witnesses who were present while the patient's memory is still fresh and details are clear.
- When counseling in the aftermath of trauma, ask the patient to describe the incident and assault, and note elements of marked distress in reporting the incident. Immediately and actively challenge any assumptions of self-blame or the emergence of increased internalized homophobia with respect to the incident (e.g., 'This wouldn't have happened if I wasn't so obviously gay').
- Explore feelings of helplessness, anger, shame, fear, and loss, applying standard crisis management protocols.
- Look for increased suicidal ideation or homicidal fantasies, and for the increased use of drug or alcohol to cope with the incident.
- Ask about past incidents of violence or trauma, which may make the individual vulnerable to developing posttraumatic stress disorder. Rule out the presence of posttraumatic stress disorder (per DSM-IV Diagnostic Criteria for Posttraumatic Stress Disorder). Refer for subspecialty gay-affirmative psychological/psychiatric care where appropriate.
- Emphasize survival rather than victimhood. Refer the individual to gay-affirmative violence support groups and/or self-defense classes.
- Look for the emergence of social withdrawal or the development of Axis I mood disorders or anxiety disorders. Refer where appropriate for subspecialty follow-up.
- If the patient is not responding to basic counseling maneuvers, refer for subspecialty care for cognitive-behavioral therapy with systematic trauma/phobia desensitization protocols. Short-term prescription of antianxiety agents may be indicated.

After a Sexual Assault

- Take a history of the specific abuse events, their context, duration, and the patient's age when the abuse started. Is the sexual interference repetitive or a one-time occurrence, coercive or forceful (rape)? Did it involve fondling/exposure or penetration/intercourse?

- Respect the client's limits in revealing details. Allow the patient to set the timing and pace. Do not press for information as this may lead to psychological decompensation. Reassert therapeutic/counseling boundaries to define safety.
- Ask about levels of shame, trust, and internalized homophobia. Abused gays or lesbians often believe that their orientation is a result of same-sex abuse. They may manifest higher levels of expressed or internalized homophobia if the perpetrator was a same-sex individual. Use education strategies to address misperceptions about the cause of sexual orientation. Explore any relationship between the abuse and avoidance of intimacy within same-sex relationships.
- Ask about current self-harm behaviors and thoughts, including suicidality.
- Refer to supportive gay-affirmative survivor groups.
- Discuss civil and criminal legal options, including the possibility of charging the perpetrator many years after the incident. Refer for legal counsel. Explore pros and cons of such an approach, but articulate that this could be the final step after the client has worked through the abuse emotionally.
- Explore all feelings about the abuse, including shame and ambivalence. Does the patient have loving or erotic feelings for the perpetrator as well as feelings of rage and betrayal? If the abuse was perpetrated by a same-sex adult, the patient may experience 'double shame' about sexual orientation and trauma.
- Consider asking the client to write a confrontational letter to the perpetrator, which may never be sent. This may allow the emergence of complex feelings that the client can then explore within counseling.
- Ask the client to articulate how the abuse has changed his or her life and feelings of safety and acceptance in the world. Challenge any self-blame aggressively within the context of therapy. Ask the patient to articulate why he or she may have been particularly vulnerable to such abuse as a child. Reinforce that gender atypicality, ostracism, neglect, or isolation may have contributed to being targeted but that 'being different' did not justify abuse.
- Encourage the client's partner or select family members to provide support when appropriate. Recognize that some clients may not be out about their sexual orientation, much less their history of abuse.
- Strategize around revealing the abuse to members of the family of

origin. Discuss the pros and cons. Be prepared for the family to discount the reports of abuse or to ascribe homophobic blame (i.e., 'You asked for it'). A family may actually deny that a member was capable of homosexual abuse of a child. Some families will 'double stigmatize' a member for being gay and bearing news about abuse. Respect the patient's decisions to act or not to act.

Treating Sexual Compulsion/Addiction

Clinicians working with lesbians and gay men will likely encounter patients who complain of an inability to control compulsive sexual behaviors. This behavior may involve high levels of risk taking, including unsafe sexual practices. Among mental health workers, there is no general consensus about the existence or definition of a clinical entity called sexual addiction. This behavior is not included in the DSM-IV, and as a result the comparative incidence in gay and lesbian communities to heterosexual communities is unknown.

Some clinicians view sexual compulsivity as a form of obsessive-compulsive disorder or anxiety disorder; others link it to Axis II diagnoses involving poor impulse control or view it as an Axis I depression variant. See 8.5 for a series of questions that help clinicians and clients identify problematic sexually compulsive behaviors.

8.5 Identifying Problematic Sexually Compulsive Behavior: A Descriptive Diagnostic Tool – Sample Handout for Patients

- Do you think of yourself as overly preoccupied or obsessed with sex?
- Do you feel driven to have sex in response to the effects of stress, anxiety, depression, or other intense emotions?
- Have serious problems developed as a result of your sexual behavior (e.g., injuries, illnesses, loss of a job, or fiscal instability)?
- Do you find yourself constantly cruising or scanning the environment for a potential sexual partner, even when you don't feel it's appropriate?
- Do you often find yourself preoccupied by the idea of making sexual contact with a particular man (woman) you've seen or heard about, even if you don't know him (her)?

- Have you repeatedly tried to stop or reduce certain sexual behaviors and been unable to do so?
- Have you missed important events in the lives of your family, friends, or life partner because of the time you spend pursuing sex?
- Do you feel yourself violating your own ethical standards or principles in sex?
- Do you worry about becoming HIV-positive, yet regularly have risky sex anyway?

And here are a few questions that need to be balanced against the realities of being gay in a largely straight world, but are still worth thinking about.

- Do you keep the extent or nature of your sexual activities hidden from friends and/or partners?
- Do your sexual encounters place you in danger of arrest for lewd conduct or public indecency?
- Do you often have sex with men or women because you're feeling aroused and later regret it?
- Has your involvement with pornography, phone sex, or online sex kept you from other kinds of intimate contact with romantic partners?
- When you have sex, do you feel depressed, guilty, or ashamed afterwards?
- Has the money you have spent on sex-related activities seriously strained your financial resources?

Adapted from Twenty Questions (Sexual Compulsive Anonymous) and educational materials from the Del Amo Hospital in California.

When working with a client with sexually compulsive behavior, consider the following approach:

- Ask the patient to describe sexual behaviors: frequency, location, risks involved, past history of arrests, previous humiliations, job loss, or relationship loss.
- Discuss the meaning the behavior seems to have for the patient at this point in his or her life. Is it related to grief, isolation, shame,

internalized homophobia, low self-esteem? Ask about attempts to stop the behavior: What has worked, what has failed, what has led to relapse?

- Ask the client to describe any rituals that precede the behavior and triggers that activate it. Establish a hierarchy of key triggers, behaviors, and rituals, and develop strategies to avoid, modify, or substitute for them.
- Develop strategies the client can use to substitute different choices.
- Look for the coexistence of an Axis I diagnosis, such as anxiety, depression, or substance abuse. Refer for appropriate physical examination for STDs, including HIV. Ask repeatedly about safe sex practices within the context of compulsive sexuality and the patient's knowledge of consequences/risk.
- Incorporate cognitive-behavioral strategies and relaxation techniques within counseling. Where appropriate, refer the client to gay/lesbian-affirmative sexual addiction or sexual compulsiveness groups (available in most urban centers). Some patients may ask for inpatient treatment, and these programs are available.
- Ask about any history of past physical/sexual abuse that may have led to self-objectification or emotional dissociation from sexual behavior.
- Assess the emotional impact of the behavior in terms of self-esteem, shame, self-hatred, and parasuicidal ideation. Ask patients to talk about risks taken, losses realized, lies they may have told to loved ones, and the impact of these lies on intimate relationships. Explore the association between internalized homophobia and self-destructive impulses. Has internalized homophobia led the patient to believe that loving, connected sexual expression with a same-sex partner is impossible?
- Consider judicious use of anxiolytics or antiobsessional agents in the serotinergic antidepressant class when indicated.

Counseling Gay and Lesbian Clients: Developmental Issues and Clinical Considerations

Regardless of their preferred model of normal human development, clinicians will find it useful to contemplate any differences in the psychological development of gays and lesbians, underscoring that difference is not deviance. The development of sexual orientation may be distinct from the development of sexual identity. Sexual orientation can be defined as a preponderance of sexual erotic feelings, thoughts, fantasies, and/or beliefs present from an early age. Sexual identity, however, is a consistent, enduring, self-recognition of the meaning that sexual orientation and sexual behavior have for the individual in his or her life (Davies et al., 1996).

Childhood

Gay men and women often report 'feeling different' as early as age 4 or 5. Throughout their lives, they are constantly exposed to usually well-defined notions of male/female behavior and expectations of eventual heterosexual compliance. When their behavior, gender, identity, or orientation is different from the prevailing norms, others may detect and respond to these differences. For example, the 'pregay' child may be ostracized for exhibiting gender atypical behaviors (e.g., gentleness in boys, roughness in girls). Richard Isay (1995) in *Being Homosexual: Gay Men and Their Development* describes how many fathers are uncomfortable with any gender atypical expression in their sons and may respond to that behavior by becoming hostile or by withdrawing emotionally. Isay argues that these trends do not cause the child to become gay, but they may complicate his successful intimate relationships with men later on. Although the feelings of being different experienced by children are described as presexual, they may be accompanied by fascinations for or crushes on same-sex individuals. Pregay children may also be drawn to the opposite sex in play activities.

Adolescence

By adolescence, feelings of difference are heightened by the emergence of physical development and same-sex physical/erotic attractions (see Chapter 5). Adolescence is a period that demands gender and social conformity, and peers may be particularly aggressive toward a gay or lesbian teen. In this homophobic environment – with no gay role models, information about same-sex dating or sexual activity, or social places to meet other gays – the teen can become isolated.

Exploring same-sex urges may seem too dangerous: it may lead to physical violence, ridicule, or expulsion from family or school. Instead, the gay youth may try to hide his or her differences by developing a 'passing self': someone who complies with gender norms of masculinity or femininity, including dating and having sex with the opposite sex. Gay youth may be hypervigilant or 'on guard' against exposure or ridicule and become even more estranged from themselves, which can affect their ability to develop real intimacy with friends and family or to develop trust across relationships. To compensate for their perceived 'inner flaw,' some teens become super students or athletes; others become depressed or suicidal or use drugs or alcohol to escape unacceptable sexual urges. In general, gay young men and women tend to have their first sexual experience at an older age than their heterosexual peers.

Adulthood

Although more gay teens and young adults are now able to negotiate coming out to themselves and to parents, schoolmates, and teachers successfully, without particular internal or external conflict, some do not consolidate the development of sexual identity in adolescence. They may continue to have same-sex attractions and fantasies but never act on them. Some may avoid sexual relationships altogether, sublimating their sexuality into work or service vocations, while others marry someone of the opposite sex and/or furtively seek out same-sex contact throughout adulthood.

As gay or lesbian youth come to explore and accept a gay or lesbian identity and their affiliation to the gay community and its social groups and agencies, they may develop an initial sense of estrangement or hostility to mainstream heterosexual culture. This phase may allow some consolidation of a lesbian, gay, or 'queer' sense of self and foster a sense of belonging to a political movement and supportive community. At this stage, the gay person's focus may be on building a supportive network and gay family of choice rather than searching for an intimate mate.

8.6 Strategies for Fitting into Mainstream Society

Lesbians and gays may use a number of different strategies to construct a social identity and fit into mainstream society. Each of these strategies can exact an unacknowledged or even unconscious price in terms of self-esteem.

1. *Capitulation.* The individual avoids all gay/lesbian impulses and settings.

2. *Passing.* The person keeps his or her personal and public worlds separate, but does not come out publicly.
3. *Covering.* The individual will come out if asked or confronted, but will otherwise try to cover sexual orientation.
4. *Blending.* The individual insists that the lesbian or gay identity is irrelevant within the world, and avoids discussing it, but will not deny it if asked.
5. *Distancing.* The individual avoids problematic situations where sexual orientation could be revealed and controls all personal information given. He or she pretends to be straight and may consciously distance from gay colleagues within the workplace.

When working with gay men and lesbians, clinicians should be aware that the ongoing negotiation of sexual identities within the family of origin and workplace can continue to be a struggle for many in the gay community. Clinicians should also be aware of some gender-related differences. For example:

• Males tend to explore their same-sex attraction sooner than females, while females may identify as lesbian before even having sex with a woman.
• Up to 90% of females have had a previous sexual experience with men, whereas the percentage of gay males who have had a previous sexual experience with women is much lower.

Chronic exposure to homophobic attitudes is a significant stressor for gays and lesbians across the developmental life cycle. Studies show that high levels of internalized homophobia correlate with overall psychological distress, depression, somatic symptoms, poor self-esteem, loneliness and poor social support, and high-risk sexual behaviors. Coming out to one's self and to others is a unique and significant component in healthy development for gays and lesbians and has been demonstrated to reduce symptoms of anxiety and depression; produce higher self-esteem; enhance relationships and a sense of community; and allow reintegration into the family of origin and the community.

Some people do experience a period of grief around the loss of their former 'heterosexual' identity, including the apparent possibility of having children, producing grandchildren for their parents, or marrying. Most gay and lesbian individuals articulate coming out to others as a continual process that happens throughout life, in new settings and with new individuals, groups, and colleagues. Because other people's response to coming out is never predictable or safe, this process can be chronically stressful.

For the 'out' gay man or lesbian, the concerns of middle adulthood seem to be the same as those of heterosexual peers: career, relationships, financial goals, and thoughts of retirement. However, the individual in mid-life who has not come to terms with sexual identity and orientation, and who delays coming out until this phase of life, may experience depression and a profound sense of grief and loss over lost time. The urban gay male community's emphasis on youthfulness and sexual attractiveness may trigger a crisis for some aging men (the emphasis on youth and looks is thought to be less significant for lesbians). See Chapter 12 for the issues associated with aging.

Models of Identity Formation

Over the last decade, the research literature has offered several models of gay and lesbian identity formation. (No similar model has been developed for bisexual identity development, and this is a key gap.) Troiden's (1988) stages are set out in 8.7. Cass (1979) articulates six similar stages in gay identity and formation, including identity confusion, identity comparison, identity tolerance, identity acceptance, identity pride, and finally identity synthesis.

8.7 Key Characteristics of Each Homosexual Identity Development Stage

1. *Sensitization.* Gender neutral or gender atypical interests; generalized feelings of marginality and difference from same-sex peers.
2. *Identity Confusion.* Same-sex arousal or activity; absence of heterosexual arousal; perceptions of sexual difference; inner turmoil and confusion.
3. *Identity Assumption.* Rewarding contacts with other gays and lesbians; self-definition as homosexual; identity tolerance and acceptance; formation of friendships and involvement/exploration in gay community; sexual experimentation.
4. *Commitment.* Homosexuality adopted as a way of life; indi-

> cated internally by integration of sexuality and emotionality;
> shifts in the meanings and value assigned the homosexual
> identity, and satisfaction with the homosexual identity; indi-
> cated externally by same-sex love relationships, identity dis-
> closure to others, and changes in stigma management and
> strategies (see also Davies et al., 1996).

Coleman (1996) summarizes the possible physical and mental health
risks associated with each of the stages of gay and lesbian identity
formation. For example, in the phase before coming out, there is the risk
of social isolation and low self-esteem. In the coming out phase, there is
risk of rejection by family and peers and the resulting shame, anxiety,
and depression. In the period of exploration of same-sex relationships,
there is the risk for drug use and alcohol use and unsafe sexual activities leading to STDs and HIV in the gay bar culture. The first serious
relationship may bring about a certain insularity from the rest of the
world and possible avoidance of medical care. Finally, integration of
the sexual identity still carries the risk of not revealing sexual orientation to medical caregivers, which can lead to substandard care. Other
authors suggest that women's identity formation is different: more
fluid and more likely to be informed by interaction with the social
environment. In addition, women may define sexual identity as different from sexual behavior (see 8.8).

8.8 Stages in Lesbian Identity Formation

Ponse (1977) describes the following phases in lesbian identity
formation:

1. A woman realizes that she has desire for women, which signi-
   fies a difference from her heterosexual peers.
2. The possibility of a lesbian identity label is entertained.
3. Lesbian identity is assumed.
4. The woman seeks out the company of lesbians.
5. She then engages in lesbian relationships.

Possible identity outcomes include:

• That she identifies as a lesbian and has lesbian sex.

- That she identifies with a lesbian identity, but has sex with men exclusively, men *and* women, or remains celibate.
- That she identifies as bisexual, but has sex with women.
- That she identifies as heterosexual, but has sex with women.

All the development stage models acknowledge the individual's early feelings of difference, self-acknowledgment of that difference, gradual disclosure to others, experimentation with and exploration of this identity alongside striving toward self-acceptance, and intimacy and consolidation of an overall holistic identity. Counselors who are familiar with these models will find it easier to identify interventions appropriate to each client's specific developmental level. However, practitioners should be aware that these models do not reflect everyone's reality. In particular, they may not reflect the experience of gays and lesbians from ethnic, minority, bisexual, transgendered, marginalized, or impoverished communities.

Guidelines for Counseling a Client on Coming Out

Because coming out may be both a personal or intrapsychic as well as sociopolitical event, counselors are advised to explore the following themes with clients contemplating coming out:

- Establish if coming out to others is the client's priority rather than the priority of someone else, such as a friend or lover.
- Establish levels of personal safety. Should the individual come out at this time in this setting? Is there the risk of violence, loss of home, support, children, livelihood?
- Encourage the individual to admit first to self about same-sex attractions, to obtain education, to meet other gay people, and to fully acknowledge and challenge his or her own negative assumptions around gay identity before coming out to others.
- Encourage selectivity at first. It is not necessary for a client to be out with everyone, everywhere, at the same time. Information about sexuality cannot be taken back once divulged.
- Suggest that a person come out in stages, usually to one person at a time (e.g., telling a best friend first, then another friend, a supportive family member, a sibling, then parents). See 8.9 for a grid for staged coming out.
- Discourage the client from coming out during a crisis or in anger, when intoxicated, or as an act of revenge.

- Suggest that coming out occur in a private place.
- Ask the client to consider both the best and worst case scenarios of coming out to a particular individual and to strategize around coping with a negative outcome.
- Provide resources, including a bibliotherapy and information on support groups such as PFLAG for family members who may initially respond to news of a gay child with shock or disdain.
- Encourage the individual to keep dialogue with friends and family open, even after a negative reaction to coming out. Point out that it may have taken the client years to accept his or her sexual orientation – it is unlikely that everyone will accept or understand it instantaneously.
- Recognize that, for some gay men, reluctance to come out and explore sexual relationships may be linked more specifically to 'AIDS-phobia' (i.e., the fear of contracting HIV). Such fears can usually be addressed with appropriate education and gay-affirmative group support, but psychiatric consultation may be required.
- Remind the individual that coming out is a lifelong process. Encourage your clients to develop supportive friendships both within and outside of the gay community that will help them process and metabolize stressful events.

8.9 Grid for Staged Coming Out – Sample Patient Handout for Use in Counseling

To Whom	Why	When	Where	Pros	Cons
Yourself					
Friend(s)					
Sibling(s)					
Parent(s)					
Colleague(s)					
Boss					
Business					
Partner					
Classmate(s)					
Acquaintances					

Guidelines for Counseling and Psychotherapy with Gays and Lesbians

The consolidation of identity and the process of coming out to one's self and to others are crucial aspects of gay and lesbian mental health, and patients may present with concerns that require counseling or psychotherapy. The Association of Gay and Lesbian Psychiatrists, a U.S. organization with international membership, has republished guidelines prepared by the American Psychological Association for psychotherapy with lesbian, gay, and bisexual clients, which are reprinted below. Although the guidelines were written for psychologists, they are relevant to all mental health professionals and the people they work with. These principles and those set out in 8.10, 8.11, and 8.12 should inform comprehensive psychosocial care of the gay or lesbian patient and enhance the therapist's basic skills.

Attitudes toward Homosexuality and Bisexuality

Guideline 1: Psychologists understand that homosexuality and bisexuality are not indicative of mental illness.

Guideline 2: Psychologists are encouraged to recognize how their attitudes and knowledge about lesbian, gay, and bisexual issues may be relevant to assessment and treatment and seek consultation or make appropriate referrals when indicated.

Guideline 3: Psychologists strive to understand the ways in which social stigmatization (i.e., prejudice, discrimination, and violence) poses risks to the mental health and well-being of lesbian, gay, and bisexual clients.

Guideline 4: Psychologists strive to understand how inaccurate or prejudicial views of homosexuality or bisexuality may affect the client's presentation in treatment and the therapeutic process.

Relationships and Families

Guideline 5: Psychologists strive to be knowledgeable about and respect the importance of lesbian, gay, and bisexual relationships.

Guideline 6: Psychologists strive to understand the particular circumstances and challenges facing lesbian, gay, and bisexual parents.

Guideline 7: Psychologists recognize that the families of lesbian, gay, and bisexual people may include people who are not legally or biologically related (i.e., 'the family of choice').

Guideline 8: Psychologists strive to understand how a person's homosexual or bisexual orientation may have an impact on his or her family of origin and the relationship to that family of origin.

Issues of Diversity

Guideline 9: Psychologists are encouraged to recognize the particular life issues or challenges experienced by lesbian, gay, and bisexual members of racial and ethnic minorities that are related to multiple and often conflicting cultural norms, values, and beliefs.

Guideline 10: Psychologists are encouraged to recognize the particular challenges experienced by bisexual individuals.

Guideline 11: Psychologists strive to understand the special problems and risks that exist for lesbian, gay, and bisexual youth.

Guideline 12: Psychologists consider generational differences within lesbian, gay, and bisexual populations, and the particular challenges that may be experienced by lesbian, gay, and bisexual older adults.

Guideline 13: Psychologists are encouraged to recognize the particular challenges experienced by lesbian, gay, and bisexual individuals with physical, sensory, and/or cognitive/emotional disabilities.

Education

Guideline 14: Psychologists support the provision of professional education and training on lesbian, gay, and bisexual issues.

Guideline 15: Psychologists are encouraged to increase their knowledge and understanding of homosexuality and bisexuality through continuing education.

8.10   Guidelines / Suggestions for Gay / Lesbian / Bisexual-Affirmative Practice

Clark (1987/1997) has developed guidelines that clinicians can use for gay-affirmative practice:

1. Be comfortable with your own feelings – including possible same-sex attractions – before working with gay clients.
2. Avoid participating in a client's program to eliminate same-sex attractions as this reinforces the notion of gay, lesbian, and bisexual identity as a pathology.
3. Explore the client's experience with repression and oppression.
4. Help your client to identify internalized stereotypes of lesbigay people and begin deprogramming negative conditioning.
5. Help the client identify and express feelings of anger about ill treatment so it can be channeled constructively.
6. Explore the relationship between the client's sense of self and body / physical impulses.
7. Encourage your client to develop a small gay, lesbian, bisexual support system that offers care and respect.
8. Foster consciousness raising. Suggest your client get involved in political or support groups or community activities.
9. Emphasize a peer relationship so the client does not feel inferior or 'second class.'
10. Ask your client to develop a personal value system as society at large may not validate the client's moral experience.
11. Explore feelings of shame and guilt around same-sex attractions and behaviors.
12. Use the weight of your professional stance to affirm the normalcy of same-sex attractions and behaviors.

8.11   When a Clinician Is New to Lesbigay Practice: Further Suggestions

Stephen Hartman, in a web educational bulletin called 'Affirming Gay and Lesbian Experience in Psychotherapy,' makes the following suggestions for counselors:

- Expose yourself to gay and lesbian culture in order to witness community patterns and norms.
- Don't profess 'acceptance' of the gay, lesbian, bisexual life as this can be patronizing. Offer affirmation instead.
- Aim for GLB cultural fluency. Read books and magazines. Attend films and plays. Provide gay-affirmative reading material in your waiting room.
- When you don't understand something, ask. Most clients will gladly explain or clarify.

8.12 Common Clinician Errors

Even clinicians who keep the above principles in mind and have extensive experience working with gay and lesbian clients frequently commit ideological or technical errors. For example:

- Some may oversimplify orientation by labeling a patient as exclusively gay or straight and failing to consider that the client may not subscribe to the label or may express sexuality in a more fluid way.
- Some overcompensate for heterosexist attitudes by stating that gay orientation is irrelevant to clinical concerns, while others determine that all psychological problems are exclusively due to either the lesbigay identity itself or to internalized homophobia.
- Some counselors profess to be comfortable with gay and lesbian clients but do not ask about sexual functioning, including same-sex practices. This may be because they are ill-equipped to answer any questions clients may have about their sexual practices.
- Some put too much emphasis on HIV and STDs rather than pursuing a timely, ongoing exploration of specific risks.
- Some may unwittingly de-emphasize or trivialize a patient's anger about experiences of homophobia by stating that such emphasis is 'negative' and should be avoided. Others may also not challenge the patient's own homophobic assumptions and sexual/social stereotypes aggressively enough, thereby unconsciously colluding with the client's internalized homophobia.

- Heterosexual counselors – particularly those working with young clients – may focus on the client's past heterosexual activity and label any gay exploration as a 'phase' or as bisexuality. This may send a message to the youth that frank discussion of same-sex attraction and experiences will not be tolerated.
- Some primary care physicians unwittingly marginalize gay and lesbian clients by referring them exclusively to gay/lesbian therapists, even though the therapist may not be competent or suitable to deal with the patient's particular clinical concerns. This often leads to a ghettoization of care.
- Some clinicians, including gay-identified professionals, may overemphasize coming out for the individual, implying that all psychological problems will somehow resolve when the client reveals his or her sexual orientation to family and friends. They may fail to perceive the real risks of rejection, violence, job loss, or family expulsion from disclosing.
- Both physicians and counselors may be reluctant to confront their clients' drug and alcohol use or unsafe sexual activities.
- Physicians and counselors may underdiagnose concurrent depression, anxiety, or posttraumatic stress disorder because they are unaware that gays and lesbians have a higher risk of developing these disorders. They may also be unaware of services/agencies providing gay-affirmative care.
- Therapists may not think to ask clients about any previous negative or homophobic experiences with a mental health care setting, particularly with attempts at conversion therapy. Not having such information may paralyze new therapeutic attempts from the start.
- The counselor who agrees to find out the psychological cause of homosexuality with his or her client is indirectly giving a message that homosexuality is a pathology. These types of questions simply do not occur with heterosexual clients.
- Some counselors trivialize the importance of their gay patients' intimate relationships by describing them as affairs or 'explorations.'
- Clinicians who have not confronted their own stereotypes around homosexuality may ask ignorant questions, such as 'Who is the dominant one in your relationship?' Counselors who lack exposure to gay-affirmative societal markers may fail to show comparable levels of enthusiasm or empathy regard-

ing gay developmental milestones (e.g., a client's moving in with a new partner). Such inadvertent cues may lead a client to withhold information or to only present information that the therapist appears to respond to or favor.

- Failure to discuss the role of religion and spirituality for the client may stall clinical progress. The client may not mention or be willing to discuss internalized negative religious messages about homosexuality unless he or she is asked about them. At the same time, the therapist should be aware of the role of spirituality and the individual's ability to achieve a sense of wholeness and worth. The exploration of existential goals may greatly enhance therapeutic gains.

From McHenry, S., & Johnson, I. (1993). Homophobia in the therapist and gay or lesbian client: Conscious and unconscious collusion in self hate. *Psychotherapy*, *301*(1), 141–9.

CHAPTER NINE

Substance Abuse

*Larry is a 30-year-old gay housepainter who comes to the doctor complaining
of fatigue, apathy, being suspicious of others, and anhedonia. His doctor considers a diagnosis of depression but asks Larry about his alcohol and drug
use. Larry explains that he smokes one or two joints during the day at work
and one in the evening to unwind. His doctor explains the role of marijuana
abuse in Larry's clinical presentation and asks how he would feel about cutting back on his use. Larry takes information about the local lesibigay drug
and alcohol treatment clinic but, as he leaves, expresses some doubt about
wanting to give up his drug use.*

*Noreen is a 50-year-old single lawyer with a past history of alcohol abuse.
She has been drinking a bottle of wine a night to cope with the stresses of
office politics. When she and her doctor discuss harm reduction, Noreen
agrees to try a lesbigay AA group.*

*After her first meeting, she returns to her doctor complaining that the
12-step program is paternalistic and overly religious. They discuss the pros
and cons of attending, and Noreen decides to express her concerns at the next
meeting. She eventually decides that the support offered by the group outweighs her ideological reservations.*

Alcohol and drug use are serious issues in the lesbian and gay communities. This chapter looks at patterns of alcohol and drug use and
discusses interventions that can be used to change addictive behaviors
and reduce risk.

Alcohol, Tobacco, and Drug Use

What is the incidence of substance use among gays, lesbians, and bisexuals? There appears to be no definitive agreement on levels of alcohol, tobacco, and drug use, and the literature provides a mix of findings, as outlined below.

Alcohol

- Gay men and lesbians account for twice as many reported alcohol problems as heterosexuals – despite similar patterns of heavy drinking in each population (McKirnan & Peterson, 1989).
- Heterosexual populations demonstrate a more marked correlation between aging and decline in alcohol consumption than homosexual populations (Skinner, 1994).
- Lesbian and heterosexual women report similar bar-going habits and comparable levels of alcohol consumption (Bloomfield, 1993).
- Lesbians report higher rates of abstention from alcohol than heterosexual women (Bloomfield, 1993).
- Gay men are more likely than heterosexual men to drink heavily or to abstain from alcohol. However, the overall quantity and frequency of consumption by these groups is comparable (Stall & Wiley, 1988).

Tobacco

- More representative studies of tobacco use indicate a significantly higher prevalence of smoking among gay men than heterosexual men (Stall et al., 1999).
- Lesbians tend to smoke more than gay men (Skinner & Otis, 1996).
- Lesbians who smoke may be at a higher risk for health problems because of their higher average body mass index and their tendency to seek health care less often. This reduces their access to overall risk factor screening (e.g., blood pressure, cholesterol) (White & Dull, 1997).

Drug Use

- Chemical dependency, homophobia, and depression may share a cyclic, synergistic interaction in which emotional and mental states,

external stressors, and substance use contribute to and perpetuate internal conditions and external outlets (Skinner & Otis, 1996).
- Marijuana, tobacco, and cocaine use is more prevalent among lesbians in particular age groups than among gay men, while gay men report higher overall rates of illicit drug use (Skinner & Otis, 1996).
- Gay men report using a more extensive variety of illicit drugs than heterosexual men, yet they do not demonstrate higher rates of dependence or addiction. Their rates of use are also similar (Stall & Wiley, 1988).
- More lesbians than heterosexual women report recreational drug use (Buenting, 1992).
- Gay men are more likely than heterosexual men to have recently used marijuana and psychedelics, and to have used barbiturates, MDMA, and amyl or butyl nitrates ('poppers') in their lifetime (Stall & Wiley, 1988; Stall et al., 1999).

Researchers explain some of the discrepancies by noting that early studies were rife with methodological errors, including the lack of clear definitions of gay and lesbian identity or of substance abuse; lack of control groups for comparison; underrepresentation of women; and faulty sampling techniques (i.e., interviewing bar patrons regarding alcohol use).

Despite these methodological weaknesses, Cabaj and Stein (1996), in the *Textbook of Homosexuality and Mental Health*, conclude that the incidence of substance abuse of all kinds is about 30% in the gay and lesbian population compared to 10% to 12% in the general population. However, these statistics have been received with caution by the gay and lesbian community, which is concerned that they could be misused by homophobic lobby groups to link patterns of substance misuse to moral or psychological flaws related to a homosexual lifestyle (Lacouture, 1998). In fact, the higher risk of alcohol and substance abuse among gays and lesbians can be attributed not to sexual orientation but to the following factors:

- Genetic, biological, and biochemical factors (Bailey et al., 1993).
- The impact of homophobia – both societal and internalized (Bailey et al., 1993). The use of mood-altering substances may be an attempt to quell high levels of internalized homophobia and self-hatred (Isay, 1995).

- Conflict around gay and lesbian identity (Isay, 1995). Psychological defense mechanisms used to deny sexual orientation, such as denial, suppression, repression, and presentation of a false or heterosexually acceptable self, may be predictors of drug and alcohol abuse in adulthood (Isay, 1995). Substance misuse invokes dissociation from sexual orientation concerns and mimics the psychologically defensive tendency to dissociate from disavowed parts of the self (Isay, 1995).
- The role of the bar as the predominant meeting place for gays and lesbians – due to the lack of other affirmative or safe venues for socializing and support (Skinner & Otis, 1996). Gay men and women in recovery or those who want to reduce their use may become socially isolated because of the lack of venues where they can socialize without consuming alcohol or drugs.
- A comorbid history of depression, anxiety, low self-esteem, and social isolation (see Chapter 8). One review showed that 70% of females and 42% of males in a substance-abusing cohort reported a history of sexual abuse (Neisen & Sandall, 1996). Coexistent posttraumatic stress disorder (PTSD) may be present.

For young gays and lesbians, peer pressure to consume may be high. They are exposed to role models who use alcohol and drugs, and individuals who are coming out may be vulnerable to higher levels of substance use (Bailey et al., 1993). Alcohol in particular is used for self-medication of anxiety and shame regarding exploring sexual orientation (Bailey et al., 1993). Drugs – especially rave drugs (discussed below) – are considered sexual enhancers and may in fact allow an individual to engage in activities he or she might otherwise be fearful of and avoid. Some gay men may use alcohol and drugs to reduce fears about acquiring HIV infection, and their use may lead to unsafe sex practices and may complicate HIV treatment (Ferrando, 1997). Some alcohol and drug use in the gay community may be driven by economics. Gay men have higher disposable incomes, and tobacco and alcohol companies actively target them as consumers (Stall & Wiley, 1988).

Part of the high rates of use may also be attributed to the difficulty many gays and lesbians have in asking for help with an addiction. Being gay and addicted creates a double stigma, making it more difficult for people to come out about either or both. It can also be difficult to find treatment for substance misuse in a nonheterosexist, nonhomophobic environment (O'Hanlan et al., 1997).

Assessing Gay and Lesbian Patients for a Substance Use Disorder

As with any patient with a history of alcohol or drug misuse, the clinician will begin by doing an appropriate assessment and gathering the information outlined in 9.1, 9.2, and 9.3.

9.1 Does Your Patient Have an Alcohol Problem?

Use the CAGE screen for diagnosis of alcoholism:

C   Thought you should cut back?
A   Felt annoyed by people criticizing your drinking?
G   Felt guilty or bad about your drinking?
E   Had a morning eye-opener to relieve hangover or nerves?

Score 2 or 3 = high index of suspicion; 4 = pathognomonic.

From Ewing, J. (1984). Detecting alcoholism: The CAGE questionnaire. *Journal of the American Medical Association, 25*(30), 1905–7.

9.2 Substance Use Disorder Assessment

Use Patterns

- Frequency and degree of intoxication
- Severity of withdrawal symptoms
- Timing and quantity of most recent dose
- Mode, frequency, duration of use
- Subjective effects of use
- List of all drugs used, including drug of choice

Medical / Psychiatric History

- Complete physical exam to observe sequelae of use, presence of current intoxication/involvement
- Psychiatric history to rule out presence of Axis I and Axis II disorders
- Mental status examination/presence of dementing illness (neuropsychological testing may be indicated)

- History of sexual, physical abuse
- Patient's observations on link between substance use and internalized homophobia, coming out process, discrimination, or history of violence

History of Substance Disorders

Past treatment:
- Setting
- History of homophobic barriers to care and degree of satisfaction
- Network used
- Duration of treatment
- Optional versus involuntary treatment
- Compliance
- Duration of outcome
- Noted improvement in social/occupational functioning after treatment
- Other efforts made in past to control use

Family History / Social History

- Current living arrangement
- Relationship status – does partner use substances
- Comfort with sexual orientation
- Stage of coming out and degree/selectivity of being out
- Relationship to family of origin
- Presence/absence of lesbigay-affirmative supports
- Experience of homophobic discrimination/violence
- Developmental history
- Substance use in family/friends
- Mental illness in family/friends
- Relationship history (friends, partners, children, parents, supports)
- Impact of substance use on relationships
- Peer relationships, loss of supports due to use
- Legal/financial complications of use
- School/occupational functioning
- Social patterns of use – with whom, where, when, how, social supports, financial means to purchase prescriptions

Blood Work

- Blood/urine screening for drug presence/levels/toxicity
- Specific tests linked to substance as indicated: CBC, electrolytes, liver and renal function tests, U/A, blood cultures, PT, PTT
- Infectious disease screen (when appropriate) for hepatitis A/B/C, HIV, TB, VDRL (note that many clients may not be psychologically ready to pursue STD testing, and this can generally be deferred until after a treatment alliance is established)
- Immune markers, nutritional markers (B12 and folate, total protein)

Motivation for Treatment

- Why now
- Individual's choice or work/family pressure to stop
- Benefits versus risks of use/stopping
- Consequences of doing nothing
- Change in physical health
- Forensic determinants (i.e., criminal charges pending)
- Goals? Harm Reduction? Abstinence?

Adapted from Expert Panel. (1995). Substance use disorders. *American Journal of Psychiatry, 152* (supplement), 11.

9.3 Substance Abuse / Dependence: Diagnostic Categories

Substance Abuse (DSM-IV)

At least one at any time during a 12-month period:

- Recurrent substance use resulting in a failure to fulfill major role obligations at work, school, or home
- Recurrent substance use in situations in which it is physically hazardous
- Recurrent substance-related legal problems

- Continued substance use despite having persistent or recurrent social or interpersonal problems

Substance Dependence (DSM-IV)

At least three of the following during a 12-month period:

- Marked tolerance (at least 50% increase needed)
- Characteristic withdrawal symptoms or substance taken to avoid withdrawal symptoms
- Substance often taken longer or in larger amounts than the person intended
- Persistent desire or unsuccessful efforts to cut or control use
- Large amount of time spent obtaining, using, or recovering from the substance
- Impaired social, recreational, or occupational functioning
- Persistent use despite knowledge of medical, psychological, or social problems

From *Diagnostic statistical manual* (DSM-IV). (1994). Washington, DC: American Psychiatric Press.

According to addiction specialists, it is important for the assessor to identify both the stage of the individual's substance use and his or her motivation for change. See 9.4 for a description of the distinct stages of addictive behaviors and possible interventions.

9.4 Stages, Motivations, and Interventions for Changing Addictive Behaviors

Stage	Associated thoughts and actions	Possible intervention
Precontemplation	No thoughts about changing habits, contrary to professional opinion	Provide objective feedback based on assessment and discuss risks associated with current drinking level or pattern.
Contemplation	Thoughts about the need to change, but no action taken yet	Explore positive and negative aspects of drinking/using and

Stage	Associated thoughts and actions	Possible intervention
		encourage the belief that change is possible. Explore options for taking action. Recommend cutting back on drinking/using or complete abstinence. Consider referral to mutual aid group or an addiction specialist.
Action	Attempts made to change drinking/ using habits	Encourage commitment to action plan and foster confidence in the ability to change. Consider 'brief intervention,' perhaps with psychopharmological antagonists, analogues (see below). Consider referral to mutual aid group or addiction specialist
Maintenance	Drinking habits have been changed, and the person is adjusting to the changes	Help develop plan to prevent relapse and continue to foster confidence in the ability to sustain changes. Continue with psychopharmological agent indicated. Consider referral to mutual aid group.
Relapse	Changes have been or are in the process of being reversed	Encourage the belief that all is not lost and explore reasons the relapse occurred. Help find other ways to cope with relapse-provoking situations. Consider alternative treatments.

From Ogborne, A.C. (2000). Identifying and treating patients with alcohol-related problems. *Canadian Medical Association Journal, 162*(12), 27.

Treating Substance Abuse

For treatment to be enduring and successful, rehabilitation must explore the patient's current difficulties, stressors, and risks. Detoxification may be the first step, but if the goal is enduring harm reduction or abstinence it is essential to have ongoing follow-up. Treatments with successful outcomes usually include the following (Gliatte, 1999):

- no less than two years of rehabilitation
- exposure to a therapeutic milieu with other people in rehabilitation
- staff with a high level of skills
- the availability of specialized counseling that emphasizes relapse prevention.

Controversy continues to exist among drug treatment experts about the benefits of abstinence (defined as complete cessation of use of the substance) versus harm reduction, which emphasizes the patient's autonomy to make decisions around use along with access to nonjudgmental care and disease prevention, including needle exchange programs. No definitive retrospective studies comparing the relative benefits of these treatment goals in gay and lesbian patients have yet been conducted or released.

When working with a gay or lesbian client, ask if he or she is interested in an individual focus, couple or family therapy, group therapy, and/or self-help modalities. Explore inpatient versus outpatient treatment options. Specify any preference for a lesbigay emphasis in treatment. Recognize that the presence of dual diagnoses (i.e., Axis I diagnosis, such as depression or bipolar disorder, as well as a substance abuse disorder) may complicate treatment and outcome. Work with the client to clarify his or her treatment goals. Discuss the feasibility of abstinence versus harm reduction and the relative advantages and risks of each approach given the client's drug use history. Discuss other goals, such as the reduction of frequency and severity of relapse, and potential improvement of overall functioning, including the ability to maintain relationships or to stay employed. Address and manage the medical risks of withdrawal and the client's fears about withdrawal (see 9.5).

9.5 Principles of Treatment Management

- Establish therapeutic alliance – monitor patient's status.
- Manage intoxication withdrawal states.

- Reduce morbidity sequelae of drug use with appropriate referral for medical care where indicated.   .
- Facilitate adherence to treatment plan.
- Strategize regarding relapse prevention.
- Provide education around risks of substance abuse.
- Diagnose and treat comorbid psychiatric disorders such as bipolar disorder, depression, anxiety, or psychosis.
- Explore pharmacological strategies as part of treatment plan (i.e., use of agonists, antagonists, substitutes, deterrents, and withdrawal treatment).
- Refer to appropriate therapy – individual programs/group-family/self-help.
- Select setting option – hospital, residential, therapeutic community, partial hospitalization, outpatient department, aftercare.

Adapted from Expert Panel. (1995). Substance use disorders. *American Journal of Psychiatry, 152* (supplement).

Many gay and lesbian clients will have had experience with Alcoholics Anonymous (AA) and its offshoots, including Cocaine Anonymous (CA) and Narcotics Anonymous (NA). Ask the client to talk about the advantages and disadvantages of these involvements and whether he or she plans to stay involved in these groups. Some clients have difficulty with the theistic premise of AA. Women, in particular, have criticized its emphasis on helplessness in the face of substance abuse. Nonetheless, AA can be a useful, initial supportive step toward recovery or an adjunct to other recovery modalities. Lesbigay-specific groups exist in most urban centers. Encourage the client to try out several to confirm the best fit in terms of support and ideology. See 9.6 for AA's 12 steps.

9.6 Alcoholics Anonymous 12 Steps

1. We admit that we were powerless over alcohol and all other mind-altering substances – that our lives had become unmanageable.
2. We came to believe that a Power greater than ourselves could restore us to sanity.

3. We made a decision to turn our will and our lives over to the care of God as we understood Him.
4. We made a searching and fearless moral inventory of ourselves.
5. We admitted to God, to ourselves, and to another human being the exact nature of our wrongs.
6. We were entirely ready to have God remove all these defects of character.
7. We humbly asked Him to remove our shortcomings.
8. We made a list of all persons we had harmed, and became willing to make amends to them all.
9. We made direct amends to such people whenever possible, except when to do so would injure them or others.
10. We continued to take personal inventory and when we were wrong promptly admitted it.
11. We sought through prayer and meditation to improve our conscious contact with God as we understood Him, praying only for knowledge of His will for us and the power to carry that out.
12. Having had a spiritual awakening as the result of these steps, we tried to carry this message to addicts, and to practice these principles in all our affairs.

From Alcoholics Anonymous website (www.aa.org).

The Impact of Substance Use

As part of the process of coming to terms with their substance use, clients may need information or education about specific substances, their addiction patterns, and the associated physical and emotional effects of using them (see 9.7 for a list of commonly misused substances, their method of use, short-term and long-term effects, and their withdrawal symptoms). The clinician may not be an expert in drug treatment, but should be familiar with current protocols so that he or she can make an appropriate referral and provide the education and preparation the client may need. For up-to-date medical protocols for managing specific intoxication, withdrawal, and abstinence treatments, see a current psychiatric, medical, or substance abuse textbook or consult online www.camh.net.

9.7 Substance Use 101

Substance	Methods of use	Short-term effect	With larger doses and longer use	Long-term effect	Withdrawal symptoms
Alcohol (booze, brew, hooch, grog)	Oral/injected.	Stimulates, then depresses. Effects vary with size, sex, metabolism, stomach contents: initial relaxation; loss of inhibitions; feeling of warmth; skin flushed; impaired coordination.	Slower reflexes and thinking; risk taking, impaired judgment; blackouts; slurred speech; staggering gait; effects magnified by other depressants; increased likelihood of accidents, sleepiness; unconsciousness; overdose may be fatal (respiratory failure).	Possible gastritis, pancreatitis, liver cirrhosis, hepatomegaly, cancers of the gastrointestinal tract, cardiomyopathy; suppression of sex hormones; loss of appetite; vitamin depletion; risk of damage to the fetus (FAS = fetal alcohol syndrome); psychological and physical dependence, recurrent physical injuries, tremor, dyspepsia, impotence, hypertension, palpitations, insomnia, polyuria.	Insomnia; headache; appetite loss; nausea; sweating; tremors; convulsions; hallucinations; may lead to death.
Amphetamines (including Biphethamine/Dexedrine, speed, ice, glass, crystal, crank, bennies, uppers, black beauties, crosses, hearts)	Oral, smoked; injected, sniffed.	Stimulates CNS (central nervous system); enhanced mood; increased energy; talkativeness; alertness; restlessness, paranoia, aggression; reduced appetite; rise in heart rate and blood pressure; dilated pupils, itchy scalp/skin.	Excitability; sense of power; aggression; delusions and hallucinations; delirium, violence; high blood pressure, dysthymia, twitching, jerking, dry mouth, fever, sweating.	Malnutrition; emaciation; susceptibility to infections; nephritis, may suppress immune system, worsens risk of hepatitis/pancreatitis, stomach ulcer, congestive heart failure.	Fatigue, irritability, depression, craving, anxiety, psychosis.

9.7 (Continued)

Substance	Methods of use	Short-term effect	With larger doses and longer use	Long-term effect	Withdrawal symptoms
Barbiturates (including Amytol, Seconal, Phenobarbital, Nembutal) (downers, barbs, blue heavens, yellow jackets, red devils)	Oral; sometimes injected.	Sedative and CNS depressant; similar to alcohol intoxication. Small dose produces mild 'high'; dizziness, lethargy; drowsiness, sedation; impaired short-term memory; nausea; abdominal pain; with large dose effects similar to alcohol; mood swings; risk taking; bad judgment; lower blood pressure, decreased motor activity/heart rate/respirations; may cause fetal damage.	Unsteady gait, slurred speech, blurred vision. Unpredictable, extreme behavior; severely impaired thinking, coordination; distorted perceptions; sleep or unconsciousness; extremely dangerous when combined with other depressants; possible death from overdose (respiratory suppression).	Tolerance/dependence develop. Impaired memory, thinking; hostility; depression; mood swings; impotence; menstrual irregularities; chronic fatigue; possible birth defects and behavioral abnormalities in infants born to users; rapid tolerance and dependence.	Temporary sleep disturbances; trembling; anxiety; weakness, dizziness; seizures; delirium; visual hallucinations; vomiting, convulsions, abdominal cramps, high temperature; possible death from cardiovascular collapse, or cerebral hemorrhage.
Cannabis (marijuana, pot, grass, hashish, hash oil, blunt, herb, weed)	Smoked in joints, pipe, or eaten. Synthetic prescription analogues exist. Used therapeutically in palliative care and outpatient settings. Legal in some countries for clinical use.	May have therapeutic role in relieving nausea, pain, improving appetite. A 'high' or happy feeling; faster pulse rate, reddened eyes; sedation; induces talkativeness, hunger, relaxation. Depth-perception and visual tracking impaired. May exacerbate psychotic symptoms in schizophrenia.	Distorts time; sharpens or distorts senses; impairs short-term memory, thinking, ability to perform complex tasks; fatigue, apathy; combining with alcohol increases effects on thinking, behavior, muscle control; hallucinations with very large doses.	Earlier presumed long-term effects (i.e., apathy, impaired judgment, psychological dependence, lower sex drive) are unsubstantiated. Reported diminished cognitive functioning was noted in small samples only. High-dose smokers develop pulmonary symptoms (bronchitis, coughing, wheezing) and invite increased pulmonary carcinoma risk.	Possible insomnia, irritability; appetite loss; anxiety.

			THC is secreted in breast milk. Marijuana may increase appetite in patients with HIV but possible increased risk of aspergillosis in late stage AIDS.	Extended but restless sleep; hunger upon wakening; possible depression.
Cocaine (crack, coke, C, blow, flake, snow, rock)	Sniffed; injected; freebase is smoked.	Stimulant. Quick 'high'; euphoria, talkativeness, energy; mental alertness; loss of appetite; decreased need for sleep; increased self-confidence; aggression; anxiety; increased heart rate, blood pressure; risk of sudden heart failure/arrhythmia.	Stronger, more frequent 'highs' followed by agitation, depression; erratic, violent behavior; paranoid psychosis; restlessness, tremors, crawling sensation under skin; vertigo; blurred vision; muscle spasms; nausea; cold sweat; shallow breathing; risk of seizures, coma, myocardial infarction, cardiovascular collapse, death.	Weight loss; restlessness; mood swings; paranoid delusions, sleep deprivation may lead to violence (reduces dopamine transport); hallucinations; depression; impotence; involuntary teeth grinding/eye rolling; risk of obstetrical complications; psychological dependence.
LSD and Other Hallucinogens. Derived synthetically from mushroom (psilocybin), from cactus (mescaline), from morning glory seeds, nutmeg, jimson weed. Is called acid, microdot, sunshine.	Oral, sniffed; or injected.	Hallucinogen. Rapid pulse; dilated pupils; raised temperature; arousal; distortions of perception, including hallucinations; 'mystical experiences,' exhilaration, or anxiety; panic; sense of power; violent behavior; occasionally convulsions.	Anxiety; panic; paranoid delusions; psychosis; 'bad trips,' injury or accidents due to delusions; increased risk of fetal abnormalities; tolerance develops rapidly. Interacts with PCP, may produce high fever, muscle spasm, erratic behavior, psychosis.	May include muscle tenseness; 'flashbacks' – brief, spontaneous recurrence of prior hallucinations; delusions, panic; profound depression; no physical dependence. Interactions with HIV drugs unknown. Possible flashbacks; anxiety.

9.7 (Concluded)

Substance	Methods of use	Short-term effect	With larger doses and longer use	Long-term effect	Withdrawal symptoms
Narcotic Analgesics (derived synthetically from Asian poppy; opium, codeine, morphine, heroin)	Oral; smoked; or injected.	Stimulates then depresses brain. Surge of pleasure, euphoria, appetite suppression; restlessness; nausea; vomiting; body warmth; limb heaviness; mouth dryness; flushed skin, nausea, vomiting, convulsions, oblivion to surroundings.	Constant drowsiness; constricted pupils; skin cold, moist, bluish; progressive respiratory depression – overdose results in death from suppressed breathing; dangerous combined with alcohol or other depressants; circulatory collapse, cardiac arrest, may lead to death.	Weight loss; reduction in sex hormones; cellulitis, abscesses, endocardial infections; heart, liver, and brain damage from unsterile injection; collapsed veins, rapid tolerance, high potential for physical and psychological dependence, pregnancy/perinatal complications. If needles are shared, high risk for HIV, hepatitis.	Anxiety; perspiration; diarrhea; fever; elevated blood pressure/pulse; abdominal and muscle cramps; yawning; goose bumps; runny nose; craving for the drug. Potential for cardiac collapse with morphine withdrawal.
Poppers (Amyl nitrate, Butyl nitrate, 'rush') Sold as liquid incense, CD/record cleaner.	Inhaled nasally.	Vasodilates, causing hypertension, heart races, blood rushes to face/head, lightheadedness, enhanced orgasm reported, anal sphincter relaxation, nasal tissue burn.		May suppress immune system, unsafe for individuals with cardiac history, dangerous when combined with other hypotensives – Viagra, MDMA. May impair judgment leading to unsafer sexual activities, including decreased sensation of rectal tear during anal sex.	None reported.

| Steroids (Testosterone) (juice, white stuff, roids) | Orally; injected, new patch delivery system. | Aggressiveness ('road rage,' 'killer instinct'); depression; mood swings; paranoia; higher sex drive; euphoria; high blood pressure; tachycardia; water retention; abdominal pain; recurring injuries; headaches; nosebleeds; insomnia. | Increased muscle strength and performance; confidence; enthusiasm. In females: increased facial and body hair; male-pattern baldness; deepened voice; acne; menstrual irregularities; infertility. In males: smaller testicles; infertility; gynecomastia; acne. | Irreversible stunting of growth in children/adolescents; myocardial infarction; stroke; hepatitis; masculinization of user's female babies; physical and psychological dependence. | Severe depression; anxiety; sweating; tremors; diarrhea. |
| Tobacco | Chewed, smoked (inhaled). | Nicotine is stimulating – short-term increase of alertness, energy, sense of well-being. | | Increased risk of MI, stroke, COPD, lung, throat, and mouth cancers, teeth staining/enamel damage, skin wrinkling, fetal abnormalities including IUGR. Rate of HIV infection may be higher in smokers due to higher risk taking in general; smoking increases HAART cardiac side effects (see Chapter 7). | Tobacco craving, irritability, anxiety, decreased concentration, GI upset, weight gain, depression, high risk of relapse. |

Adapted from Canadian Aids Society. (1997). Under the influence: Making the connection between HIV/AIDS and substance use: A guide for ASO workers who provide support to persons living with HIV/AIDS. Ottawa: Canadian Aids Society.

Rave / Circuit Party Drugs

Raves are all-night parties attended by thousands – gay, straight, or mixed – who dance to electronic music (see also Chapter 10). Recreational drug use is widespread at these events. In addition, some gay men travel to large events, called 'circuit parties,' organized in large urban centers, often on a monthly basis. There is controversy within the lesbigay community about the merits and risks of these parties. On the one hand, they are a celebration of lesbigay identity. On the other hand, their emphasis on drug use and focus on the 'perfect body' may lead to risky behavior. Because of the risks, for some gays and lesbians these events may be oppressive. See 9.8 for information on the drugs used at raves and circuit parties, their clinical features, and how to manage their toxicities.

Viagra

Sildenafil citrate, also called 'poke' or 'boner pill,' has emerged as a recreational drug among gay men, who may use it as a sexual enhancement rather than for treatment of erectile dysfunction. Use is contraindicated in men with cardiac history. Risk of stroke/death due to hypertension has been reported due to interactions with amyl nitrate, crystal methamphetamine, and protease inhibitors.

Enhancing Treatment Outcomes: Why Gay-Specific Treatment Matters

Anderson (1996) emphasizes the position shared by many substance counselors who work with the gay and lesbian population: rehabilitation strategies must focus on substance use as one of the manifestations of internalized homophobia. This means that, for gay and lesbian clients, acceptance of their gay identity is one of the steps of recovery from substance abuse. When assessing gay or lesbian clients for alcohol or substance use, the clinician should also include their developmental stage, degree of internalized homophobia, stage of coming out, current supports and relationship to the gay/lesbian community, relationship to family and culture of origin and access to support there, health status including HIV, and comfort level with sexual expression. It is also essential to detect any comorbid diagnoses such as depression, anxiety, or posttraumatic stress disorder (Amico, 1997).

9.8 Party Drugs, Their Features and Toxicities

Drug	Street names	Class	Mechanism	Features	Toxicities
3, 4-Methylenedioxy-methamphetamine (MDMA, ecstasy)*	E, X, XTC, Love, Adam	Hallucinogenic amphetamine	5-HT release	Heightened perception and sensual awareness, mydriasis, sympathomimetic, bruxism, jaw tension, ataxia	Dysrhythmias, hyperthermia, rhabdomyolysis, disseminated, intravascular coagulation hyponatremia, seizures, death
Lysergic aciddiethylamide (LSD)	Acid, Hits, Blotters	Hallucinogen	5-HT2 receptor agonist	Mydriasis, sympathomimetic, nausea, muscle tension, visual hallucinations, agitation	Persistent psychosis, hallucinations, persisting perception disorder, 'flashbacks'
Ketamine*	Kit-kat, Special K	Anesthetic	NMDA receptor agonist	Nystagmus, increased tone, purposeful movements, amnesia, hallucinations, sympathomimetic	Loss of consciousness, respiratory depression, catatonia, highly addictive
Phencyclidine (PCP)	Angel dust, Peace	Anesthetic	Glutamate, agonist at NMDA receptor	Miosis, nystagmus, hypertension, sympathomimetic, cholinergic symptoms	Coma, seizures, hyperthermia rhabdomyolysis, hypoglycemia, hypertension
Crystal methamphetamine	Speed, Crystal, Crys, Jib, Meth	Amphetamine	Enhances release and blocks uptake of catecholamines	Tachycardia, tachypnea, hyptertension, hyperthermia, mydriasis, diaphoresis	Dysrhythmias, seizures, hypertension, hyperthermia, encephalopathy

9.8 (Concluded)

Drug	Street names	Class	Mechanism	Features	Toxicities
Gamma-hydroxybutyrate (GHB)*	G, Liquid	Anesthetic	Biphasic dopamine response	Agitation, nystagmus, ataxia, sedation, amnesia, hypotonia, vomiting, muscle spasms	Seizures, apnea, sudden reverse coma with abrupt awakening, violence, bradycardia, death
Cannabis Oil-resin = hashish Oil-herb = marijuana	Pot, Weed, Grass, Herb	Mild hallucinogen, relaxant	Binds to cannaboid receptor	Mild hallucinations, paranoia, appetite stimulant, tachycardia, conjunctival infection	Rare
Cocaine	Coke, Dust, Blow, Snow, Flake	Stimulant	Inhibits uptake of catecholamines	Tachycardia, hypertension, pyrexia, mydriasis, ataxia, diaphoresis, agitation, delusions, rapid euphoria	Hyperthermia, hallucinations, seizures, death

Note: 5-HT = serotonin, NMDA = N-methly-D-aspartate.
Street names provided by TRIP. Primary source: Tintinalli et al.
*Note: Protease inhibitors may dangerously increase levels of MDMA, Ketamine. There have been reported deaths when alcohol was used with MDMA and GHB. MDMA use with poppers or Viagra led to compounded hypotension: MDMA used with MAO inhibitors may lead to death. Impact of party drug use on safer sex habits should be explored. Long-term use of ecstasy may reduce 5HT (serotonin) levels. Permanent structural damage in serotonin receptors and in serotonin synthesis is postulated; (2000). Psychiatry rounds. *CAMH, 4*(5).

From Weir, E. (2000). Raves: A review of the culture, the drugs and the prevention of harm. *Canadian Medical Association Journal, 162*(13), 1843. Reprinted with permission.

Referring clients to a traditional center that does not recognize or acknowledge issues of racism, coming out, homophobia, heterosexism, and other gay and lesbian concerns may lead to experiences of discrimination. The client may continue to assume a false self, pretending to be heterosexual 'to fit in' with the treatment milieu and perpetuating secrets by re-entering the closet. The Pride Institute, a gay/lesbian-specific treatment center in the United States, describes several gradations of drug treatment centers based on their acknowledgment of gay and lesbian clients (see 9.9).

9.9 Attitudes of Substance Abuse Treatment Centers to Lesbigay Needs

Antigay: Treaters are antagonistic to gay and lesbian clients.

Traditional: The center has no gay sensitivity but is not antagonistic. Heterosexist assumptions, however, prevail.

Gay naive: The center or program realizes that it has gay and lesbian clients, but no official policy or specific approach is in place.

Gay tolerant: Gay concerns may be raised individually, but not in the group setting.

Gay sensitive: Gay-specific workshops are organized, gay staff are engaged, there are groups for gay and lesbian clients, but programs are generally mixed as gay and straight.

Gay affirmative: All programs are designed specifically for gay, lesbian, and bisexual individuals and their particular concerns.

From the Pride Institute website (www.pride-institute.com).

Working with Gays and Lesbians with a Substance Disorder

To enhance treatment protocols, practitioners should consider the following guidelines when working with gay and lesbian patients with a substance disorder.

- Keep a list of gay-sensitive and gay-affirmative resources for individual and group drug treatment.
- When appropriate, refer the client to gay-identified AA, CA, or NA programs.

- Encourage clients of color to seek out programs where lesbigay visible minorities have been successfully received and treated so that cultural isolation does not compound sexual isolation.
- Discuss the advantages of referral to a gay-affirmative program, even if your client is not fully out. Explain to patients that their boundaries will be respected, but issues linking nonacceptance of their orientation with their drug/alcohol problem will be respectfully explored.
- Keep in mind that lesbians have specific challenges, including lower income, responsibility for children, and access to day care. Careful timing in terms of identifying and planning treatment options and recruiting family supports may be essential.
- When possible, provide a range of options for treatment and involve the patient in the selection process.
- Inquire about supports the client can recruit. Is the family of origin supportive or estranged?
- Offer to include the client's same-sex partner, friends, or family of choice in treatment planning.
- With all lesbians and gay men or bisexuals, explore the risks associated with alcohol and drug use (getting high) and unsafe sex practices that may lead to transmission of HIV and other STDs.
- Be prepared for 'double denial.' The client may not acknowledge either sexual orientation or a drinking or drug problem.
- Ask about a history of sexual abuse and, if timely, arrange an appropriate psychotherapy referral.
- Avoid oversimplifying the drug problem as the result of internalized homophobia. Other personality, Axis I, and psychosocial issues may be significant.
- Ask how the client uses alcohol or drugs to deal with issues of discomfort around sex, HIV-phobia, or fears of sexual dysfunction.
- Look for the coexistence of other compulsive behaviors, such as gambling or compulsive sexual activity.
- When working with families and friends of a gay or lesbian patient, make it clear that homosexuality does not cause addiction but that the addiction may be a manifestation of homophobic discrimination.
- Avoid delving deeply into family of origin issues or history of sexual abuse until the client feels stable and comfortable with these treatment goals. Premature or aggressive exploration of these issues may lead to relapse. Help clients learn basic self-care and grounding skills in order to cope better with difficult memories or feelings.
- Keep in mind that Alcoholics Anonymous programs may be helpful

to your patient but that these programs downplay the individual's uniqueness. The emphasis on God and helplessness may also alienate some gay and lesbian patients. Encourage clients to select a group with messages that best support their goals.

- Although clients may prefer gay and lesbian settings, mention that studies assessing the outcome of treatment in gay centers versus traditional centers are currently unavailable. Some authors argue that integration into a mixed heterosexual/gay program may be more representative of the pressures of the real world in a heterosexual society.
- Explore clients' fear that referral to a gay-identified center may be tantamount to coming out to friends and family when they have not yet done so.
- Keep in mind that studies regarding alcohol use in gay men and lesbians reveal that intake may not decrease with age as it does in the heterosexual population.
- Remember that, for women clients, being in a relationship may not reduce their risk of increased drinking.
- Use the models of coming out in Chapters 5 and 8 to identify links between patterns of drug and alcohol abuse and the client's developmental level. For example, clients in the early phase of identity confusion may use drugs or alcohol as a disinhibitor: to allow them to have sexual activity and socialize, or to allow them to dissociate from making any decision regarding orientation.

9.10 Addictions Treatment: A Client Checklist

The Pride Institute (www.pride-institute.com), a multicenter gay-specific treatment facility in the United States, provides the following checklist to potential clients, which specifically addresses gay and lesbian concerns. Review these questions with your clients when planning treatment strategies. Clients can also access the Lesbigay Service at the Centre for Addiction and Mental Health in Toronto (www.camh.net/lesbigay), a gay-affirmative program with multiple resources.

1. Can you help me decide whether treatment is the answer for my problem?
2. Do I have options about how and where I receive treatment?

3. Can treatment address HIV and behavioral health problems as well as chemical dependency?
4. Will I be able to talk openly about my sexual orientation and my sexual identity?
5. I have already been through a heterosexual treatment program. Is there really a difference?
6. Will the staff understand where I'm coming from as a gay, lesbian, or bisexual person?
7. Is the treatment center accredited regarding insurance coverage?
8. Will the center be discreet in its communications with others who may not know that I am gay?
9. Can my partner or family members or friends be involved in treatment?
10. Will the program provide transition care and after care?
11. What is the philosophical approach of treatment (i.e., 12-step or other)?
12. How realistic is the program in terms of integrating mind, body, and spiritual elements?

CHAPTER TEN

The Body

Alain is a 33-year-old gay male who wants to join your practice. He doesn't practice anal intercourse and has been in a stable relationship with his male partner for seven years. His most significant health risks relate to anabolic steroid use. He attends the gym six days a week for several hours each day and has been preparing for a local weightlifting competition. He has used testosterone for the past three years and likes the changes in his body and the speed with which his weightlifting capacity has increased. Alain is not interested in stopping the testosterone. He wants you to monitor his liver every three months and to write him a script for clean needles and syringes.

Andrea, a 38-year-old single woman who self-identifies as lesbian, is the executive director of a local women's shelter. Although Andrea's BMI is 34, she is active and fit. She works out at the gym four times a week during the winter and spends summer weekends hiking and canoeing at her cottage. Her blood pressure and lipids are in the low range of normal. She is happy with her body, eats a balanced diet, and is able to take on any physical challenge she chooses.

Recently, Andrea has begun to dread her annual trips to the health clinic where she receives her Pap smears. At every visit, she is given advice on losing weight and offered appointments with the nutritionist. One nurse practitioner, who didn't know her well, warned her that if she didn't do something soon, she would never have a hope of finding a husband.

For many lesbians and gay men, body image is part of their personal and sexual identity. This chapter looks at body image and body modifications.

Lesbian Body Image

Lesbian women are significantly heavier, have a significantly higher weight ideal, and aspire less to thinness than do heterosexual women (Herzog et al., 1992). Heterosexual women tend to be more concerned with appearance and weight, have higher levels of weight-related anxiety, and are more likely to diet than their lesbian counterparts (Gettleman & Thompson, 1993). Normal-weight lesbians demonstrate a higher level of body satisfaction than normal-weight heterosexual women (Herzog et al., 1992). Lesbians are also less likely to suffer from eating disorders. According to a 1994 study, 4.2% of lesbians reported a clinical eating disorder compared with 14% of heterosexual women (Siever, 1994).

In general, lesbians are more accepting of their bodies. Some lesbians achieve this acceptance through supportive friendship networks, the establishment of lesbian identities, and processes of self-discovery (Rothblum, 1994). Those who have primarily lesbian friends tend to report greater body acceptance than those who have mostly heterosexual women or men or gay men as friends. This implies an association between lesbian subcultural values and less emphasis on thinness and smallness (Beren et al., 1996). Values emphasized within lesbian subculture may reduce body dissatisfaction by contradicting societal messages regarding body image (Brown, 1987). A greater level of involvement in the lesbian community may result in a corresponding drop in weight concern (Hefferman, 1996). Therefore, the more lesbian women are involved in lesbian-focused activities, the less likely they are to be concerned about weight and the more likely they are to accept their bodies.

Despite the differences in body image between lesbians and heterosexual women, there is actually a stronger correlation between body satisfaction and gender than body satisfaction and sexual orientation (Brand et al., 1992). Among both heterosexual and lesbian women, feminine women tend to be less satisfied with their bodies while masculine and androgynous women demonstrate higher levels of body acceptance (Jackson et al., 1988). Feminine lesbians more closely resemble society's image of an appropriate female and may therefore experience greater pressure to conform to an ideal. Through the experience of accepting themselves as different from society's ideal, masculine and androgynous women may also resolve issues related to body size and shape (Brown, 1987).

Gay Male Body Image

Gay men report significantly higher levels of body dissatisfaction and related psychosocial distress than heterosexual men (Beren et al., 1996). Studies indicate that, in terms of body image satisfaction, gay men are similar to heterosexual women. One study explored and confirmed the hypothesis that gay men and heterosexual women are vulnerable to eating disorders and dissatisfied with their bodies because of a shared emphasis on physical attractiveness that is based on a desire to attract and please men (Siever, 1994).

Beginning as early as adolescence, sociocultural ideals of the perfect body (i.e., thin and athletic) place gay men at high risk of body dissatisfaction and eating disorders (Silberstein et al., 1989; Hefferman, 1994). In the Minnesota Adolescent Health Survey of 30,000 adolescents in grades 7 to 12, homosexual boys were more likely than heterosexual boys to report a poor body image (28% vs. 12%), frequent dieting (9% vs. 6%), binge eating (25% vs. 11%), and purging behaviors such as vomiting (12% vs. 4%) (French et al., 1996). Sexual orientation has been found to be a significant predictor of eating disorders among men, but not among women. Of the 135 men treated for eating disorders at the Massachusetts General Hospital from 1980 to 1994, 27% reported a gay sexual orientation (Carlat et al., 1997).

10.1 Strategies for Working with Gays and Lesbians with Body Image Issues

- Make a point of asking about physical self-esteem/body satisfaction. Does the client have a history of eating disorders, food restriction/purging/laxative use, fad dieting, or excessive use of exercise/weight loss supplements/anabolic steroids? Elaborate diagnosis per DSM-lV criteria for eating disorders.
- Remember that teens and young adults presenting with an eating disorder may have an underlying conflict related to sexual abuse or orientation.
- Ask about the client's perceptions of an ideal body type. Are there pressures within the GLB community to conform to a certain notion of physical beauty?
- Ask the patient to record dietary intake, measures used to control weight, and repeated behaviors such as meal avoid-

ance, frequent weighing, or checking in the mirror. This inventory will help you establish the severity of the problem.
- For cases of lesser severity, offer psycho-education or refer to a dietitian to correct misinformation about weight control or physical training.
- In more severe cases, diagnose and treat coexisting suicidality and mood/anxiety/substance use disorders. Where appropriate, refer to GLB-affirmative subspecialty care for medical/psychiatric admission or outpatient treatment.

Conditions that Affect Body Image

Gynecomastia

Between 40% and 70% of men will experience enlargement of their breasts at some point in their lives. For the majority, the gynecomastia will be associated with puberty and will resolve within four to twenty months. For others, the cause may be steroid use, obesity, tumors, genetic disorders, chronic liver disease, medication side effects, Klinefelter's syndrome, or aging. Many cases are idiopathic.

Men at any age often experience a profound self-consciousness and distress associated with having a 'female-appearing' chest. They are often embarrassed to wear bathing suits or form-fitting clothing. Shame and embarrassment may also interfere with seeking medical attention for gynecomastia. When caring for patients with gynecomastia, clinicians should observe the following:

- Reassure adolescents that a certain amount of breast enlargement is normal. If it persists for more than two years, refer for a surgical opinion. Pubertal breast enlargement is often quite tender.
- Screen men over age 30 who experience a sudden enlargement for an organic cause (think medications first). Ask about steroid and supplement use. Be aware that male breast cancer represents 1% of all breast cancer cases (0.2% of all male malignancies).
- Don't underestimate the psychological morbidity associated with gynecomastia.
- When appropriate, refer patients to a surgeon familiar with cosmetic

techniques and the treatment of male gynecomastia. The standard breast incisions used in women will have disastrous effects if used on men.

Lipodystrophy

Lipodystrophy is a syndrome associated with a loss of fat in the arms, legs, and face (similar to the effects of 'wasting syndrome') and with deposits of fat in the neck ('buffalo hump'), abdomen, and – in women – breasts. Lipodystrophy was originally thought to be a side effect of protease inhibitors, but it is now being seen in men and women on protease-sparing regimes and in HIV-positive people taking no medications at all.

The mechanism of the syndrome is still not understood. Metabolic complications associated with physical changes include hypercholesterolemia, hyperglycemia, hypertriglyceridemia, and insulin resistance. The metabolic changes often have less impact than the changes in body image. Because of its characteristic appearance, lipodystrophy can be an unwanted announcement of one's HIV status. The stigma attached to having the 'HIV look' can influence relationships, career opportunities, and self-esteem. Treatment of lipodystrophy has been disappointing. Surgical options include liposuctioning of unwanted deposits on the neck (fat that has been redistributed abdominally is too deep to remove) and depositing fat or collagen in areas that have wasted, but these treatments rarely maintain the desired effect. Medication changes may help stop the progression of lipodystrophy.

When treating patients with lipodystrophy or at risk for the syndrome:

- Be aware of the risk associated with protease inhibitors (PIs) and the possible adverse effects of antiretroviral therapy (ART). Although the relationship between lipodystrophy, protease inhibitors, and antiretroviral therapy is not understood, there is an association between the length of time a patient is on ART and the degree to which he or she develops lipodystrophy (Schultheiss, 1998).
- Ask patients on long-term antiretroviral therapy about any changes in appearance, and screen for metabolic abnormalities. A detectable change in appearance may also precipitate·a change in the patient's compliance with medication or make it necessary to switch to a different regime.

214 Caring for Lesbian and Gay People

For patients who need to remain on PI therapy, there is growing evidence to support the use of medications to lower the risk of diabetes and heart disease. An HIV specialist should be consulted (Hadigan et al., 2000).

Fitness and Nutrition

Eating well and getting regular exercise are health practices that can lower risks of many chronic diseases and improve well-being (see 10.2). However, gay men and lesbians are at risk of taking a quest for fitness to an extreme. When counseling gay, lesbian, and bisexual patients about their fitness and nutrition goals, it's important for clinicians to help clients find the balance between health and 'obsession.'

Gay men and lesbians most at risk of obsessional behavior are those whose image and self-esteem depend on physical appearance. Gay male culture in particular has valued physical beauty and youth for centuries. Instead of merely exercising for health reasons, some gay men may use extreme fitness, weightlifting, anabolic steroids, and cosmetic surgery to maintain a body that fits an impossible ideal. There are parallels between the legacy of eating disorders, diet pills, and distorted body image uncovered by the feminist movement in the past twenty years and gay men's obsession with buff bodies and fitness. In addition to a cultural ideal that idolizes physical beauty, gay men are subject to a phenomenon that affects all North Americans: the intense marketing of health, fitness, and nutrition.

10.2 Ten Evidence-Based Lifestyle Tips for Healthy Living

Bandolier, a British evidence-based medicine group, has distilled evidence surrounding lifestyle changes and their impact on health into ten tips for healthier living. Bandolier suggests these tips be distributed as patient handouts (www.ebandolier.com).

1. Eat whole grain foods (bread, rice, or pasta) four times a week. This will reduce the chance of having almost any cancer by 40%. Given that cancer gets about one in three of us in a lifetime, that's big advice.
2. Don't smoke. If you do smoke, stop. Nicotine patches, gum, or inhalers won't help much, and acupuncture won't help at

all. Try to reduce your smoking, as there is a profound dose response (the more you smoke, the more likely you are to have cancer or heart or respiratory disease). So cut down to below five cigarettes a day and leave long portions of the day without a cigarette.

3. Eat at least five portions of vegetables and fruit a day – especially tomatoes (including ketchup), red grapes, and the like, as well as salad all year. This protects against a whole variety of different nasty things:

    • It reduces the risk of stroke dramatically.
    • It reduces the risk of diabetes considerably.
    • It will reduce the risk of heart disease and cancer.

4. Use Benecol or something similar instead of butter or margarine. It really does reduce cholesterol, and reducing cholesterol will reduce the risk of heart attack and stroke even in those whose cholesterol is not particularly high. Benecol contains a stanol ester that prevents cholesterol from reaching the liver. It is not yet available in all countries.

5. Drink alcohol regularly but in moderation. The type of alcohol probably doesn't matter too much, but the equivalent of one to two glasses of wine a day or one to two beers is a good thing. The odd day without alcohol won't hurt either. Think of it as medicine. Men should consume no more than fourteen drinks per week; women no more than ten.

6. Eat fish. Eating fish once a week won't stop you having a heart attack in itself, but it reduces the likelihood of you dying from it by half.

7. Take a multivitamin tablet every day, but be sure that it is one with at least 200 micrograms of folate. The evidence is that this can substantially reduce chances of heart disease in some people, and it has been shown to reduce colon cancer by over 85%. It may also reduce the likelihood of developing dementia. Folate is essential in any woman contemplating pregnancy because it will reduce the chance of some birth defects.

8. If you are pregnant or have high blood pressure, minimize the amount of coffee you drink. For the rest of us, drinking up to four cups of coffee or tea a day is likely to reduce our chances of getting colon cancer and Parkinson's disease.

9. Get breathless more often. You don't have to go to a gym or be an Olympic marathon runner. Simply walking a mile a

day or taking reasonable exercise three times a week (enough to make you sweat or glow) will substantially reduce the risk of heart disease. If you walk, don't dawdle. Make it a brisk pace. One of the benefits of regular exercise is that it strengthens bones and keeps them strong. Breaking a hip when elderly is a very serious thing.

10. Check your height and weight on a chart to see if you are overweight for your height. Your body mass index is the weight in kilograms divided by the height in meters squared: for preference it should be below 25. There are health risks associated with having a BMI over 25. Fortunately, there are also many things you can do to lower those risks.

Losing weight is an option for some. There is no good evidence on simple ways to lose weight that work. Crash diets don't work. Take it one step at a time, do the things that are possible now, and combine some calorie limitation with increased exercise. In a few years' time we may have some appetite suppressants to make it easier for some people.

All people, regardless of their BMI, need to incorporate regular physical activity into their routine. This is especially important for those who are overweight. Regular aerobic and conditioning exercise may go a long way to mitigating the health risks that are associated with obesity. Being 'fat' has nothing to do with being 'fit.' Fitness is the number one priority.

What Is the Role of the Physician?

Practitioners should ask about exercise behaviors during the health review: What are the client's reasons for exercising? How many hours per week are spent at the gym? Does exercise interfere with other aspects of life (e.g., friendships)? Is the client unhappy with his or her physical appearance? Does the patient ever use anabolic steroids or steroid supplements to help change body appearance? How about other supplements? Lesbians and gay men are frequent consumers of supplements and herbal products. An abridged guide to supplements and their purported benefits is provided in 10.3. This summary is not intended as evidence of therapeutic effectiveness but rather as a starting point for shared understanding between caregivers and their patients.

10.3 Commonly Used Supplements and Their Proposed Benefits and Side Effects

Product name	Scientific name	Proposed action/ benefit	Side effects/ interactions/warnings	Dosage/duration/ frequency
Androstenedione	Same	Similar function and properties as anabolic steroids (muscle builder)	Has variable muscle building effect yet same health risks as anabolic steroids (heart disease, hormonal imbalance, acne, liver tumors, infertility)	Dosage varies according to body mass and duration of use
Antioxidants	Includes vitamins A, C, E, trace elements: zinc, selenium	Minimizes free radical damage	Use caution when supplementing single micronutrients to avoid creating broad-spectrum imbalance	RDA of each vitamin and trace element
Bitter melon	Momordica charantia	May inhibit HIV; treatment of diabetes (lowers blood sugar); psoriasis (treats skin infection)	In excess, causes abdominal pain and diarrhea; avoid if hypoglycemic or if diabetic and taking hypoglycemic drugs or insulin	50 mL fresh juice once daily, or 5 mL tincture, 2–3 times daily
Chromium picolinate	Chromium + picolinic acid	Lowers LDL cholesterol; regulates glucose tolerance; encourages fat loss and muscle gain	Enhanced dream activity/ recall; depleted by refined sugars and grains; absorption inhibited by calcium carbonate (antacids)	200–600 mcg/daily
Co-enzyme q10	Ubiquinone	Treats cardiovascular diseases; weight-loss aid; antioxidant properties – enhances immune function; enhances muscular performance	Do not use if pregnant/ lactating; negatively affected by drugs – supplementation can prevent deficiency and alleviate drug-related side effects	50–150 mg/daily

10.3 (*Continued*)

Product name	Scientific name	Proposed action/benefit	Side effects/interactions/warnings	Dosage/duration/frequency
Creatine	Methyl guanidine-acetic acid	Helps convert ADP to ATP; muscle volumization; buffers lactic acid buildup; enhances protein synthesis	Dehydration; do not use in presence of kidney disorders	10–20 g/daily first four days; 3–5 g/daily thereafter (determined according to body weight)
DHEA	Dehydro-epiandrosterone	Enhances immune function; weight-loss agent (calories burned, not stored); blocks enzyme that promotes cancer cell growth	Avoid if pregnant or breast-feeding, or at onset of menopause, or if afflicted with adrenal, ovarian, or thyroid tumors	Use only under supervision of allopathic doctor/naturopath; will vary according to naturally occurring levels in each patient
Echinacea	E. purpurea/angustifolia	Blood purifier; prevents colds and alleviates cold symptoms; enhances immune function	Avoid with high blood pressure; works synergistically with goldenseal; potentially harmful in HIV (not yet known)	10–15 drops tincture 3 times daily; take only in presence of symptoms (may develop tolerance to product)
Ephedra	Ephedra sinica/ephedrae herba/ma huang	Weight loss; treatment of respiratory conditions	Not safe for unsupervised use; causes magnesium depletion, heart palpitations; avoid if pregnant; may cause anxiety	Safe dosage varies (not recommended for use)
Essential fatty acids (efas)	Linoleic and gama-linolenic acids (omega-6); alpha-linolenic and eicosa-pentaenoic acids (omega-3)	Hormone regulators; essential for tissue integrity and numerous metabolic processes	No known interactions; optimal ratio of omega-3 to omega-6 varies	Sources include: flax seed oil, evening primrose, cold-water fish, walnuts, avocado

Product name	Scientific name	Proposed action/ benefit	Side effects/ interactions/warnings	Dosage/duration/ frequency
Feverfew	Tanacetum parthenium	Alleviates migraines; may alleviate amenorrhea	Do not use during pregnancy; may inhibit blood coagulation	Dosage will vary according to needs of patient and purpose of supplementation
Garlic	Chrysanthemum parthenium allium sativum	Treats cardiovascular disease; antifungal properties (treats yeast overgrowth); cleanses colon (esp. with ginger)	In excess may cause irritation of digestive tract; may affect blood coagulation and/or glucose tolerance	Equivalent to 4000 mg fresh garlic daily
Ginko biloba	Gingko biloba	Treats Alzheimer's disease; enhances memory recall	Side effects rare; no known interactions	80 mg 3 times daily
Ginseng	Panax ginseng/ eleutherococcus senticosus	Energizing; treats stress, fatigue	Panax ginseng; no known interactions; Siberian ginseng: avoid if patient has high blood pressure; no known drug interactions	Panax: 1–2 g/daily Siberian: 2–3 g/daily
Goldenseal	Hydrastis canadenis	Blood purifier; similar properties to echinacea; anti-inflammatory, antibacterial	Works synergistically with echinacea; avoid if pregnant; in excess, causes diarrhea, vaginal irritation, tissue inflammation; avoid with high blood pressure; may inhibit vitamin B absorption	Limit use as with echinacea; dosage same as for echinacea (preparations available in combination)
HGH	Human growth hormone	Therapeutic use includes treatment of growth disorders and develop-mental problems; illicit use includes muscle and strength enhancement in athletes	In adolescents, causes pre-mature fusion of growth plates; numerous other side effects (vary between individuals)	Not available without prescription

10.3 (*Continued*)

Product name	Scientific name	Proposed action/benefit	Side effects/interactions/warnings	Dosage/duration/frequency
HMB	Beta-hydroxy beta-methylbutyrate	Protein-sparing action may help build muscle and reduce muscle wasting; potentially cuts body fat while building lean body mass	None known	Varies by individual (no standard dosage)
L-carnitine	Individual amino acid	May help build lean body mass and reduce lactic acid buildup in muscles	Supplemental forms are rarely pure; body manufactures L-carnitine as required; therefore impure supplements will impair proper function of naturally occurring amino acid	Individual amino acids are not available without prescription in Canada; in U.S. availability may vary (take only under medical supervision)
Licorice root	Glycyrrhiza glabra	Destroys free radicals, enhances detoxification by liver by increasing glutathione content; colon cleanser; inhibits HIV infection (transfer between cells)	Water retention; edema; hypertension; may cause headache; avoid if pregnant (increases aldosterone production)	Tea: 1 oz root in 8 oz water, 2 times daily
Melatonin	Same	Antioxidant properties; stimulates antioxidant enzyme glutathione peroxidase; protects cell nucleus from free radical damage; stimulates hormone production and immune system; used to treat sleep disorders	Avoid use if pregnant or nursing, or in presence of autoimmune conditions or severe allergies, if suffering from immune-related cancers (leukemia, lymphoma); may function as contraceptive; avoid if taking mao inhibitor prescriptions	Dose best utilized if taken within two hours of bedtime; reduce intake if while taking melatonin you awaken "groggy"; average dosage: 2.5–3 mg/daily

Product name	Scientific name	Proposed action/benefit	Side effects/interactions/warnings	Dosage/duration/frequency
Milk thistle	Silybum marianum	Enhances liver and kidney integrity and function; treats disorders of these organs; antioxidant properties	No known interactions; increases bile, which may change stool consistency	70–210 mg 3 times daily; is synergistic with curcumin (turmeric)
Probiotics	Lactobacillus acidophilus/bifidobacterium bifidus	Treats yeast overgrowth due to antibiotic use, cancer, AIDS; supports intestinal and vaginal flora	No known interactions; negatively affected by sugar, alcohol, antibiotics	1–10 billion active cells 3 times daily
Protein supplements	Usually soy-based products (capsules, powders, beverages, etc.)	Promote muscle gain; prevent muscle wasting	Avoid creating nutrient imbalance; except in cases of therapeutic use (e.g., muscle wasting) do not use as food replacement	Varies according to product and purpose of consumption
St John's wort	Hypericum perforatum	Alleviates anxiety, depression, sleep disorders; inhibits viral infection (antibacterial)	May decrease protease inhibitor levels; do not combine with prescription antidepressants; increases sun sensitivity; allergic reaction is indicated by migraine-like headaches; may elevate blood pressure	300 mg 3 times daily
Saw palmetto	Sabal serrulata/eleutherococcus senticosus	Treats/prevents prostate enlargement (urinary antiseptic, diuretic; improves urinary flow)	Pregnant or lactating women should not use; in excess, causes diarrhea; no known drug interactions	160 mg/daily
Spirulina	Strain of bluegreen algae	Antioxidant properties; may support immune function in presence of HIV/AIDS; source of easily digestible protein	No contraindications; avoid in presence of candida albicans overgrowth (potentially present in AIDS, cancer)	1 tsp–1 tbsp daily

10.3 (*Concluded*)

Product name	Scientific name	Proposed action/ benefit	Side effects/ interactions/warnings	Dosage/duration/ frequency
Spv-30	Buxus semperviren	Strong antioxidant; may treat HIV/AIDS, tuberculosis, severe immunosuppression	Avoid if pregnant or lactating; no known drug interactions but use with caution if taking other medication as research is still pending	330 mg, 2–3 times daily (use under supervision of allopath or naturopath)
Tea tree oil	Melaleuca alternifolia	Antibacterial properties (warts, cuts, burns, skin infections, acne)	Sensitive skin may not tolerate	Apply sparingly to affected area, as needed (external use only)
Turmeric	Curcuma longa	Anticarcinogenic; antiinflammatory; promotes digestive processes; cleanses liver, gall bladder; inhibits platelet aggregation	In excess, may cause ulcers	350 mg, 1–3 times daily; is synergistic with milk thistle
Valerian	Valeriana officinalis	Sedative (treats insomnia, anxiety disorders)	May evoke spaced-out sensation; use with caution in presence of cardiovascular disorders (may alter heart rate and/or blood pressure)	150–300 mg, 30–45 minutes prior to bedtime

Circuit Parties

Circuit parties are an important phenomenon in gay culture and provide a backdrop for some of the health risks associated with the urban gay 'scene.' They are events, usually held in an urban North American location, that last between two and seven days and attract up to 20,000 gay men. The central activity is a dance party (similar to a rave), which features high-energy techno music and nonstop dancing.

The stereotypic circuit party attender is a gay/bisexual, upper-middle-class white male who spends hours in the gym during the week preparing his body for the inevitable display of physique during the weekend party. First-person accounts of the circuit party scene describe an intense atmosphere of competition for the 'best body.' Men whose bodies don't match desired standards are shunned or ridiculed and denied access to private, exclusive parties offered to the most buff and trim (Signorile, 1997).

The party scene, like raves, also features a great deal of recreational drug use, particularly MDMA (ecstasy), gamma hydroxybutyrate (GHB), ketamine (K), and crystal methamphetamine. These drugs, taken to heighten emotional experience and serve as an aphrodisiac, place users at risk of adverse reactions such as hyperthermia and fatal overdoses (see Chapter 9). The 'flight of reason' associated with recreational drugs and the intensity of the party may also put gay men at risk for unsafe sexual practices (Guzman, 2000).

Despite the criticisms of circuit parties, many find them a source of significant social, recreational, and spiritual renewal. Gay men have traditionally had few safe places to celebrate openly and in large numbers. Clinicians with clients who participate in circuit parties will likely find a risk-reduction approach more effective than punitive or judgmental measures. The goal is to help gay men stay safe and encourage them to build their sense of self and community.

Body Modification

For centuries, human beings have adorned or physically altered their bodies. In North American culture, people spend billions of dollars a year on everything from hair care products and makeup to elaborate tattoos, piercing, and cosmetic surgery to express their individuality through their outward appearance. 'Customizing' one's body is not confined to gay and lesbian subcultures. However, as an act of self-expression, body modification is becoming increasingly popular within certain segments of the gay and lesbian community, especially in urban settings.

Irrevocably changing one's body can be a true gift to one's self or an absolute disaster. While health care practitioners are not in the position to judge their patients' choice, it may be worthwhile for them to ask patients who are considering nonreversible surgery or adornment a few key questions, such as:

- Are you sure this is what you really want?
- Are you doing this for yourself – or for someone else?
- How will you feel if people react negatively to your choice?
- How will you feel about this decision a year from now? Five years? Ten years?

Plastic Surgery

Although the majority of cosmetic surgery is purchased by hetero-sexual women, cosmetic surgery is becoming an increasingly popular choice for gay men and lesbians as well. The most popular procedures for lesbians and gay men are highlighted in 10.4. An overview of plastic surgery procedures, including techniques and risks, can be found online (www.plasticsurgery.org).

10.4 Gays' and Lesbians' Most Commonly Requested Cosmetic Surgery Procedures and Their Price (in $US)

1. Eye lift: $1,700–$3,000
   Benefit: Erases the sagging skin and weakened muscles that create droopy upper eyelids and lower lid bagging.
2. Botox injections: $30 per treatment (lasts 4–6 months)
   Benefit: Erases forehead and frown lines through the injection of small amounts of the botulism toxin to weaken muscles.
3. Collagen injections: $400
   Benefit: Reduces or erases wrinkles around the mouth and cheeks via the injection of bovine collagen.
4. Laser skin resurfacing: $1,300–$2,800
   Benefit: Uses a wand of controlled light to tighten loose skin and erase wrinkles, skin folds, and brown spots.

---

5. Breast reduction: $5,500 for women, $2,800 for men
   Benefit: Reduces chronic back, neck, shoulder, and breast pain caused by large breasts. Often covered by insurance for women. Performed on men who suffer gynecomastia.
6. Pectoral and calf implants: $6,000
   Benefit: The implanting of soft solid silicone creates a muscle-like appearance.
7. Liposuction: $1,900 per site
   Benefit: The procedure is most commonly performed to remove unwanted fat on the abdomen and flanks, but is also done on hips, buttocks, thighs, knees, upper arms, chin, cheeks, and neck.
8. Liposculpture: $3,000
   Benefit: Used to carve grooves into the abdominal muscles to make the fat on top of them have a rippled 'six-pack' look.
9. Tummy tuck: $4,000
   Benefit: Flattens the abdomen by lifting the loose abdominal skin, removing excess skin and fat, and tightening the muscles. Requires the construction of a new navel to replace the original, which is removed during the surgery.

From Woog, Dan. (1999). Plastic made perfect. *The Advocate*, December 21.

Foreskin Restoration

A man's decision to restore his foreskin is not necessarily related to sexual orientation. It may be related to political belief, personal preference about the appearance of his penis, or a belief that it will increase sexual pleasure. There are two approaches to foreskin restoration: surgery and gradual traction. Surgical foreskin restoration is practiced less than methods using gradual traction (Schultheiss, 1998). Traction uses tape, rings, or weights to restore the foreskin. Although there are few scientific studies, proponents claim that over time (one to three years) traction will result in enough skin growth to cover the glans and create a cosmetically 'uncircumcised' appearance. For more information, contact the Circumcision Information and Resource Pages (www.cirp.org/).

Penis Enlargement Surgery

The wish to 'enhance' penile length or girth may lead to behaviors that cause relatively little harm. Mail order pumps, vacuums, creams, and herbal products have all touted the capacity to add inches. Of greater concern is another intervention that costs a great deal of money and has the potential to cause far more harm: penile enlargement surgery. This surgery is not approved by any official plastic surgery or urology organization in the world and is targeted at men who feel shame about their penis size or are unhappy with the shape, length, or circumference. Unfortunately, they are far more likely to end up with a disfigured penis than a larger one. Penis enlargement surgery involves the following process:

- *Step one:* Cut the penile suspensory ligament, which holds the penis to the pubic bone. When this ligament is cut, the penis falls away, giving the base of the penis greater exposure and the illusion of increasing length. *Complications:* By cutting the ligament, the penis also loses its 'anchor.' During erections, the penis points down, which can create difficulty for maintaining erections. The other danger is damage to the sensory nerves, which run through the suspensory ligament.
- *Step two:* Add skin to the base where the suspensory ligament was cut. A 'Y,' 'Z,' or 'V'-shaped incision is made and then sewn to cover the original cut. *Complications:* Scarring, loss of pubic hair, disfiguring keloids.
- *Step three:* Add fat under penile skin (offered to those wishing to enhance girth). *Complications:* If the injection method is used, the patient ends up with a lumpy, irregularly shaped penis. If the method of harvesting fat from one part of the body and sewing it onto the penis shaft is used, then the skin of the penis must be 'peeled' back and forth to sew the fat on. Significant scarring may result. With both methods, the body will resorb some of the fat and leave the rest. This will result in more lumps and bumps.
- *Final step:* Prepubic liposuction to give the impression of a larger penis in contrast to a flatter stomach completes the optical illusion. *Complications:* Depending how far down the prepubic area the procedure is done, there can be significant nerve damage.

10.5 Facts about Penis Size

- Average size of an adult penis: 6 inches.
- 95% of men fall between 5.0 and 7.9 inches.

- Measurements from the base of the penis vary widely according to how much pressure is placed on the skin/fat at the pubic region.

Body Piercings

Health Canada has published extensive infection control guidelines for practitioners who perform body piercing (Health Canada, 1999). Piercings are done using sterile, hollow needles of varying gauges. In contrast to the 'guns' typically used by estheticians to pierce ear lobes, these needles cut through the skin, rather than forcing the skin apart to make a hole. Generally, a qualified piercing professional will never use a piercing gun, even for ear lobes. Any equipment (tools, jewelry) that comes into contact with the piercee should also be sterilized using an autoclave as HIV and hepatitis transmission have been documented. Sterile gloves (latex or nitrile) should be worn, and work spaces should be cleaned between clients.

The piercing site is sterilized and dried, then marked to ensure accuracy of entry and exit points. In most cases, surgical clamps are used to stretch the skin taught. When piercing tongues, genitals, and other delicate regions, clamps are applied loosely, intended to reduce mobility and minimize the risk of injury due to flinching. Once the needle passes through the marked site, the clamps are removed to free up the area for jewelry insertion. Appropriate surgical steel or gold jewelry is then slipped through the hollow end of the needle, which is then slowly drawn free from the piercing site while the jewelry is simultaneously slipped through in its place. The length of time a piercing takes from setup to jewelry insertion varies depending on location, choice of jewelry, and the piercer's skill (see also Weir, 2001).

10.6 Client Guidelines for Piercing Aftercare

- Piercings may bleed slightly immediately after and, in some cases, for a few days after being done.
- All piercings should be left exposed to the air, unconstrained by tight clothing or synthetic fibers to minimize the risk of infection.
- Antibacterial solutions are not recommended as most contain

alcohol or similar irritating compounds that dry the area, leaving it prone to cracking and abrasion. Instead, use warm water and mild saltwater soaks to clean fresh or infected piercings.

- Gently swab the area twice daily to remove any accumulated plasma, lymph, and dead cells.
- A solution of one teaspoon of salt in eight ounces of water, used once daily for one or two minutes as a soak, is a highly beneficial and nonirritating means to free up matter accumulated inside the piercing or encrusted on the jewelry.
- It is possible to overclean a piercing. With this in mind, cleaning more than twice daily is discouraged.
- Hands should be washed before coming into contact with a fresh or infected piercing, and paper products or fresh cloths/towels should be used to prevent the transfer of bacteria.

Oral Piercings

Oral piercings heal comparatively fast, taking on average three to seven days to reach a 'manageable' state of sensitivity and another two to six weeks to heal completely. They should be flushed with an alcohol-free mouthwash or sea salt solution morning and evening and after eating or drinking fluids other than water. The same ratio of salt to water as for general piercing soaks should be used. If the mouth becomes irritated from frequent cleaning, dilute the rinsing solution.

Toothbrushes should be replaced often to avoid transfer of accumulated bacteria. During the inflammatory reaction to a new oral piercing there is an increased risk of transmitting blood-borne infections through contact with infected body fluids. It is normal for oral piercings to bleed on and off for the first two or three days. Swelling may be extreme and may be uncomfortable particularly when patients first rise in the morning (due to overnight dehydration) and when eating or talking. The swelling and associated discomfort should subside within two weeks.

It is normal for a fresh oral piercing to secrete lymphatic fluid and plasma. In the case of tongue piercings, it is also common for a thread of muscle tissue to work its way out over the first few weeks. This is not a sign of infection or complication. Once swelling has subsided and the piercing is healed, jewelry needs to be fitted to prevent any damage to teeth or interference with speech. Oral piercings, especially those through the tongue, can close up within minutes of the jewelry being removed, so any jewelry should be replaced quickly.

10.7 Client Care Guidelines for Oral Piercings

During healing period avoid:

- smoking, alcohol, caffeine
- sharing utensils or drinking glasses
- recreational drugs
- undue stress
- chewing gum
- placing foreign objects into mouth (e.g., pencils, fingers, eye-glass arms)
- spicy/salty foods
- acidic or hot beverages or food
- oral sex, 'French' kissing, transfer of body fluids into the mouth.

Avoid playing with the piercing between the teeth (e.g., pinching, clicking), even once it is healed, as these activities may cause extensive dental damage. Contact your doctor if you develop a fever. A professionally executed oral piercing, fitted with proper jewelry, poses minimal risk of permanent dental damage provided its owner follows this advice.

Other Piercings

A list of the different body sites that can be pierced is provided in 10.9. Average healing time for common piercings is outlined in 10.10. A piercing may appear bruised, bleed slightly, or swell during the initial period following its insertion. These are all normal symptoms and do not indicate complication or infection.

Extreme heat, redness, and radical swelling do indicate an infection. If these symptoms persist, it may be necessary for the patient to seek medical attention. Jewelry should not be removed until the infection has drained as the hole may close over with bacteria and pus trapped inside, resulting in a more serious condition or systemic infection. When a patient does develop an infection at the piercing site, he or she should continue the regular cleaning regimen, using saltwater soaks and ensuring that bedding, clothing, and any objects that come into contact with the piercing – including the patient's hands – are clean. If the patient develops a fever or the infection persists, antibiotics may be necessary. The organisms that usually cause infection are skin pathogens such as streptococcus and staphylococcus, which are best treated with cloxacillin.

Clients with body piercings should be aware of some general risks and precautions, including:

- *Allergies:* Titanium, silver, and zinc jewelry may cause an allergic reaction. Use surgical steel or gold until healed, then experiment with caution.
- *Scarring:* Some people are prone to scarring and tissue accumulation at the site of wounds (keloids). They may wish to avoid piercing, including 'play' piercing (temporary piercing performed for erotic purposes).
- *HIV and hepatitis:* Ensure all equipment is adequately sterilized and that needles and jewelry are new, sterile pieces.

10.8 Client Care Guidelines for Other Piercings

During healing period avoid:

- activities that bring into contact the piercing and another person's body fluids; this includes oral sex, kissing, etc.
- alcohol, smoking, caffeine, aspirin
- ointments (neosporin, etc.) – these smother the wound and prevent air flow; they may also collect debris and bacteria
- overcleaning
- rough handling of a fresh or infected piercing/undue contact with the piercing
- bandaging or dressing the piercing
- tight, restrictive clothing or synthetic fibers, which reduce air flow and trap bacteria against skin.

10.9 Piercing Sites (by Location on Body)

Ear

- Conch: through cartilage at base of auricle (near beginning of lobe)

- Lobe: through noncartilage base of ear
- Rim: any location around outer edge above the lobe
- Rook/doth: through cartilage folds adjacent to opening of ear canal
- Scaffold: through cartilage of auricle
- Tragus: through nub of cartilage adjacent to cheek bone

Genitals: Female

- Clitoris: directly through the clitoris; is a rare piercing; usually fitted with 'barbell' jewelry (a post with small balls threaded on each end)
- Hood/prepuce: more common than clitoral piercing; passes through hood of skin above the clitoris; usually fitted with hoop jewelry
- Inner labia: passes through labia minora; usually fitted with hoop jewelry
- Outer labia: passes through labia majora; usually fitted with hoop jewelry
- Pubic: through the skin above the genitals; hoop jewelry worn

Genitals: Male

- Ampallang: passes through head of penis horizontally, crossing urethra; barbell jewelry used
- Apadrayva: through head of penis vertically, crossing urethra; barbell jewelry used
- Dydo: pierces the rim of the penis head, parallel to its shaft, most commonly on the side (left, right); usually barbell jewelry
- Foreskin: through any location around the end of the foreskin flap; fitted with a ring
- Frenum: through web of skin that attaches the foreskin to penis head; fitted with a ring
- Guiche: at base of scrotum (perineum); fitted with a ring
- Hafada: pierces any location on the scrotum, frequently above and to one side of the testicles; fitted with a ring
- Lorum: passes horizontally through the skin at the point where the scrotum meets the base of the penis; also through the skin along the underside of the penis; fitted with a ring or barbell jewelry, depending on location

- Prince Albert: a ring that enters the urethra from the underside of the penis head
- Pubic: through the skin above the genitals; usually hoop jewelry

Mouth

- Labret: centered below the lower lip; fitted with 'labret' jewelry (a post with a ball on the exterior point and a flat disc on the inside of the mouth)
- Lip: any location along the outer edge of the lips; may be fitted with hoop, barbell, or labret jewelry
- Madonna: to one side of the upper lip; mimics a 'beauty mark'; labret jewelry worn
- Tongue: through the center or any location along the outer edge of the tongue; through center – barbell or labret jewelry; through tip – usually hoop jewelry

Neck

- Madison: pierces the soft indentation between the collar bones (above the manubrium of the sternum); hoop jewelry worn
- Nuchae: centered on the back of the neck above the shoulder blades; hoop jewelry worn

Nose

- Earl: through the bridge of the nose, between the eyes; most commonly fitted with barbell jewelry
- Nostril: passes through the nostril; usually fitted with hoop jewelry or a hooked stud
- Septum: through the soft tissue below cartilage between the nostrils; hoop, barbell, or 'retainer' jewelry (discreet monofilament nylon plug)

Torso

- Navel: pierces flap of skin, usually at the top of the navel, occasionally below; may be fitted with hoop or barbell jewelry
- Nipple: through nipple; one of the most difficult to heal, prone to complications; fitted with hoop or barbell jewelry

10.10 Average Healing Time for Common Piercings

Location	Healing Time
Ear lobe	6 to 8 weeks
Ear cartilage	3 months to 1 year
Eyebrow	6 to 8 weeks
Genitals: – clitoris/hood – labia – ampallang/apadrayva/dydo	6 to 8 weeks 6 to 8 weeks 6 months to 1 year
Foreskin: – frenum – guiche	6 weeks to 2 months 3 months to 1 year 3 months to 1 year
Prince Albert	6 to 8 weeks
Lip (any location)	6 to 8 weeks
Tongue	2 to 6 weeks
Navel	3 months to 1 year
Nipples	3 months to 2 years

Tattooing

How safe is tattooing? According to CDC data, there have been no documented cases of HIV transmission associated with tattooing in the United States (Centers for Disease Control and Prevention, 1997). Although exposure to HIV and hepatitis B during tattooing procedures is possible, adherence to proper health and safety standards minimizes the risk to the client and the tattooist. In fact, there is a 300% greater incidence of hepatitis B transmission during dental procedures than through tattooing (Centers for Disease Control and Prevention, 1996).

With tattooing, bacterial infection can occur at the site of a newly acquired tattoo if a client fails to follow care guidelines or if conditions at the point of tattooing are unsterile. The area to be tattooed should be prepared using a surgical soap wash. Safety precautions for tattooing are as follows:

- Only new, sterilized needles should be used.
- Needles should be removed from packaging in the presence of the client. Workstations should be clean. Ink receptacles, latex surgical gloves, and other materials that come into contact with the client's body should be disposed of.
- Surfaces touched by the client should be washed down using medical-grade disinfectant soap (Levins, 2000).
- When selecting a tattooist, clients should ensure that reusable equipment is sterilized in an autoclave; needles, ink receptacles, and other single-use items are sterile and safely disposed of; latex gloves are worn by the tattooist throughout the procedure, and any health concerns are discussed.

10.11 Client Care Guidelines for Tattooing

- Keep a new tattoo bandaged with a sterile dressing for two to 24 hours, depending on size and location of the tattoo and the client lifestyle (i.e., if the area is likely to be subjected to abrasion, repetitive motion, including clothing chafing, it should remain covered longer).
- Once the dressing is removed, wash the tattoo gently yet thoroughly using a mild or antibacterial soap and warm water. Avoid scrubbing or direct pressurized water.
- Pat the area dry; then cover with a thin coating of antibacterial ointment or hypoallergenic moisturizer.
- Whenever the tattoo is exposed to water, treat it in the above manner until it is completely healed.

During the healing period, a tattoo will scab lightly. Heavy scabbing is not uncommon and may occur at points of friction or movement (e.g., joints, over large muscles, points of clothing abrasion). Once scabbing ceases, light, flaky scales may cover the area for several weeks. Keep the tattoo dry until it is free of scabbing. Although application of ointment or moisturizer minimizes cracking and itching, avoid overmoisturizing the area as this may cause localized irritation and inhibit the skin's natural

---

healing processes. Guard against direct sun exposure in order to minimize fading and to avoid damaging vulnerable skin. Apply sunblock before prolonged exposure to the sun.

From *Care of new tattoos*. (2000). Available online (www.cs.ruu.nl/wais/html/ na-dir/bodyart/tattoo-faq/part6.html).

Tattoo Removal

Despite ongoing developments in cosmetic surgery, clients should not assume that a tattoo can be removed or that having a tattoo removed will produce satisfactory results. There are three methods for removing tattoos: excision, laser removal, and dermabrasion.

- *Excision* involves surgically removing the tattooed skin and then closing the area with sutures. Although this procedure is quicker and more complete than laser removal, it requires general anesthetic and can cause extensive scarring.
- *Laser removal* procedures are performed over a series of two to ten sessions, depending on the location, color, and size of the tattoo. They require local anesthetic, produce highly variable results, and often fail to achieve complete eradication of the tattoo. Potential side effects include permanent scarring and skin discoloration.
- *Dermabrasion* and *salabrasion* produce results comparable to laser removal techniques. The process causes scarring and extensive skin damage, and results tend to be inconsistent (Popkow, 2000).

CHAPTER ELEVEN

Relationships

Alex, a 43-year-old stockbroker in a Toronto firm, and John, his partner, have been together for four years. Alex is hoping for a promotion within his Bay Street firm, but acknowledges that public knowledge of his same-sex relationship would likely reduce his chances. This has led to what John calls 'covering behavior.' For example, Alex brings their closest female friend to business functions as a 'girlfriend,' or he refers to John as a roommate rather than his partner when he and John encounter people from work publicly. Alex is also not 'out' to his family.

John requests couple counseling around these issues, which have intensified over the last year. John expresses doubts about continuing in the relationship, as his own individual psychotherapy has led him to be more assertive about his gay orientation in all settings. He is concerned that Alex's career advancement and presentation of a public self will take priority over their life as a couple and love for each other.

Rachel, age 32, sees her family physician for an annual checkup. During the physical examination, the doctor notices multiple bruises along Rachel's left arm and back, which look like punch marks. The physician is aware that Rachel lives with her 4-year-old son Sam and her lover, a younger woman named Sarah. The physician asks Rachel directly how she got the bruises, and Rachel becomes quite defensive. She explains that she and Sarah have been drinking more heavily lately and that this sometimes leads to arguments and 'pushing.' Three days ago, in an incident witnessed by Sam, Sarah became enraged and hit Rachel repeatedly about the arm and back. Rachel pleads with the physician not 'to make a big deal of it' because she feels ashamed for not being patient enough with her younger, somewhat impetuous partner. She also expresses fear that their friends might find out – she and Sarah are perceived as a 'model couple' – and that Sam's father might push for full custody.

The physician completes the physical examination and then requests that they meet for a session in a few days to talk further about what's happening in Rachel's couple and family life. They agree to explore what meaning the escalation of violence may have on the health and future of the couple's relationship and its psychological impact on Sam.

Like all other people, lesbians and gay men must negotiate personal identity in the context of a series of relationships. This chapter looks specifically at the issues associated with same-sex couples, abusive relationships, workplace relationships, gay and lesbian friendships, and parenting and relationships with children.

Same-Sex Couples: What Is the Same? What Is Different?

Between 45% and 80% of lesbians and 40% and 60% of gay men are in steady relationships. Although these figures are quite high, they may underestimate the actual numbers of gays and lesbians in long-term couples because they are based on studies of a younger cohort ('Same-Sex Couples,' n.d.). Gay and lesbian couples struggle with the same relationship issues as heterosexual couples: conflict, communication, extended family, money, sex, career, and power. See 11.1 for a list of the most common reasons that same-sex couples consult therapists (Simon, 1996).

11.1 Why Do Same-Sex Couples Consult Therapists?

- Increased conflict
- Decreased communication
- Negotiation of space
- Third partner involvement
- Monogamy issues
- Cohabitation disputes
- Parenting problems/blended family issues
- Change in frequency of sexual relations
- Emergence of violence
- Disputes around finances
- Property

- Power shifts
- Health changes, including depression, substance abuse in a partner
- Discordant stages of intimacy
- Differing levels of being out to colleagues, friends, family
- Long-distance relationship concerns
- Religious/cultural issues

From Simon, Gail. (1996). Working with people in relationships. In D. Davies et al. (Eds.), *Pink therapy: A guide for counselors and therapists working with gay and bisexual clients*. Philadelphia: Open University Press.

Most practitioners have some experience working with heterosexual couples around these types of issues. However, those who want to work with same-sex couples may have common misperceptions (see 11.2) about gay relationships that may shape their attitudes and affect the quality of care they provide (Simon, 1996).

11.2 Common Misperceptions about Same-Sex Relationships

- There is an absence of power differential between two women or two men.
- Physical and sexual abuse do not occur within same-sex relationships.
- Women communicate better than men.
- One member of the couple is dominant sexually or in terms of personality.
- Lesbians choose women as partners because of assaultive experiences with men.
- Gay relationships are short-lived.
- Gay and lesbian relationships become sexualized too quickly and generally overemphasize sexual behavior.
- Fear of intimacy represents intrinsic or individual pathology rather than a learned response to homophobic injury.

From Gay, Diana. (1996). Balancing autonomy and intimacy in lesbian and gay relationships. In G. Alexander (Ed.), *Gay and lesbian mental health: A sourcebook for practitioners*. New York: Harrington Park Press.

While some of these perceived differences do not exist, the physician or counselor should be aware of other key differences in same-sex relationships that can affect intimacy and the way conflict is expressed. Same-sex relationships differ primarily in how they are structured, the attitudes and expectations of the people involved, and their acceptance in society. For example:

- Same-sex couples lack visible role models of successful pairing and so must 'reinvent the wheel' each time. Even choosing what to call the same-sex partner (spouse, significant other, lover, partner, companion, husband, wife) can be an issue.
- Each member brings to the relationship his or her own internalized homophobia, which has the potential to sabotage self-esteem and intimacy. For example, one member of the couple may be deeply but unconsciously convinced that same-sex intimacy and commitment are doomed to failure and may sabotage any move toward lasting commitment. One member may be more comfortable with being out than the other, which makes it more difficult to construct a public notion of couplehood.
- Very few jurisdictions in North America sanction gay or lesbian unions or marriages, which means that gay couples do not have the same societal and legal rights and supports as heterosexual couples. Gay partners may not be included in workplace spousal benefit contracts, and same-sex partners are often disinherited after the death of a partner.
- In day-to-day life, the division of tasks and responsibilities may be less structured around traditional sex roles and may require more negotiation than in a heterosexual relationship.
- Same-sex couples often face stresses that can affect their quality of life and their relationship, including threats of homophobic violence, rejection by their families of origin, lack of support, loss of parental rights, lack of access to a sick partner or spouse in the hospital setting, and job loss.
- Male couples may face the added burden of HIV infection. In some cases, both partners may be ill; in others, one partner is infected and the other is not (discordant couple); both partners may have lost many friends to HIV.
- A same-sex couple may have a serious relationship but not live together or even live in the same city.
- In a same-sex couple with an intimate relationship, one partner may also be married to someone of the opposite sex.

- Monogamy may not be a given for male or female couples. Either one or both members of the couple may explore other intimate and/or sexual relationships alongside the primary union.
- When a relationship ends, support in the workplace or in the social circle is seldom provided or available because the relationship may not have been revealed, discussed, or seen as legitimate by others in the first place.

About Male Couples

About one million male couples cohabit in the United States (Mason, 2001). Over the last twenty years, there has been more study of the patterns and qualities of male partnering. McWhirter and Mathieson (1996), in a study of 150 male couples conducted prior to the AIDS epidemic, described six stages in the formation of male couples, summarized in 11.3.

11.3 Stages in Formation of Male Couples

Stage	Timing	Characteristics
1. Blending	Year 1	Characterized by the wish to merge with the partner. High levels of romantic preoccupation and frequent sexual activity prevail. Both members maintain equality in tasks, finances, and shared responsibilities.
2. Nesting	Years 2 to 3	Formation of a home base and ongoing exploration of compatibility. Romantic idealization and preoccupation decline, and perception of imperfections in the partner lead to increased ambivalence around the relationship.
3. Maintaining	Years 4 to 5	Both individuals pursue a balance between being an autonomous individual and being a partner. Need for separation may be expressed through sexual liaisons outside the relationship and the formulation of new friendships. This may lead to conflict, which calls for elaboration of new shared problem-solving approaches. The couple continues to build shared traditions, which leads to a sense of permanence, stability, and shared history.

Stage	Timing	Characteristics
4. Building	Years 6 to 10	Continue to collaborate on shared concerns while establishing independence in terms of their own career paths. Tolerance of conflict and clarity around personal and shared boundaries are enhanced.
5. Releasing	Years 11 to 20	Deepening of trust phase characterized by less possessiveness and, for many, the pooling of financial resources. Both partners may have a tendency to take the other for granted, which may lead to feelings of neglect.
6. Renewing	Year 20+	The couple share career and financial successes and have a renewed sense of belonging to one other. Although age-related health concerns emerge, partners believe that they will be together until death. Reminiscence and remembering are indulged. Of note is the fact that the rate of relationship breakup in couples together for more than ten years has been determined in one study to be 6% for lesbians, 4% for gay men, and 4% for heterosexual couples.

From McWhirter, David, & Mathieson, Andrew. (1996). Male couples. In R.P. Cabaj & T.S. Stein (Eds.), *Textbook of homosexuality and mental health*. Washington, DC: American Psychiatric Press.

Stage theories seldom reflect the actual evolution of intimacy. Any analysis of the development of intimacy must acknowledge the obstacles that two men face when they choose to cohabit or to commit to one another. For example, each partner has been socialized by the predominating heterosexist and homophobic culture. One man may have been socialized to be nurturing, the other to be 'masculine' in terms of prevailing social gender norms and, therefore, to not communicate feeling. One partner may have had previous relationships, while the other may be newly divorced, newly 'out,' or new to same-sex dating and gay sexual expression. It is not uncommon for the partners' differing levels of acceptance of homosexuality and internalized homophobia to lead to a discordance in how 'out' the couple may be publicly.

McWhirter and Mathieson (1996) found that most male relationships began as monogamous, but few remained so. It is important to remember, however, that this analysis was done in the mid-1970s before the emergence of the HIV epidemic. This trend toward open relationships may have diminished somewhat due to fear of HIV contagion through extramarital sexual relationships. McWhirter and Mathieson also discovered that, for two men, differences in age, culture, race, and background may actually be predictors of success in couple life, given the lack of contrast provided by socialized gender differences. For some couples, however, these differences can also lead to significant conflicts. The authors explain that the capacity for each member of the couple to commit, or each partner's perception of the couple's stage of intimacy, may differ significantly, and this can lead to pronounced frustration and discordance – a frequent reason for gay men to consult couple counselors.

In the absence of legally recognized domestic unions, male couples can face significant stress points in terms of their commitment, including cohabitation, the purchase of property, the pooling of finances, a commitment ceremony, or the decision to adopt a child. As laws governing same-sex domestic unions evolve, couples may have to redefine previous financial accommodations, which can intensify conflict (see Chapter 14).

For gay couples, the threat of HIV infection, real or imagined, hovers over sexual expression both within and outside the relationship. For some couples, this leads to a greater expectation of sexual exclusivity and a greater motivation to stay together 'because of what's out there.' For others, it may mean that some HIV-positive men stay in unsatisfying or abusive relationships because of fears of abandonment or of being or dying alone. 'AIDS-phobia' and unresolved grief around AIDS-related losses may lead some men to be fearful of sexual expression or avoid attempts at developing a lasting union.

11.4 Nonmonogamous Relationships

Although many couple counselors use a heterosexual model of marriage (i.e., where sex outside the couple is by definition a sign of dissatisfaction or lack of commitment and trust in the couple), this may or may not be the case for gay or lesbian couples. Many same-sex couples disavow monogamy, describing it as inappropriate to their union. However, they may set out specific parameters for sexual relationships alongside the couple life, which allow them to remain committed emotionally. These 'rules' may include:

- Whether repeat contact with a third party is permitted, and if so, how many times.
- Whether contact is to be discussed or not discussed. Some couples adopt a 'don't ask, don't tell' approach, while others eroticize third party contact to recharge their own sexual exchanges.
- Whether sexual contact is to be shared within the couple (i.e., as a threesome).
- Where the sexual liaison may or may not occur (i.e., not in our city/home/bed/social circle).
- Safe sex requirements (i.e., no anal penetration, no receptive oral intercourse) or contraception if an opposite-sex partner is involved, with agreement to reveal any safe sex lapses or condom failure and to be tested for STDs at certain intervals.
- How to process emerging jealousy and when to revisit the couple's need for sexual exclusivity.

See also Polyamory in Chapter 3.

About Female Couples

Although there have been fewer studies on lesbian relationships than on gay relationships, researchers note that female couples differ both from male-female couples and from male couples and exhibit some specific trends (Klinger, 1996). For example:

- Lesbians are more likely to be parents than gay men, and it is more common for them to develop shared households.
- Women are more likely to be involved in an exclusive relationship, but these relationships may be of a shorter duration than those of gay men and heterosexuals. This is often referred to as 'serial monogamy.'
- Women are more likely to be sexually monogamous but may experience the development of emotional closeness for one member outside the couple to be more threatening.
- Women have genital sex less often than men and may be more satisfied with other expressions of physical closeness such as hug-

ging. The gradual dissipation of genital sexual contact within some female couples has been called 'lesbian bed death.' However, lesbian researchers believe this construct overemphasizes genital contact and ignores the meaning of other forms of intimate expression within lesbian relationships.

- As with male couples, differences along the lines of age, race, background, and past sexual relationships may be predictors of longevity.
- Women may be more sensitive to the delineation of household tasks, which are traditionally predetermined culturally based on gender.
- Unlike gay men, most women have had relationships with the opposite sex, and their sense of sexual identity and self-definition may be more fluid (see Chapter 3). This may lead to political conflicts between partners or within their community about the validity of bisexual expression.
- Some people believe that women in lesbian couples are more likely to merge or blur boundaries than two men or a man and a woman because women are conditioned to care for others and lose themselves in the process. However, this is a misconception (Clunis, 1988).

Like male couples, female couples may face homophobic violence and discrimination – although women living together may be ostracized less in some countries than others. Lesbian couples also face issues with property rights, child custody rights, and the ability to marry, which some couples will find stressful or defeating.

11.5 Guide to Assessing / Working with Lesbian and Gay Couples

- Build on your experience in conflict management and communication skills from working with families and heterosexual couples, but be aware of significant differences.
- Allow the couple to define their notion of couplehood, keeping in mind that it may not conform to your own notion of partnership, cohabitation, monogamy, or marriage.
- Be sensitive to the partners' differing or discordant levels of comfort with their orientation and differing levels of internalized homophobia, as these may be significant but not articulated in couple conflict.

- Examine your own assumptions about the fragility or non-endurance of same-sex relationships. Find out how deeply such assumptions are held by each member of the couple.
- Find out which members in the families of origin are supportive or critical of the relationship. What does the couple do about holiday visits? Do they travel together or separately? How do they handle nondisclosure or hostility within one partner's family?
- Ask about plans to marry or to have a commitment ceremony. Inquire about the status of prenuptial agreements concerning shared property and any plans for having or adopting children. When appropriate, refer the couple to a lawyer familiar with gay-specific issues who can provide updates on same-sex marriage, spousal rights and benefits, and child custody as these laws evolve (see Chapter 14).
- Be sensitive to how internalized homophobia can sabotage intimacy for one or both partners. Ask each member of the couple to identify the presence and degree of internalized homophobia in himself or herself, and then in the partner (e.g., one partner may feel incapable of public displays of affection due to years of hiding same-sex attraction and fear of ridicule or violence).
- Find out about social supports. Who are the people who acknowledge and honor the clients' couple life? In which social or work settings is the couple 'out' and in which settings are they secretive about their union? How have these decisions been reached and accepted by each partner?
- Ask about the influence of institutionalized homophobia and how it affects their couple life (e.g., housing, work, spousal benefit rights, and church attendance). Have the partners experienced any physical or verbal violence as a couple or as individuals?
- Inquire about each partner's drug and alcohol use. Does it represent a problem for one or both partners?
- Ask how the couple resolves conflicts. What happens in a dispute? Has there been any physical or verbal abuse in the couple's history?
- Ask about how chores are allocated at home. How is the couple's power differential expressed around money, job prestige, age, physical size?

- Ask about the couple's sexual life and sexual intimacy. Be open to hear about the couple's sex life, including any decision to involve a third party. Some male and female couples express dissatisfaction with the pattern of who gets to be a 'top' or a 'bottom,' and this may be significant in terms of sexual counseling. Lesbians may report diminishing genital connection, and the meaning of this should be explored without assuming that it is a sign of lessening intimacy.
- Look for signs of merger or boundary blurring. Has the couple achieved a boundary between autonomy and intimacy?
- Remember that both members of the couple may attempt to conform to what they think you want them to say or may withhold conflicting information for fear you will judge them (i.e., projected homophobia).
- Ask if they have a role model – gay or straight – for marriage, intimacy, and functioning as a couple. What do they aspire to as a couple?
- If you don't understand something, ask. Be open. Avoid pathologizing labels. See each couple as unique and in search of their own specific compromises.
- If you become stuck or uncomfortable assessing a couple or providing same-sex counseling, seek supervision or a second opinion, or refer the couple to a colleague who is more experienced in couple psychotherapy.

Domestic Violence in Same-Sex Relationships

Because incidents of violence within gay and lesbian relationships are often not reported, it is difficult to accurately assess the incidence of domestic violence among same-sex couples (Island, 1991). The unwillingness to report violent incidents is due to a number of factors, including:

- The abused individual's fear of having his or her complaint dismissed, being discriminated against, or facing the 'double shame' or stigma of being both gay and abused.
- The abused partner not being out about his or her sexual orientation.
- The tendency to attribute male-to-male violence as normal male physicality or brawling.

- A tendency on the part of the gay press to downplay or deny male-male and female-female incidents of violence for fear the information will be misconstrued homophobically by right-wing interest groups (Island, 1991).

As a result of these factors only 10% to 20% of violent incidents within same-sex relationships are reported. About 10% to 20% of abused men and about 25% of abused women actually report the abuse (Island, 1991).

11.6 What Is Abuse?

Abuse is:

- direct physical harm
- threat of harm
- forced sexual activity
- psychologically demeaning comments
- destruction of a partner's cherished possessions
- exertion of excessive control over a partner (i.e., not letting the partner manage his or her own money or choose his or her own friends)
- harassment after the relationship has ended.

www.gaypartnerabuseproject.org

11.7 Myths about Same-Sex Abuse

- Abuse does not occur because same-sex partners have healthier distributions of power.
- Women don't abuse because of female nonviolent tendencies.
- Only one member of the couple abuses, and this is usually the more dominant member of the couple.
- Abuse is less common because same-sex partners tend to be the same size physically.
- Violence occurs mostly in 'femme-butch' relationships among women, or in 'passive-dependent' relationships among men.

- Violence perpetrated in same-sex conflict is different than that in heterosexual couples (i.e., women don't rape or use guns).
- The gay community is generally supportive of individuals who have been abused.
- Financial dependence is less often an issue in same-sex couples because of shared equality.

From 519 Community Resource Centre (Toronto). (1998). *Abuse in lesbian relationships.*

Is Abuse Different in Same-Sex Relationships?

The etiology of violence within gay or lesbian couples varies, just as it does in heterosexual couples. It may have its roots in a history of physical or sexual child abuse in the family of the abusing partner, or in drug or alcohol abuse, power differentials, or feelings of dependency and/or jealousy. In general, same-sex abuse differs from heterosexual domestic violence in three ways:

1. *The power differential.* In heterosexual abuse, it is usually the stronger or more powerful partner (physically or financially) who is the abuser. In same-sex relationships, the less powerful partner in the relationship in terms of finances or physical strength may be the abuser, or both partners may be abusive to each other.
2. *Lack of social support.* Often victims of violence in same-sex relationships cannot ask families or friends for help or support because they are not 'out' about their sexual orientation and they fear being rejected. In some cases, the battering spouse may actually use homophobic threats of 'outing' the partner to others in order to control behavior. Even within the gay community, people who are abused may not receive the support they need. In some cases, gay and lesbian friends may be less than supportive because the abuse becomes politicized or friends take sides, which can lead to a schism within the support community.
3. *Lack of professional support.* For many gays and lesbians, reporting the violence to external authorities is tantamount to 'coming out' when the individual may not be psychologically ready to do so. Victims fear they will be blamed for the abuse, or for being gay/lesbian. This fear may reflect the victim's projected homophobia, or it may be a

realistic assessment of risk in specific cities, families, or communities. Detection and treatment of same-sex domestic abuse is complicated by the fact that professional caregivers, including police, doctors, and clergy, are generally unaware of the problem. In many cases, professionals may not even know the victim they are seeing is in a same-sex relationship. If they do uncover a history of domestic same-sex abuse, access to gay or lesbian-affirmative shelters is limited in most communities. In fact, shelter workers may be unwilling to work with gay clients.

11.8   Tips for Working with Victims of Same-Sex Domestic Violence

- Have posters and pamphlets about domestic abuse, including same-sex abuse, available in your waiting room.
- Always include questions about verbal, physical, or sexual abuse in your couple history on assessment.
- If performing a physical examination, look for signs of injury and abuse in all patients, male and female, gay and straight, regardless of age.
- When a client discloses abuse, avoid providing couple counseling or confronting the perpetrator. This may cause the violence to escalate. An individual assessment for both partners is essential.
- Deal with safety issues first. Check for the potential for suicidal ideation or fear of homicide if the abuse is disclosed.
- If continuing to counsel the abused partner yourself, be sure to challenge feelings of self-blame or responsibility for the abuse as well as attempts to deny or trivialize the abuse. Determine how internalized homophobia and low self-esteem may lead the battered individual to believe that he or she deserves abuse or that 'this is all that can be expected' in same-sex relationships.
- Monitor the abused partner for increased use of drugs or alcohol and for increased risk of depression and suicide. Take a step-wise, cautious approach to exploring the abuse. Have the patient admit that abuse is going on, then ask him or her to tell select trusted individuals about the abuse. Tell the client about legal options for stalking or violent partners, including re-

straining orders. Encourage the client to find a safe place to go to (e.g., a friend's house or a shelter). Map out strategies for an urgent departure, including keeping a packed bag ready, establishing a separate postal box and bank account, organizing a supply of short-term funds, and gathering together important telephone numbers and documents. Remind the client not to return to the apartment or house to fetch his or her things, but to go with police, if necessary.

- Keep a list of lesbigay-affirmative shelters, resources, and emergency phone numbers.

When a Relationship Ends: Gay and Lesbian Separation, Divorce, and Widowhood

Although the incidence of failure of long-term gay relationships is thought to be comparable to failures in straight relationships, counselors working with same-sex couples should be aware of some key differences when gay or lesbian relationships end. For example:

- Some same-sex couples may continue to cohabit or to remain close, supportive friends when their relationships end, while others may become involved in long, acrimonious court battles over shared property and assets. This situation is often aggravated by the fact that there are few legal precedents for sharing or dividing assets in same-sex relationships. In general, however, it is quite common for same-sex partners to remain in a friendship after their relationship ends.
- A same-sex breakup can lead to schisms within the partners' family of choice or within the gay community, which may dramatically reduce one partner's access to supportive friends who fully accept his or her orientation. This may lead to profound isolation.
- 'Divorced' gay and lesbian partners may not receive the customary support from family members or colleagues – either because the relationship was secret or because friends and family did not understand or acknowledge its intimacy or significance. In most cases, formal compassionate leave is not available for same-sex separation or divorce.

For men and women who lose a same-sex partner to death, there is often a link between how 'out' they are about their orientation and relationship and their capacity to grieve the loss in a healthy way (Schernoff, 1998; Deevey, 2000). If the significance of the individual's relationship is not perceived or acknowledged, the grief may become 'disenfranchised.' As a result, the depth of the person's grief goes unrecognized. Bereavement in this community is often 'invisible': there is no lesbian or gay word equivalent to 'widow' or 'widower' to describe the loss of a same-sex partner and to allow a public recognition of bereavement. It is also important to realize that the bereaved gay individual has to negotiate his or her loss in several communities, including the heterosexual community at large, and then in each of his or her gay or lesbian social circles. The discordance in what can be revealed in each of these circles may lead to much anger and confusion. For example:

- Heterosexual friends and family who respect boundaries established by the bereaved may be reluctant to ask about the loss or to offer support, while those who are homophobic may trivialize the relationship and the loss.
- In the workplace, the loss may go completely unnoticed. Some gays and lesbians may not discuss the loss at work because they don't wish to reveal the importance of their same-sex relationship – for fear of losing their job. Even if they do reveal their personal situation, most companies have no policy for formal bereavement leave for same-sex partners and may not offer the usual compassionate response to any job absences for employees caring for a dying same-sex partner or coping with bereavement.
- Because same-sex relationships are not always legally recognized, men and women who lose a same-sex partner may face legal battles with the dead partner's heirs. Surviving partners may be disinherited or even evicted from the homes they shared with their partners, or scorned, ostracized, or blamed by the dead partner's family.
- When the death is due to AIDS, the surviving partner may face more issues. For gay men in particular, the AIDS epidemic has produced two generations of widowers whose losses may be misunderstood or judged morally. People may ask stigmatizing questions about the deceased partner's sexual or drug-using habits, or draw conclusions about guilt or irresponsibility. In some cases, people's persistent, unfounded fears of contagion may prevent them from visiting the survivor's home as they would do for anyone else who had lost a spouse.
- For the individual who has lost a partner to HIV, this may be another

in a long list of HIV-related deaths to be grieved (see Chapter 7). He may have to deal with feelings of survivor guilt or, if he is HIV-positive, cope with fears about treatment and his own illness and death.

After an acute loss, the surviving partner may experience a resurgence of internalized homophobia and feelings that gay unions 'only lead to loss.' It may be important for the counselor to refer the client to a gay and lesbian bereavement group. In the case of a sudden death or death due to HIV, rule out the emergence of posttraumatic stress disorder. Monitor patients for signs of depression, anxiety disorders, or heavy substance use, and refer for medical treatment when appropriate. Individual grief counseling may help the surviving partner to explore the personal, cultural, and community meanings of his or her loss in a safe, nonhomophobic setting.

Workplace Relationships

Workplaces are not always easy settings for lesbians and gays. In North American workplaces, lesbians and gays commonly suffer from harassment, physical and verbal violence, social ostracism, and even blackmail. Although unions, workplaces, provinces, and states may have policies that prohibit discrimination on the basis of sexual orientation, many workers are afraid to file a complaint for fear of job loss or retribution. Much has also been written about the 'glass ceiling' that thwarts many gay and lesbian executives' efforts at career advancement or promotion.

Many gay and lesbian workers choose to hide their sexual orientation at work. However, over time, some find 'passing' as heterosexual increasingly unbearable or they simply wish to be open about their home life and relationships – just as their heterosexual colleagues are (Slezak, 2000). However, choosing to come out in the workplace can be a complex and difficult decision. See 11.9 for tips on counseling clients about coming out in the workplace.

11.9 Coming Out in the Workplace: Counseling Tips

- Consider physical safety first. Is there the possibility of violence or physical retribution after coming out?

- Consider job safety second. Can revealing your sexual orientation lead to dismissal, demotion, or nonpromotion?
- Consider the pros and cons. Make a list of the advantages and disadvantages of being 'out' in the workplace, including expected reactions from specific coworkers and supervisors.
- Find out about precedents regarding conflicts related to sexual orientation in the specific workplace and how they were resolved. Do not use e-mail for personal messaging or for accessing sexualized sites, as this may be grounds for dismissal. Gay men should be prepared for 'AIDS-phobia' (i.e., a preoccupation with HIV issues and HIV contagion) as well as potential homophobia once they've come out.
- Look for potential allies within the workplace, including other gay individuals and colleagues who seem supportive.
- Prepare for a variety of responses, including positive reactions, subtle rejection, shunning, and outright hostility. Document any threatening behavior or comments.
- When coming out to a new colleague, be matter-of-fact and don't offer lengthy explanations. For example, a lesbian could casually say, 'My partner Bev and I,' or a man could use rapid correction in conversation, such as, 'Oh! Didn't you know I was gay?'
- Feel free to respond to homophobic jokes and comments in the workplace. Respond calmly and firmly, pointing out that that kind of remark about another minority group would be unacceptable.

From Slezak, Michael. (2000). Coming out at work. Available online (www.gayhealth.com/iowa-robot/society/?record=32).

The Importance of Lesbian and Gay Friendships

No discussion of gay and lesbian relationships would be complete without mentioning the importance of gay-affirmative friendships and how these friendships lead to the construction of a 'family of choice.' One of the greatest fears of gay and lesbian youth and young adults is being rejected by family and friends or being physically injured or ridiculed after revealing they are homosexual. On the other hand, as discussed in Chapter 8, revealing the 'true' gay self – rather than the guarded, publicly accepted self – can be affirming and liberating. Gays and lesbians universally describe the experience of coming out to a friend and being accepted as a step in deepening that friendship and establishing a model for trust and intimate disclosure in other relationships. It can facilitate other forms of disclosure around vulnerability, anger, tenderness, playfulness, sexual fantasy, gender atypicality, and outrageousness.

The building of a supportive gay-affirmative network is essential to the formation of a healthy sense of self-esteem about one's sexual orientation and sense of wholeness. Within the safe confines of supportive relationships with other lesbigay friends or with gay-affirmative friends, gays and lesbians can fully explore their orientation and its links to their deepening sense of self. These nurturing friendships can help to compensate for or cope with the homophobic discrimination and losses they experience in other settings.

When caring for gay or lesbian clients, it is important that the physician or professional caregiver understand the patient's family of choice or support group. Ask about friendships and relationships. Clients may reveal that they are 'out' with some friends but not others – although they may still value their relationship with people in the latter group and consider them intimate friends. For clients who are socially isolated, have recently relocated, or are recently separated or widowed, the physician may be asked to provide information on support groups, social venues, and alternatives to night clubs and bars; online resources can be found at www.glbcare.com.

Lesbian and Gay Parenting

Between six and 14 million gay men and lesbians in the United States are presently raising children (Patterson, 1996). The actual number is difficult to document because many gay and lesbian parents do not disclose their sexual orientation for fear that they may lose custody, have their visitation rights limited, or face discrimination (Havemann, 1997).

The invisibility of gay and lesbian families in research and statistics contributes to the erroneous assumption that gay men and lesbians are not, and do not wish to be, parents (Levy, 1996). At the same time, gay and lesbian parenting continues to be a source of contention for policy makers, litigators, and those caring for the children of such unions. Homosexual orientation has been routinely deemed an 'unfit' parental quality (Dean et al., 2000). There has been fear that children raised in gay or lesbian households will grow up to be homosexual, develop improper sex-role behavior or sexual conflicts, and may be sexually abused. There has also been concern that children raised by gay or lesbian parents will be stigmatized and have conflicts with their peer group, thus threatening their psychological health, self-esteem, and social relationships.

A growing body of literature has begun to examine the nature of lesbian and gay parenting and elucidate the similarities to and differences from traditional families. Most of that research has focused on whether children of gay men and lesbians suffer adverse effects of their parents' sexual orientation. The findings can be summarized as follows:

- Research has failed to demonstrate that children are negatively affected by their parents' homosexuality. As Gold et al. (1994) summarize in 'Children of Gay or Lesbian Parents': 'There are no data to suggest that children who have gay or lesbian parents are different in any aspects of psychological, social, and sexual development from children in heterosexual families ... These fears and concerns (i.e., that children will develop improper sex-role behavior or sexual conflicts or be stigmatized) have not been substantiated by research. Pediatricians can facilitate the health care and development of these children by being aware of these and their own attitudes, by educating themselves about special concerns of gay or lesbian parents, and by being a resource and an advocate for children who have homosexual parents.'
- There is no evidence to support claims that children of gay men or lesbians are more likely to become homosexual themselves (Patterson & Chan, 1996).
- Many gay and lesbian families struggle with a number of psychosocial issues, including recognition/status of the nonbiological parent, reactions from extended family, status of and interaction with a surrogate mother or known-donor father, what to tell children about donors, and how to provide children with peers with a similar family structure (Dean et al., 2000).
- Past heterosexual relationships are the most common means through which gay men and lesbians become parents. However, a growing number of gay men and lesbians are turning to other means to become parents, including alternative insemination or surrogate mothering, foster care, adoption, and co-parenting (Brotman et al., 2000).
- When asked their reasons for becoming a mother, lesbians commonly

cite the desire to experience pregnancy and motherhood, the importance of mother–child bonds, the desire to raise a newborn, and
barriers to adoption (Harvey et al., 1989).

- Studies suggest that children raised in lesbian families experience
  greater mother–child interaction than those raised in heterosexual
  families (Golombok et al., 1997).

- Most lesbians seeking access to conception services receive inadequate information or referral services from their physicians (Harvey
  et al., 1989). Poor communication between lesbians and health care
  providers may result in a reduced level of care and screening. Anec-
  dotally, fertility clinic practitioners often deny services to lesbians,
  particularly in regions where equal access is not protected by law.

- Lesbian women seeking access to alternative insemination may confront such barriers as heterosexism, homophobia, and insensitivity
  toward or ignorance of lesbian health issues.

- Lesbians who employ the services of midwives report higher rates of
  satisfaction than women under the care of a physician (Harvey et al.,
  1989).

- The sole legally recognized role of known sperm donors is that of
  parent, which has potentially unsatisfactory implications for both the
  donor and the mothers raising the child (Bernstein, 1998).

- At present, most gay fathers became parents during heterosexual
  marriage and did not come out until after the birth of their children
  (Brotman et al., 2000). The other means through which gay men
  become fathers include surrogacy, adoption, and co-parenting arrangements with female friends, single women, and lesbian couples.
  However, these arrangements tend to be emotionally and logistically
  complicated (Shernoff, 1996).

Discrimination and Legal Issues

Gays and lesbians who wish to become parents and those who are
parents may experience discrimination and struggle with a number of
legal issues. For example, lesbian mothers may confront systemic discrimination at fertility clinics, prenatal classes, and during interaction
with medical practitioners, heterosexual couples, and the lesbian community (Levy, 1996).

Systemic barriers to care and custody of children confronted by gay
and lesbian families include: exclusion of same-sex partners from spousal

health coverage; hostility in school systems; and discrimination and hostility in health care settings (Allen & Burrel, 1996). Courts typically rule in favor of biological parents (Dean et al., 2000), and gay and lesbian families have limited, if any, legal protection. In fact, one-third of the gay and lesbian respondents to a 1999 survey reported experiencing custody problems, and gay fathers experience more custody problems than lesbian mothers (Frederiksen, 1999).

11.10 Working with Gay and Lesbian Parents and Potential Parents

When working with gay and lesbian parents, or same-sex couples that wish to parent, the clinician should observe the following:

- Ask all gay and lesbian patients about their wish to be parents, which options they have considered, and what barriers they perceive or have already encountered.
- Review all clinic intake forms to provide a category that can encompass same-sex parents (i.e., names of parents vs. 'mother/father.'
- When interviewing a new parent, ask 'Who else cares for your child?' or 'Who else makes up your family?'
- In the case of a divorced or separated parent, ask about custody arrangements and any conflicts posed by the gay parents' sexuality.
- Ask about the family's unique stressors, including exposure to homophobic/heterosexist assumptions at the child's day care, school, or church.
- Find out who supports the family, and do not assume that members of the family of origin support the parents or children.
- Document the child's legal guardian with respect to medical decisions. Ask to meet and include the other parent in medical care discussions.
- Ask what else would make your same-sex patients and their children more comfortable in your clinical setting and share this feedback with other clinic staff.

11.11 Helping Parents Come Out to Their Children: A Client Guide

Coming out to their children may be an issue for some gay and lesbian parents, particularly if the children were born as part of a heterosexual relationship and the parent has only recently started to self-identify as gay. Mental health professionals can offer the following practical suggestions that may be helpful for gay parents and their children.

1. Come to terms with your own sexual orientation before disclosing to children. This is crucial. The parent who feels negatively about homosexuality or is ashamed of it is much more likely to have children who also react negatively. The parent must create a setting of acceptance by first accepting himself or herself. If disclosure takes place when the parent is ready and comfortable, it is more likely to be a positive experience for everyone.

2. Children are never too young to be told. They will absorb only as much as they are capable of understanding. Use words appropriate to the age of the child. Details may be added as they grow older.

3. Discuss your sexual orientation with children before they know or suspect. When children discover their parents' sexual orientation from someone other than the parent, they are often upset that their mother or father did not trust them sufficiently to share the information with them. It is exceedingly difficult for children to initiate the subject, and they will not bring it up even if they want to.

4. Disclosure should be planned. Children should not find out about a parent's homosexuality by default or discover it accidentally or during an argument between their parents.

5. Disclose in a quiet setting where interruptions are unlikely to occur. Tell each child separately.

6. Inform, don't confess. The disclosure should not be heavy or maudlin but positive and sincere. The child is more likely to accept information provided in a simple, natural, or matter-of-fact manner when the parent is ready. If possible, discuss

or rehearse what to say to children with someone who has already had a similar experience.

7. Inform the children that relationships with them will not change as a result of disclosure. Disclosure will, however, allow the parent to be more honest. Children may need reassurance that their mother or father is the same person as before. Younger children may need repeated reassurance.

8. Be prepared for questions:
   - *Why are you telling me this?* Because my personal life is important and I want to share it with you. I am not ashamed of being gay or lesbian, and you shouldn't be ashamed of me either.
   - *What does being gay mean?* It means being attracted to someone of the same sex so that you might fall in love with a person and express your love physically and sexually.
   - *What makes a person gay?* No one knows, although there are a lot of theories. (These questions may be a child's way of asking if she or he will also be gay.)
   - *Will I be gay, too?* You won't be gay just because I'm gay. It's not contagious, and it doesn't appear to be hereditary. You will be whatever you are going to be.
   - *Don't you like men/women?* (The child might be asking, 'Don't you like Mom?' or 'Do you hate Dad?' Explain that preferring one gender sexually does not mean that you have stopped loving people of the other gender. If this question is asked by a child of the opposite sex it may also mean, 'Don't you like me?' or 'Do you hate me?')

9. Children's responses may vary from relief to silence to anger to confrontation. Be prepared for each. Respond calmly and keep the door open for new questions.

10. Help identify supports for yourself as a parent and for your children, including a doctor, minister, or family friend, so that communication can be facilitated if required.

Adapted from Barret, Robert L., & Robinson, Bryan E. (1990). *Gay fathers.* Available online (www.domani.net/richard/cotk.html).

CHAPTER TWELVE

Special Populations

Rona, a 33-year-old single lesbian with cerebral palsy and spastic paraplegia, lives in supportive housing and works as an administrator in disabled housing. She uses an electric wheelchair to navigate but requires assistance with transfers, bathing, and personal care. Although Rona is not currently involved with a partner, a rumor circulates about her sexuality after an attendant discovers a lesbian magazine in Rona's filing cabinet.

Rona reports to her therapist that her attendants have started to wear rubber gloves when transferring her and often delay responding to her calls for transfer or help to the bathroom. She has discussed her observations to no avail with the faculty's administrator and reports that transfer to a new center could take eighteen months. She asks her therapist how best to deal with discrimination from people she relies on for physical assistance.

Mark, a 23-year-old college student and athlete, started seeing a college psychiatrist about conflicts with his father. In the course of their sessions, Mark reveals that he has been having sex with men and women. When the psychiatrist uses the term bisexual in a session, Mark grows angry at being labeled. He reminds the therapist that labels may be convenient shorthand but that they do not reflect his reality. The psychiatrist agrees, and the work proceeds around issues of intimacy and conflict management in personal relationships.

Physicians and other health care workers treating gay and lesbian patients often make a common error: they assume that the experience of being gay is similar for all and that progression through developmental milestones and responses to mainstream societal influences are fixed or shared. However, there is no one way to formulate a gay identity or self-concept. Color, race, religion, political milieu, family dynamics, gender, stature, able-bodiedness, and family obligations all play a role in sexual and societal affiliation. Yet mainstream urban gay culture does little to challenge this notion of a common gay identity. Community newspapers, magazines, even pornography seldom show images of the aging gay or lesbian individual, ethnic minorities, or individuals with disabilities. Much has been written about 'pink capitalism': the notion that gays and lesbians are a significant consumer population that responds to images of youth, sexiness, and affluence. Most media and marketing images are of young, athletic Caucasian men and women.

Older adults, youth, immigrants, or individuals with a less than perfect physique will not find themselves reflected in gay culture and indeed may experience a second layer of discrimination from the very community they wish to embrace. For example, if a member of a visible minority seeks gay-affirmative counseling, the practitioner may begin with an underlying assumption that the client's cultural conceptualization of homosexuality is 'backward' or repressive. This often leads to a not-so-subtle form of cultural-sexual colonialism or condescension. As a result, 'double minorities' may be ghettoized within a ghetto, which affects their ability to blend multiple identities into a congruent notion of self and of community. For some, the ethnocultural and sexual identities are never reconciled.

Not surprisingly, gay minorities of all types are an understudied population in gay and lesbian academic research. This chapter summarizes key research findings on some of these groups – lesbian and gay ethnoracial minorities, Aboriginals, elders, the disabled, rural individuals, bisexuals, married gays and lesbians, and transsexual and transgendered individuals – and provides useful clinical strategies for working with each of these populations.

Working with Gay Ethnoracial Minorities

Minimal research has been done to document the ethnoracial minority experience of homosexuality, particularly of men and women living in Canada (Brotman et al., 2000). Due to lack of random sampling, most research studies predominantly include middle-class white gay men and exclude gay men of color – and by extension, issues and behaviors that reflect the experiences of this population (Icard et al., 1996).

When working with gay ethnoracial minorities, practitioners should be aware of the research that does exist and how culture and race affect the experience of being gay or lesbian.

- Ethnoracial groups each experience and address issues pertaining to coming out, spirituality, multiple identities, and sex roles differently (Rodriguez, 1998).
- The struggle to reconcile ethnic and homosexual identities, particularly when their cultural communities are homophobic or ethnocentric, instills in many lesbians feelings of isolation and loss (Brotman & Kraniou, 1999).
- In addition to an understanding of distinct ethnoracial experiences of homosexuality within the gay community, practitioners must consider the degree of tolerance each ethnoracial community affords homosexuality (Zamora-Hernandez & Patterson, 1996).
- To serve lesbians from ethnoracial communities adequately, white practitioners must have an awareness of key issues such as racism, sexism, homophobia, and heterosexism; knowledge of ethnoracial experiences of lesbianism; and the ability to address the multiple issues associated with coming out, being a woman of color who must negotiate roles, empowerment, and class struggle (Swigonski, 1995).
- The coming out process has an influence on the social condition and state of health of members of ethnoracial communities (Brotman et al., 2000).
- The majority of African-American lesbians report coming out first to gay men or lesbians from other ethnoracial communities (Jackson & Brown, 1996).
- Black gay men and lesbians struggle with issues of religion, family, community of origin, education, social status, stereotypes, development of homosexual identity, racism, discrimination, homophobia, and sexism (Adams & Kimmel, 1997).
- Asian gay men and lesbians struggle with philosophical and religious influences, racism, homophobia, discrimination, family, community of origin, and development of homosexual identity (Lopez & Traung, 1998).
- Latin American lesbians and gay men struggle with issues of family, sexuality, sex roles, stereotypes, machismo, religion and spirituality, acculturation, immigration, homophobia, community of origin, and development of homosexual identity (Gonzalez & Espin, 1996).
- Jewish lesbians may experience twofold marginalization: from their Jewish identity and from the cultural stigma of failing to bear chil-

dren to ensure the survival of the Jewish people (Dworkin, 1997). They also bear the cultural stigma of failing to be a male.

12.1 Race, Ethnicity, and Culture

According to a 1997 survey of sexual minorities and their experience with the health care and social service systems, it appears that gay ethnoracial minorities living in Ontario:

- are overrepresented at the bottom of the income scale
- are no more likely to be receiving social assistance
- are more likely to be students and unemployed
- have a slightly higher percentage of bisexuals
- have a slightly higher percentage of those who identified themselves as 'other' rather than lesbian, gay, bisexual, or heterosexual.

About 80% of the gays, lesbians, and bisexuals from minority communities had been in counseling or therapy at some time; 27% of those felt their lives were neither understood nor respected by the person they saw. About 66% cited coming out, loneliness, and isolation issues; 42% identified racism as a problem for them; and 33% had entered into counseling or therapy to deal with the resulting problems.

From Coalition for Lesbian and Gay Rights in Ontario. (1997). *Systems failure.* CLGRO Project Affirmation. Toronto.

12.2 Guide to Working with Gay, Lesbian, and Bisexual Cultural Minorities

- Find out about the importance of family and extended family to your client. The clinical tendency may be to promote autonomy and separation from family, but this advice may not reflect the interdependence so highly valued by certain minorities.
- Ask about cultural determinations of sex roles. They may be

fluid or solidly fixed, as in the machismo noted in certain male Latin cultures.

- Ask about the culture's attitudes toward sexuality in general. Sex may not be discussed at all, much less homosexuality. As a result, counseling that emphasizes disclosure may not be timely or helpful.
- Find out about any cultural pressures to marry and have children or to produce an heir. Some cultures value having children above all other endeavors.
- Do not oversimplify ethnicity. Find out about your patient's country of origin and its cultural distinctions. For instance, Chinese attitudes to homosexuality may differ substantially from Korean, Vietnamese, Indonesian, or other Asian cultures. Within a culture, class and socioeconomic factors can also play a role in determining whether gay or lesbian sexuality is tolerated or invisible.
- New immigrants or individuals from visible minorities may be economically disadvantaged or experience higher levels of workplace discrimination or urban violence. Find out how clients have experienced the neighborhood where they live and the quality of medical care they have received in clinical settings.
- Some cultures have a 'don't ask, don't tell' compromise about same-sex activity, which allows some flexibility in negotiating identities. Find out about your client's comfort with this attitude.
- Certain attitudes, such as duty to the group versus the fostering of individual autonomy, can differ dramatically across cultures. White, upwardly mobile patients may be driven by autonomy, while a Japanese-Canadian patient may have a greater sense of duty and obligation to her family and community.
- Religion may play a fundamental role in the individual's cultural identity. Ask about the client's notions of sin and shame with respect to sexuality, homosexuality, and sexual behavior. Consider referring clients who seek to reconcile sexual and religious identities to chapters of specific gay-affirmative religious denominations.
- Discuss how the cultural community punishes nonconformity. Is it through isolation, violence, or exclusion from leadership roles? Which sanctions has your patient experienced so far?

- Ask about the client's experience of mainstream gay culture. Does he or she feel excluded by the predominance of white middle-class imagery? Has the client been stigmatized or fetishized? Certain myths about particular racial types abound in both mainstream and gay culture (e.g., that an Asian lover is soft-spoken, exotic, compliant, and sexually submissive; that a black male lover is macho, virile, and endowed with a large penis). Ask about such experiences and about what accommodations the client has made to fit into mainstream, white urban lesbian and gay culture.
- If you're not a member of the same minority as your patient, be open to learning about particular cultural experiences. Emphasize, however, that you want to learn about the individual's response to these experiences. If you are a member of the same minority, don't assume you know everything. You may risk oversimplifying the patient's experience or colluding with particular projections of mainstream, gay, or minority culture.
- Ask about ethnic interpretations of homosexuality. What words, if any, are used to describe it in the culture? Some cultures may insist that homosexuality does not exist. Others may view it as a 'sellout' to Western decadence, or as a frank disavowal of traditional cultural principles.
- Find out where the individual feels safest openly expressing cultural and sexual identity. Is it in a particular social club, bar, or volunteer group? Where possible, refer to appropriate support and resources.
- Ask about the dilemma between choosing culture over sexual identity. How does the client make these decisions? To whom is the individual out in his or her social circle (e.g., sister, parent, friend, coworker, minister)?
- Some individuals will be married with children but have a same-sex partner. In some cases, their heterosexual spouse will be aware of but not acknowledge the same-sex partner; in others, the spouse will be completely unaware. Avoid moralizing as this may represent an individual's best compromise between cultural, family, and sexual identities. Explore the stressors of maintaining these two lives. Review knowledge of safer sex practices. Couple counseling or individual counseling by partners may be requested. (See the sections on bisexuals and married gays and lesbians later in this chapter.)

> • When working with refugees or immigrants from violent set-
> tings, be sure to ask about clinical features of posttraumatic
> stress disorder and gay-specific violence.

Working with Aboriginal Gay Men and Lesbians

Historically, most North American Aboriginal tribes had specific terminology for gay relations, and a few had terminology for lesbians. Many
cultures honored what was called Two-Spiritedness – a melding of
male and female spirit – and Two-Spirited people were often leaders,
teachers, or healers within the community (Brotman et al., 2000). However, this acceptance within Aboriginal communities has largely eroded.
Gay and lesbian Aboriginals living in urban settings find themselves
divorced from cultures of origin and are doubly stigmatized by the
white and Aboriginal communities where they seek to live.

Although Aboriginal populations in Canada and the United States
are another understudied cohort, research that has been done (Brotman
et al., 2000) indicates the following:

• Health issues of primary significance among Aboriginal communities include alcoholism, homelessness, and cultural discontinuity.
• Aboriginal men and women on reserves and in urban centers are
underserved by social services and health care systems.
• Historically, homosexual presence within North American Aboriginal societies has been inaccurately documented and subjected to
distortion through biased accounts and research.
• Christian evangelization introduced the concepts of internalized sin
and, by extension, homophobia into Aboriginal societies previously
unaffected by heterosexism.
• Two-Spirited people have been subjected to homophobia, violence,
exclusion, and murder at the hands of European colonizers and
Christian missionaries who viewed the Aboriginal world as abnormal.
• Degrees of acceptance and tolerance of homosexuality vary between
tribes.
• Negative attitudes toward homosexuality are more prevalent among
acculturated Aboriginal populations than in traditional societies,
which are often accepting or reverent of same-sex sexual relations
(Williams, 1984).

- Coming out experiences of urban-dwelling Aboriginals vary significantly; their identities are often comparable to those of other gay men and lesbians (Jacobs & Brown, 1997).
- Language of identification is a contentious issue for Aboriginal gay men and lesbians. Terms such as gay, lesbian, and homosexual are inadequate because they fail to encompass the distinct identities of such persons. Two-Spirited is generally considered acceptable (Tafoya, 1997).
- Research identifies six alternative American Indian genders: men, women, not-men, not-women, lesbians, and gay men. Specifically, not-men are biological women who adopt masculine roles, and not-women are their male counterparts (Brown, 1999).
- Mental health care providers should refrain from equating not-man and not-woman identities with gender identity disorder as defined by the DSM-IV, as Aboriginal societies do not regard these identities as disorders or disturbances (Crow et al., 1997).
- Mental health research typically excludes gay and lesbian Aboriginals (Brotman et al., 2000).

12.3 About Aboriginal Gays and Lesbians

According to a 1997 survey of sexual minorities, Aboriginal or First Nations gays and lesbians are mainly from urban settings and are less likely to have graduate or undergraduate degrees.

- Only 54% said it was safe to be out in their communities.
- 12% had experienced inappropriate treatment plans from doctors, 12% had experienced inappropriate assumptions, and 6% had experienced inappropriate comments within the clinical context.
- About 22% saw a traditional native healer. Only 16% of these had disclosed their sexual orientation to their healers, and 47% reported that native healers need more sensitivity and knowledge about sexual orientation.
- 78% had been in counseling or therapy at some point; 54% had sought counseling or therapy for issues related to coming out; 66% felt lonely and isolated.
- 62% had experienced self-esteem difficulties, and 58% of this group had sought counseling or therapy.

- 35% reported negative experiences with welfare services; 30% reported negative experiences with family benefit assistance.
- Women cited childhood sexual abuse as their second most common problem; this was also cited by a significant number of men.

Summary from Coalition for Lesbian and Gay Rights in Ontario. (1997). A First-Nations people. *Systems failure*. CLGRO Project Affirmation. Toronto.

12.4 Guide to Working with Aboriginal Gays and Lesbians

Much of the advice about working with ethnoracial minorities (see 12.2) also applies to Aboriginal patients. Here are some other suggestions:

- Ask about the experience of being gay and Aboriginal. How do these identities conflict? How have they come together? Provide some information about the proud history of Two-Spiritedness in most North American tribes to help counter the modern stigma related to Indian interpretations of homosexuality.
- Wherever possible, refer clients to organizations that will be supportive of their efforts to explore issues of sexuality and Aboriginal identity.
- Ask about the client's preferred use of language. Has the client maintained his or her Aboriginal dialect?
- Be sure to ask about certain experiences, such as living on a reserve, attending a residential school, being adopted or placed with a foster family, as well as any history of alcohol and drug use, violence, incest, or sexual abuse.
- Ask about experiences with double racism (i.e., being gay/bisexual/lesbian, and Aboriginal).
- Explore repatriation options to more supportive Aboriginal communities, if appropriate.
- Inquire about finances, employment, housing, and poverty. Unemployment and poverty may be more pressing problems for urban dislocated Aboriginals than sexuality.
- Keep in mind that Aboriginal people may not utilize main-

stream gay organizations out of fear of rejection or discrimination. Many have also had negative experiences within Aboriginal organizations because of nonacceptance of homosexuality or gender atypicality.

- Ask about any experience with negative stereotypes, such as, 'Aboriginals are lazy, drink excessively, or live chaotic lifestyles.' Find out if these beliefs have been internalized.
- Ask about specific experiences of discrimination in employment and health care settings, including emergency rooms. Look for the impact of both racism and internalized homophobia on self-esteem.

Working with Gay and Lesbian Elders

Aging lesbians and gay men face the same issues as anyone who is growing older, including isolation, changes in physical and cognitive functioning, retirement, loss of career, change in financial status, and societal stigma. In addition, they must deal with some issues that are specific to gays and lesbians. Although the experiences of older gay men and lesbians are rarely discussed in research publications or mainstream journalism (Berger & Kelly, 1996), the following trends have been documented:

- Elderly lesbians and gay men are rendered invisible by ageism within their community. They often willfully adopt that invisibility as a means of avoiding discrimination (Connolly, 1996).
- The main concerns of elderly gays and lesbians are income, stress, loneliness, and age discrimination from within the homosexual community and society at large (Jacobs et al., 1999).
- Depression is the most prevalent mental health concern in older gays and lesbians (Berger & Kelly, 1996).
- Gays' and lesbians' experience of aging is affected by economic status, race, culture, the presence or absence of children and family life, living environment, and their developmental phase in the coming out process (Kertzner & Sved, 1996).
- Elderly gays and lesbians confront specific health care problems, including age-related anxiety and stress, homophobia, discontentment with their sexual orientation, loneliness, and sexuality issues, including changes in sexual functioning (McDougall, 1993).

- Most gerontological and other health care providers typically perceive all elderly people as heterosexual and relatively sexually inactive. They tend to underestimate their health needs, and are unprepared to provide services that meet their needs (Berger & Kelly, 1996; Faria, 1997).
- Most health care and social services systems generally fail to provide resources, housing, respite, and emotional support for aging lesbians and gay men (Mellor, 1996).
- Because they have already experienced stigmatization as homosexuals, most gay men and lesbians may be *better* able to face the transition into old age than their heterosexual peers (Berger & Kelly, 1996).
- Certain factors, such as community involvement, peer support, and access to appropriate housing resources, can make it easier for gay men and lesbians to accept their aging (Quam & Whitford, 1992).
- Gay men of all ages tend to be more community-oriented (i.e., frequenting gay-identified establishments) than lesbians and to frequent bars more often (Beeler et al., 1999).

Within the gay community, there are some common myths about aging that may make it more difficult for older gays and lesbians. For example, lesbians are thought to be less affected than gay men by the process of aging because their community is less physically competitive (McDougall, 1993). Gay men are thought to age more quickly than heterosexual men, prefer only younger men, become depressive and sexually frustrated, and ultimately end their days alone in isolation (McDougall, 1993). This perception is reinforced by the focus on the physical desirability of youth in gay and mainstream culture (Ehrenberg, 1996). Many people also assume that homosexuality compounds problems as a person ages (McDougall, 1993).

Aging Lesbians

According to the research, lesbians do tend to approach aging with a more positive attitude than gay men (Beeler et al., 1999), although aging is experienced differently by lesbians who are out compared to those who are in the closet. The majority of older lesbians live in a couple relationship, have limited involvement with the lesbian community at large, and attend fewer evening outings with friends (Beeler et al., 1999). Their greatest health risks are related to irregular breast self-examination, high alcohol consumption, weight control, and mistrust of conventional health care. Many elderly lesbians use different terms than younger women to describe themselves. For example, they rarely use terms such as dyke, lesbian, queer, or homosexual. Practitioners caring for older lesbians should take this into account (Simkin, 1998).

Aging Gay Men

Elderly gay men who do not fit the urban, white, socially active, educated, intellectually and physically able model are largely overlooked by researchers, the gay community, and health and social services (Ehrenberg, 1996). It is a common belief that, as gay men enter their forties, their appearance and desirability decline. Yet, it is during this period that men tend to reinforce their supportive friendship networks (Kertzner & Sved, 1996). Gay men who have not disclosed their sexual orientation experience a higher degree of anxiety about aging and death than those who have (Berger, 1982).

The present cohort of gay men aged 40 to 50 is markedly smaller than past generations due to the AIDS pandemic. Many older gay men have had multiple, significant AIDS-related losses (Berger & Kelly, 1996), and the AIDS epidemic has reinforced the misconception that it is impossible for gay men to maintain good health beyond their forties (Kertzner & Sved, 1996).

12.5 Experience of Older Lesbians, Gay Men, and Bisexuals with Physicians

According to a survey of older lesbians, gay men, and bisexuals in Ontario concerning their experience with physicians and the health care system:

- 59% of the doctors hadn't asked about safer sex practices, and 74% offered no instruction around safer sex.
- 23% of doctors were described as silent about sexual orientation even when their patients came out to them.
- 29% of doctors asked if their patients had a partner.
- Only 19% of doctors asked if a partner was to be included in major treatment decisions or if a partner was to be present in hospital.

From Coalition for Lesbian and Gay Rights in Ontario. (1997). *Systems failure.* CLGRO Project Affirmation. Toronto.

12.6 Guide to Working with Gay Elders

- Don't assume that an unmarried older person or individual living alone is either single or heterosexual. Ask about sexual orientation, keeping in mind that older people may not use current terminology, such as lesbian, gay, homosexual, or queer. They may acknowledge a history of loving relationships with same-sex partners but choose not to identify with the gay community at large.
- Inquire about experiences of ageism in general, as well as any past experience of homophobia in the workplace or clinical care setting. Remember that some older gays and lesbians have sought out reparative therapy, including electroconvulsive therapy or psychoanalysis, in an attempt to obliterate same-sex attraction. This may have caused considerable damage to self-esteem and identity consolidation.
- Avoid imposing a modern political identity on their issues. Ask about past homophobic experiences, including forced hospitalizations, job loss, blackmail, or family rejection because of sexual orientation.
- Ask about sexual functioning and any specific sexuality concerns. Discuss safer sex practices. How consistent is your patient with safer sex? Older men may be less informed about HIV prevention or new to dating after the end of a lengthy relationship.
- Keep in mind that your gay or lesbian patient may have come out only recently or incompletely. Don't assume that issues related to internalized homophobia and heterosexism have been resolved or worked through simply because of advanced age.
- Find out about your client's current supports. Are they lesbigay or straight individuals? How connected is your client to family of origin, including siblings, surviving parents, and children from previous marriages? Older gays and lesbians are more likely to have been married and to have had children.
- Encourage gay elders, where appropriate, to teach gay and lesbian youth about gay history and the history of the gay rights movement. Several successful mentoring programs have matched lesbigay elders with gay youth in mutually helpful,

nonexploitative contacts. Encourage other forms of volunteerism such as literacy teaching.

- Keep a list of resources for gay and lesbian elders, such as Prime Timers or SAGE (Senior Action in a Gay Environment). Do the retirement homes have gay-affirmative policies? Do they plan to develop them? Be prepared to advocate for your gay and lesbian patients living in traditional retirement communities.
- Display photos of older individuals and couples, including same-sex couples, in your office to counter any impression of invisibility or ageism.
- Find out about gay-sensitive senior services. Some patients may be more receptive to these than to gay-specific agencies.

Working with Disabled Gays and Lesbians

There are no accurate statistics on the numbers of gays, lesbians, or bisexuals who are physically disabled – research studies have not systematically asked the question. This gap may reflect homophobic attitudes, but it may also reflect ableism or the assumption that disabled individuals are not sexual or do not have sexual relationships. It may be useful to assume that there is the same incidence of homosexuality in the disabled population as in the general population.

Disabled gays and lesbians face a number of specific challenges (Ryan & Futterman, 1998), including:

- *Double discrimination.* Disabled individuals may experience discrimination from the population at large because of their physical differences and also from the mainstream gay culture, which appears to overvalue youthful, athletic bodies.
- *Assumptions about their sexuality.* There may be a tendency to assume that the disabled person is not sexual at all, much less gay or lesbian-identified. Disabled women may be perceived as invisible because they may not be capable of reproducing or do not fit social conventions of beauty or sexual attractiveness.
- *Homophobia.* Disabled gays and lesbians who live in care facilities or group homes may rely on physical assistance from homophobic or heterosexist professional caregivers and support staff. Because they are physically dependent, they may feel that acknowledging their

sexual identity or gender could result in neglect, physical punishment, or sexual exploitation.

- *Abuse.* The risk of physical and sexual abuse among severely disabled
  individuals has been noted to be higher than that of the general
  population.
- *Lack of confidentiality.* Disabled individuals may be reluctant to come
  out about their sexuality because of breaches of confidentiality and
  lack of respect for appropriate worker–client physical boundaries.
  This may be compounded by fears about confidentiality, documentation, or who in the care team has access to their chart.
- *Invisibility.* Disabled gays and lesbians are invisible in mainstream
  gay culture. They do not appear in media ads and are not targeted as
  a consumer audience. Bars, clubs, and dance floors seldom are
  equipped with access ramps. Information phone lines about safer sex
  or gay community resources are seldom equipped for the deaf, and
  pamphlets are rarely produced in braille. In some cases, particular
  physical differences may be fetishized (e.g., a fascination with
  amputees), which results in the objectification of the difference rather
  than real acceptance of the person.
- *Health changes.* New onset disabilities resulting from illness, trauma,
  or a recent medical diagnosis, including HIV/AIDS, may cause re-
  gression in identity integration and affect ego-wholeness, sexuality,
  and body image. In some instances, the client may see the physical
  change as punishment for sexual orientation and experience a dramatic resurgence of internalized homophobia.

12.7 Guide to Working with Disabled Gays and Lesbians

- Always do a complete medical and psychological history with
  a disabled individual. Do not overemphasize the physical
  limitation. Take a proper sexual history, including questions
  about sexual functioning, sexual abuse, comfort with sexual
  orientation, and knowledge about safer sex. Safer sex campaigns have not generally targeted disabled populations so
  disabled clients may have a significant need for confidential,
  updated information.
- Ask when the disability or loss of functioning occurred and the
  effects it has had on the person's sense of wholeness and
  sexual attractiveness.

- Stress that all information about sexual orientation is kept confidential in a clinical setting. Reassure the patient that the office is a safe place where anything can be discussed, including dissatisfaction with professional caregivers. Check to see whether the client wants information about sexual orientation recorded on the chart, where support staff may read it and accidental outing may occur.
- Provide information on resources and transportation, including volunteers who might confidentially drive the individual to gay-identified meetings or social events. (Wheelchair transport operators may divulge where clients travel, adding to their anxiety about exploring gay venues.) Keep a list of website resources, chat lines, and telephone lines, as these may allow a disabled individual to explore issues of homosexuality confidentially. Keep an up-to-date list of resources for gay, lesbian, and bisexually disabled individuals, as well as a list of advocacy groups dealing with general disability issues.
- Offer to discuss with the individual's partner various issues, such as the need for education around the illness/disability, ableism, fear of disease progression, and ways of accessing available supports.

Working with Rural Gays and Lesbians

Because of lack of research, accurate statistics on the proportion of gay, lesbian, and bisexual individuals currently living in rural rather than urban centers are unavailable, and the needs of this population are undocumented. Efforts to assess the size and needs of this population are complicated by the fact that gay men and lesbians in rural communities often conceal their identities out of fear of social ostracism. Small communities are often ten years behind urban centers in terms of attitudes toward minorities, including gay and lesbian individuals. Much of rural gay culture is still underground ('Urban versus Rural,' 1998), although some bars and restaurants may have unofficial gay events on specific nights, and occasional support group meetings may provide places for gays and lesbians to congregate. Many rural gays and lesbians do not disclose or live that part of their lives within their community. Instead, they visit an urban center for social support or sexual expression.

The consequence of hiding sexual identity to avoid rejection or violence can lead some men and women to marry in order to pass in the community. Others absorb shame-based community messages about deviance and immorality and experience intense internalized homophobia. This can lead to self-destructive behaviors, including alcohol and substance abuse. According to the research that has been done on rural gays and lesbians:

- The nonacceptance faced by many urban gay men and lesbians, and characterized by hostility and awareness of one's differences, is particularly evident in rural regions (Foster, 1997).
- The common manifestations of homophobia in rural areas are physical and psychological violence, varying degrees of social rejection, physical threats, and verbal harassment (Bonneau, 1998).
- Homophobic threats force individuals to gauge the impact visibility would have upon their relationships and day-to-day living. This heightens social isolation and hampers the development of more integrated gay and lesbian identities (Brotman et al., 2000).
- Many rural-dwelling lesbians and gays are selectively out to relatives and friends but remain invisible in the workplace and in public (Bonneau, 1998).
- The most significant problem encountered by rural gay men is isolation when coming out (Cody & Welch, 1997).
- Social and geographic isolation are prominent barriers for many rural gay men and lesbians, who often need support in the coming out process (Lindhorst, 1997).
- Establishing gay and lesbian community bonds in rural areas often requires discretion and may be impeded by geographic isolation (Brotman et al., 2000).
- It is essential that rural health care practitioners extend acceptance to homosexual clients (Foster, 1997).

Recent Trends

Over the last ten to fifteen years, a significant number of gay men who lived in urban areas and developed HIV infection have returned to their homes in rural communities to be cared for by family or to die. Because of the double stigma of being gay and having AIDS in a small town and the lack of local expertise, these men often have difficulty locating competent, trained medical and social supports (O'Rourke, 1997).

Another more recent phenomenon is the growing number of urban gays and lesbians retiring or moving to rural settings in search of a less stressful lifestyle. Often they reconnect with other former city-dwellers and form social cliques with like-minded gay and straight neighbors. Some are out; others use a 'don't ask, don't tell' approach to fit into the community, having determined that such a compromise may be worthwhile given the other advantages of living in a rural setting.

12.8 Guide to Working with Rural Lesbians and Gays

- If you struggle with your own attitudes regarding homosexuality, seek education, mentoring, or telephone supervision from an urban center, or refer the client to a more supportive colleague.
- Don't assume that because you know a patient socially you know about his or her sexual life or orientation. The family man may have sex with men, the mother of three may have a female lover. Neither may identify as gay or lesbian. Ask questions about sexual behaviors discretely, and ensure confidentiality.
- Reinforce the need for confidentiality with support staff and receptionists, particularly around the ordering of STD tests, to keep this information from traveling beyond the confines of your office.
- Find out about local resources, and keep a list of colleagues in the nearest urban center who are gay affirmative. Provide your patient with a helpful website (www.ruralgay.com), which explores the pros and cons of living in small towns, provides links to other web and health resources, and allows patients private access to information.
- As with all patients, screen for alcohol and drug use. Discuss the role that substances play in either masking same-sex urges or allowing their expression.
- Do not attempt to manage HIV infection unless you are treating a significant number of patients or you have an ongoing supervision and co-following arrangement with a subspecialist.
- Consider organizing a rural clinic, community center, or hospital rounds to provide education sessions on the health care needs of gay and lesbian consumers. Contact the lesbian/gay physicians' group or community center in the city nearest you for the names of potential volunteer guest speakers.
- Remember that rural men in particular may repress sexual

experience but use travel as a way of sexual bingeing or exploration. Always emphasize safe sex education and harm-reduction strategies before each trip.

- Ask about stigma, fears, ostracism, and explore issues related to internalized homophobia within the community. Where necessary, offer ongoing supportive counseling or referral to gay-affirmative psychotherapy.

- Inquire about supports in the family of choice. What methods has the client tried to connect with the gay or lesbian community? Keep in mind that some rural dwellers may disavow or be suspicious of city life or urban resources.

- Be particularly sensitive to the needs of gay or lesbian youth, or youth exploring sexual orientation, as the degree of stigmatization in rural schools may be higher than in urban centers. Acknowledge the teen's dilemma and offer confidential support. Do not push youth to declare their orientation until they are ready.

- Be aware of patient concerns/fears of a breach of confidentiality about HIV status or orientation in small communities. AIDS-phobia often coexists with homophobia in rural settings. An openly gay man may be shunned socially or in the workplace because of the assumption that he is HIV-infected because he is gay.

- If your patient is a parent and living with a partner, ask about available family supports. How have the neighbors and the children's school reacted to the same-sex partnership?

- Rural doctors may be open-minded but inexperienced around specific health-related issues and risk management for gay and lesbian patients. As a result, they may try to minimize differences to emphasize their nondiscriminatory stance (e.g., 'I'll treat you the same as all my patients'). This approach may preclude candid discussion of gay-specific health and prevention concerns. See Chapters 3, 4, and 7 for information on population-appropriate care and counseling.

Working with Bisexuals

A bisexual is someone who is sexually and emotionally attracted to both men and women. Bisexual expression is more common than most people realize. For example, one educational pamphlet suggests that one in three sexually active heterosexual people has admitted to having had same-sex experiences over his or her lifetime (University of Ottawa, 1999, 'Assume Nothing'). Everything that applies to the medical and psychological care of homosexual and heterosexual patients applies to bisexual patients. The clinician should be sensitive to the impact of 'bi-phobia,' as illustrated by the myths about bisexuals (see 12.9). It is particularly important to note that the gay community may be as unaccepting, unsupportive, or suspicious of bisexuals as the heterosexual community.

12.9 Common Myths about Bisexuals

- Bisexuals are really gay individuals who are fearful of leaving the closet.
- Bisexuals are really straights who like to dabble as a form of sexual rebellion.
- Bisexuals are indecisive or unreliable.
- Bisexuals are sexual predators.
- Bisexuals are traitors to the gay and lesbian political cause.
- Bisexuals will always revert to heterosexuality.
- Bisexuals are confused.
- Bisexuals spread diseases, including HIV, to their unsuspecting heterosexual partners, husbands, or wives.
- Bisexuals are incapable of commitment.
- Bisexuals are apolitical and can have the luxury of pretending to be straight if it suits them.

The clinician should anticipate the patient's discomfort at disclosing bisexual behavior. When a married person confesses to same-sex relationships outside of the marriage, the clinician, who assumed the patient was heterosexual and monogamous, often responds in a moralizing way. The patient who describes even a casual same-sex relationship may be prematurely labeled as homosexual, and the caregiver may not anticipate more fluid expressions of sexuality across the individual's life.

12.10 Guide to Working with Bisexuals

All the suggestions about conducting sensitive histories and comprehensive physical examinations listed in Chapter 2 apply with bisexual patients. In addition:

- Use the same medical standards of care relevant to all men and women, based on age group and risk/predisposition assessment.
- Avoid making assumptions regarding a patient's sexuality. Same-sex or opposite-sex sexual relationships can emerge in a person's life at any age.
- Some patients identify themselves as bisexual as a defense against coming out as homosexual. It is important to respect patients' desire to avoid labels until they are clear about orientation and have worked on self-acceptance.
- Be aware that some bisexuals may resent the label. Find out what language your patient uses to describe the way he or she lives.
- Ask about your patient's primary intimate relationship. Often people who are bisexual describe falling in love with an individual rather than a gender. Ask about this person.
- Avoid oversimplifying sexuality or insisting that a patient choose a primary sexual orientation. Reinforce the notion that sexuality is a continuum and may change over time.
- Do not assume that your patient is monogamous. Some bisexuals describe themselves as 'polyamorous.' Find out about that choice.
- Review safer sex information for patients of both genders, and anticipate questions and needs regarding contraception. Concentrate on specific sexual behaviors rather than orientation.
- Compile a list of bisexual-specific resources in your community. Because of hostility to bisexuals within the lesbian and gay community, your bisexual patients may not be comfortable using gay resources.

Working with Married Gays and Lesbians

Up to 20% of gay men either have been married or may currently be married – that is, in a heterosexual relationship (www.bisexual.org). At some point in their practice, clinicians are likely to encounter a gay or lesbian client who is married and, at the same time, engages in same-sex exploration or has a same-sex partner. Working with a married client who identifies openly, privately, or secretly as gay or lesbian can pose an ethical and moral dilemma, particularly if the doctor treats the client's spouse or children. The clinician may tend to moralize based on cultural norms for monogamy and marriage and may feel uncomfortable with what is perceived as duplicitous behavior. With a male client, the clinician may allow AIDS-phobia to affect judgment, make safer sex the priority, and encourage the client to disclose same-sex activity to his female partner even when the male patient's sexual activities are low-risk.

12.11 Guide to Working with Married Gays and Lesbians

- Don't force disclosure within the family until the patient has explored and articulated the meaning of his or her sexual exploration. If you feel ill at ease continuing to treat the client and his or her spouse and children, refer family members to colleagues. Avoid punitively discharging your gay or lesbian patient from your care.
- Review safer sex practices. Some married men who are in denial about their sexual orientation may use alcohol or drugs to disinhibit themselves in sexual encounters and, as a result, may be at high risk for exposure to HIV. Others may be extremely careful around safe sex practices and engage in low-risk activities only. Discuss STD risk with each patient. Focus on individual risks, not the fact that the client may be part of 'a high-risk group.'
- Avoid making assumptions about the quality of the patient's marriage. Your patient may have truly loving feelings for his or her spouse and may be reluctant to leave the spouse to come out as a gay or lesbian person.
- Be aware that many people may be reluctant to leave a marriage out of fear of losing access to their children or facing legal retaliation or hostile treatment by the courts. Refer your patient to gay-affirmative legal services to explore legal rights and obligations.
- Be prepared to have your patient experience, as his or her sexual identity emerges, a tremendous sense of lost opportunity and youth. Screen for depression, anxiety, and substance abuse, where appropriate. Provide counseling or refer to a

skilled counselor to help the patient explore careful, well-thought-out decisions about the future of the marriage. While it is unwise to rush patients to leave a marriage, it may be useful to set some time-limited goals for making specific decisions.

- When a patient does disclose to his or her straight partner, be prepared for some married couples to achieve a compromise where their relationship is redefined or 'opens up' sexually, or where both partners embrace a 'don't ask, don't tell' policy regarding extramarital sex. It is not the clinician's role to judge these compromises. Recognize that the people involved may consider family affiliation and parenting more of a priority than sexual identity.
- When a gay or lesbian patient does disclose, the straight spouse may experience feelings of self-blame, betrayal, loss, rage, and fear of contagion with HIV or STDs, and may need counseling. If providing that counseling conflicts with your care of the gay spouse, refer the straight spouse to an appropriate colleague. The straight spouse can also contact Parents and Friends of Lesbians and Gays (PFLAG), which has resources and support groups for spouses who have just discovered that their partner is gay.
- Discuss disclosing to children. When is the most appropriate time? If the marriage is over, children may have to deal with both the stress of a divorce and the stress of disclosure. Can they cope with both revelations at the same time? Should the client wait to disclose his or her sexual orientation? See Chapter 11 for suggestions about coming out to children.

Working with Transsexual and Transgendered Individuals

'Transsexual' is a commonly used term to describe biological males or females who identify over time as the opposite gender. The term 'transgendered' is a broader nomenclature that includes cross-dressers or transvestites, transsexuals, and the intersexed, including hermaphrodites. Transsexual and transgendered generally refer to states of gender identity and affiliation that are distinct from sexual orientation.

It is important to understand that being transsexual or transgendered is different than identifying as lesbian or gay. Consider persons whose genetic assignment is male but whose gender identity is female. It is quite possible that these persons' sexual attractions and behaviors will be with other men – they would likely be labeled gay or 'homosexual.' However, if they seek and receive successful gender reassignment treatment to become morphologically female, the same persons may then travel through the world as 'heterosexual.' Sorting out identities, behaviors, and morphology can be tricky – the key is in asking and listening to patients describe their experiences and identities. It is essential to not make assumptions or jump to conclusions too quickly.

In terms of diagnosing gender discordance, the DSM-IV defines an entity called gender identity disorder (GID), which has come to replace the term transsexualism. GID in adults and adolescents is characterized by a strong, enduring cross-gender identification (i.e., the wish to be of or live as the opposite sex), persistent discomfort with the gender of birth (including displeasure with primary/secondary sex characteristics), absence of a biological intersex state (such as hermaphrodism), and persistent disturbance in psychosocial and occupational functioning due to such gender dissonance.

The diagnosis of GID should always be rendered by a qualified mental health professional. Transsexual individuals frequently seek primary care from family physicians who are unfamiliar with the various steps and challenges of transitioning, including prescription of hormones. Concurrent individual or group psychotherapy or involvement in a gender-reassignment program is not uncommon due to the day-to-day complications of living as the opposite sex, coping with 'trans-phobia' (even within gay, lesbian, and bisexual communities), and preparing for eventual gender-reassignment surgery.

Overall, Lombardi (2001) emphasizes that transgendered individuals (including transsexuals) are at high risk for violence, harassment, and economic discrimination. HIV seroprevalence rates in California for this population exceed 20% and may be as high as 60% among African Americans. Factors contributing to such risk for HIV infection in the transpopulation include risky sexual behaviors, sex-trade involvement, sharing of needles for estrogen injection, and nonaccessing of prevention services due to previous discriminatory health care encounters. Some individuals find standard clinical guidelines for transitioning (such as the Harry Benjamin protocol) to be politically insensitive, overly rigid, or restrictive and discriminatory to adolescents. Some individuals do not wish sex-reassignment surgery but request hormonal intervention for aesthetic effect. It is noted that those rejected for hormonal or surgical treatment may take risks or seek unsafe treatment methods. Even within conventional clinical settings, most doctors have received no training in providing comprehensive care for transsexual patients and may be uncomfortable with their requests.

Standards of Care

The physician meeting a transsexual (GID) patient for the first time should perform a history and physical that emphasizes the following:

- in the context of requests for hormone therapy, any history of hypertension, angina, cerebrovascular illness, thrombotic irregularities, liver/kidney dysfunction, migraine, diabetes, hyperlipidemia, and psychiatric diagnoses including depression
- substance use profile
- HIV serostatus or STD risk
- psychosocial history, including a review of the challenges of living in an opposite-sex role
- assessment of social supports
- history of economic/social discrimination or physical/sexual abuse
- plans for/obstacles to gender-reassignment surgery
- physical exam of a preoperative female to male (FTM), pelvic/Pap/ breast exams; for the preoperative male to female (MTF) over 40, a digital rectal exam
- lab work: CBC electrolytes, BUN, creatinine, glucose, TSH, urinalysis, lipid profile and liver/renal function tests, and baseline-free testosterone/prolactin for MTF patients.

More detailed medical, surgical, and psychological standards of care for gender identity disorders have been prepared by the Harry Benjamin International Gender Dysphoria Association and are available online (www.hbigda.org).

The most common reason transsexual individuals consult primary care physicians is for provision of hormonal therapies. Patient education information regarding hormone therapy is outlined in 12.12 (MTF) and 12.13 (FTM). Their reprinting is authorized in the excellent review article 'Medical Care of Transsexual Patients' (Oriel, 2000) for physicians interested in providing care to transsexuals. Although physicians unfamiliar with hormonal regimes fear significant side effects and risks for their patients, most patients use hormones and transition without significant complications. Researchers have found no increased mortality in MTF/FTM patients using hormones (Van Kestefen et al., 1997).

12.12 Patient Handout: Guidelines for Hormone Therapy: Male-to-Female

The process of changing one's gender is a serious, important, and potentially dangerous project. The normal process of going through puberty is a gradual one, and to transform a male body to a female one also takes time. There are several things you can do to achieve optimum results both physically and psychologically in a safe manner.

In our program, we have some general principles that we address with you numerous times. They may be different from things you may hear from friends, on the Internet, or from other doctors. However, in reviewing the medical literature, communicating with other gender centers, and following patients for years, we have found them to be sound principles that result in safer transitions with excellent results.

Principles

1. Gender change is a gradual change both physically and psychologically. Your body and mind need time to adjust in a healthy manner. It takes approximately five years to complete the process.
2. Living in your chosen role is the single most important thing that you can do in this process. For a variety of reasons, some transsexual individuals are not able or willing to live in their chosen role. Your physician may still prescribe hormones in these cases, assuming you continue psychotherapy. Your doctor will have ongoing discussions with you about your thoughts on this process.
3. Hormones are potent medications with potentially serious side effects. They must be used carefully and with regular monitoring.

4. We will work with you to optimize your health in all areas, not just specific to gender. We will have frank discussions about how cigarettes, alcohol, illicit drugs, and obesity may have an impact on your health and gender transition.

Guidelines

We ask that you agree to and follow these guidelines as you go through your treatment:

1. Because living in the role is an important step, we prefer that you have a defined plan to make this change. In most cases, it is preferable that you complete this transition within two years. If you do not complete this step, we may need to re-evaluate the appropriateness of hormone therapy. We will continue to check in about your plan and may request permission to talk to your therapist.
2. Our goal is to give you the best clinical results in the safest manner possible. Larger hormone doses may be associated with more side effects than smaller ones, some of which are dangerous.
3. It is important that you take the hormones and medications as prescribed by your physician. Violation of this may mean termination from hormone therapy.
4. Cigarette smoking and estrogen are a dangerous mix. If you choose to smoke, your physician may choose not to prescribe hormones or do so with lower doses.
5. Abuse of alcohol and other drugs must be dealt with before any other therapy is initiated.
6. We strongly recommend a continued relationship with a therapist who is experienced with transgendered issues. In many cases, hormonal therapy is contingent on a continued relationship with a therapist. If you need assistance finding a therapist, we can help.
7. You are responsible for your medical bills. Many insurance plans do not pay for gender change. Your insurance company may ask for your medical records. We cannot falsify records to suggest another diagnosis. In general, the cost for initial consultation, physical exam, and laboratory testing is very expensive. Follow-up visits at three and six months and at one year tend to be less costly, with fewer laboratory studies.

8. Our highest priority is the medical safety of persons receiving hormone therapy.

12.13 Patient Handout: Guidelines for Hormone Therapy: Female-to-Male

Principles and guidelines in 12.12 apply for female-to-male hormone therapy with the following two guideline substitutions:

2. We will work to use the smallest dose of testosterone that gives you the best physical and psychological results. Hormone levels may need to be followed when decisions on dosing are made. Larger hormone doses may be associated with more side effects.
4. Testosterone increases risk of heart disease, as does cigarette smoking. If you choose to smoke, your physician may choose not to prescribe hormones or do so with lower doses. It is important to decrease other risk factors for heart disease, such as controlling cholesterol, maintaining normal body weight, and exercising.

Clinical expectations, side effects, and risks of hormonal therapy should be reviewed with each patient (and with documentations of informed consent). Specific sample dosing regimes for both FTM and MTF patients are summarized in 12.14. For testosterone therapy for FTM patients, side effects and risks include:

- *Side effects*: acne, oily skin, weight gain, hair loss, fluid retention, headaches, mood swings.
- *Risks*: hepatic toxicity, lipid profile changes (decreased/increased HDL), insulin resistance, theoretical concern regarding breast/endometrial cancer (testosterone is metabolized to estrogen) and polycystic ovary disease.

According to Oriel (2000), FTM monitoring should occur at three, six, and twelve months for the first year and twice yearly thereafter. Satisfaction with treatment should be reviewed, including concerns regarding side effects. CBC, LFTs, glucose, and lipid panel should be drawn at three, six, and twelve months and yearly thereafter. Standard gender-appropriate care and counseling discussed in Chapters 3 and 4 should continue until oophorectomy, hysterectomy, and mastectomy are performed.

12.14 Sample Hormonal Regimens for Transsexual Patients

	Medication	Starting dose	Subsequent dose	When to change doses
Female to Male	Testosterone enanthate or testosterone cypionate	200 mg IM q 2 weeks	100–150 mg IM q 2 weeks	After masculinization complete and/ or oophorectomy/ hysterectomy.
	Transdermal testosterone (Testoderm TTS, Andro-derm)	5 mg to skin QD	Usually stays the same	Little data available on efficacy. Transdermal testosterone effective for maintenance and may be less efficacious during transition.
Male to Female	Conjugate estrogen (Premarin^R)	1.25 mg per day 0.625 mg per day (smoker)	2.5 mg per day Do not increase in smokers	To obtain best clinical results, or if testosterone is not suppressed.
	or Estradiol (Estrace^R) or Transdermal estradiol (Climara^R)	1 mg per day 0.1 mg patch per week	2 mg per day Two 0.1 mg patches per week	After sexual reassignment surgery, dose may be decreased without losing secondary sexual characteristics.
	Spironolactone	200 mg per day	May discontinue	After sexual reassignment surgery.
	Medroxyprogesterone (Provera)	10 mg per day	May increase to 20–40 mg (usually not needed)	If testosterone is not suppressed and patient/doctor does not want to increase estrogen.
	or micronized progesterone (Prometrium)	100 mg BID	May discontinue after breast development complete	Micronized progesterone is more costly but may lessen side effects of anxiety as compared with medroxyprogesterone.

For MTF hormonal regimens, several agents are commonly used. Estrogen is used to induce feminization/secondary sex characteristics, and progesterone is sometimes used to stimulate breast growth. Spironolactone and cyproterone are used to reduce androgenic effects. Clinical actions and side effects/risks are summarized in 12.15. Oriel (2000) emphasizes that MTF follow-up visits should be scheduled for three, six, and twelve months after initiation of hormones and twice yearly thereafter. Inquiry should cover satisfaction with body changes/breast growth and side effects, including changes in mood. Lab investigation should include LFTs, serum potassium at three and six months, and prolactin after six months for the first year and at twelve months for three years thereafter. Serum testosterone and lipid profiles can be done yearly. Standard health care maintenance should include STD screening, review of safe sex practices, and a global assessment of functioning. Mammography is recommended after ten years of hormone therapy.

12.15 MTF Hormonal Regimens: Clinical Actions and Side Effects / Risks

Hormone	Desired effect	Side effects	Risks
Estrogen	breast development, body fat redistribution, testicular atrophy, loss of erectile functioning	galactorrhea, elevated prolactin, abnormal LFTs	stroke, pulmonary embolism, myocardial infarction, breast cancer, hepatic adenoma/cysts
Spironolactone	decreased beard growth, decreased male-pattern hair loss, allows use of lower-dose estrogen	hypotension, hyperkalemia	few
Progesterone	antiandrogen, breast development	anxiety, irritability, weight gain, headaches	few

Primary care of the transsexual patient does not end with successful hormonal intervention or subspecialty referral for psychotherapy or surgical reassignment. Lombardi (2001) provides public health suggestions, outlined in 12.16, for improving the health of all transgendered individuals. For more information geared toward patients and their concerns, the following websites can be consulted: Ontario Female to Male Network (www.webhome.idirect.com/~martybear/index.htm);

Standards of Care for Gender Identity Disorders, prepared by the Harry Benjamin International Gender Dysphoria Association (www.hbigda. org); TG/TS Resources and Links (www.3dcom.com/tgfr.html); also see www.glbcare.com.

12.16 Guide to Working with Transgendered Individuals

1. Acknowledge the authenticity of transgender individuals' identities and lives in all areas (policy, research, and clinical practice). When in doubt, inquire in a respectful manner. Allow for complexities; people may not fall into neat categories. Do not become overly fixated upon the technical-medical aspects found in the *Diagnostic and Statistical Manual of Mental Disorders* or the Harry Benjamin International Gender Dysphoria Association standards of care.
2. Promote the view that discrimination and denial of services to transgender men and women will not be tolerated.
3. Allow young people some flexibility in questioning their gender identity.
4. Advocate for increased and better access to health care resources. This includes public and private third-party coverage of hormones and surgeries needed for people to change their legal sex, greater input of transgender individuals in their own care, and more education on transgender health care issues.
5. Advocate for cultural relevancy within research, policy, education and prevention programs, and direct care contexts. One strategy is to contact and develop partnerships with individuals and organizations within the local transgender community.
6. Advocate for more and better promotion of transgender-related research and for more innovation within transgender health care practices.
7. Advocate for greater awareness of intersexed individuals and against the practice of surgically altering children and infants for solely aesthetic reasons. This would include conducting more research on the effects (both short- and long-term) of medical interventions on intersexed infants and children and taking a critical stand against surgically altering children and infants purely for aesthetic reasons.

From Lombardi, Emily. (2001). Enhancing transgender health care. *American Journal of Public Health, 91*(6), 869–71.

CHAPTER THIRTEEN

Professional and Training Issues

Albert, a 29-year-old psychiatry resident, has recently come out to himself and a few close friends. During his psychotherapy practicum, he meets a young man, Simon, who began having severe panic attacks at the age of 19. During the first assessment it becomes clear the panic attacks are related to Simon's anxiety about revealing his newly considered gay sexual orientation.

Albert approaches his psychotherapy supervisor, a well-known senior psychiatrist, for some help in providing therapy to Simon. He is told that brief therapy would be impossible in this case because Simon's 'psycho-pathologies' as a gay man are 'too deeply ingrained to change.'

Elizabeth is a 38-year-old internist and a full-time university faculty member. Since joining the faculty, she has played a leadership role in renewing the medical school's curriculum on sexual minorities, started a thriving mentorship program, and published several papers in educational journals about challenging heterosexism and using small group learning to change attitudes about lesbian and gay patients. The volume of her academic work compares well with peers at a similar level.

At her promotion and tenure appearance, Elizabeth is denied promotion to associate professor. The committee tells her that her work is 'narrow, self-serving, and too political' and doesn't reflect the academic interests of the university.

The health care system's ability to care for lesbian, gay, and bisexual patients is shaped by the training system, the practice environment, and the research agenda. This chapter explores the issues the health professions face in their collective mission to train skilled and compassionate caregivers, support their gay, lesbian, and bisexual colleagues, and conduct research relevant to the populations they serve.

The Training System

Health care professionals spend many years in training. During those years, they learn much of the content they need to practice within their discipline, and they develop attitudes and values that will shape how they practice. The content of health professional training is overt and transparent. It can be found within the curriculums and learning objectives of any training program. Attitudes and values, however, are shaped not by formal course work but by the so-called 'hidden' curriculum: the broad social and cultural milieu in which the training and education occurs.

Currently, neither training content nor culture will necessarily prepare physicians to work with lesbian, gay, or bisexual clients. In terms of curriculum, medical schools spend relatively little time teaching students about sexual health or the health care needs of gay, lesbian, and bisexual patients. At the same time, the culture remains largely indifferent, if not hostile, to the experience of lesbian, gay, or bisexual trainees and practitioners. According to one survey, 10% of medical students and 29% of residents reported that homosexuality was completely excluded from their curriculum (Townsend et al., 1993). In the curriculum of many medical schools, a student's only exposure to a gay or lesbian patient will be in the context of HIV infection. To assume that gay patients will only present with HIV infection is a gross distortion of reality and an example of extreme stereotyping. To help prepare students to work with lesbian, gay, and bisexual patients, the education system should provide opportunities to systematically and critically assess myths and stereotypes about homosexuality (see 13.1).

13.1 Common Myths and Misconceptions about Homosexuality

- I have never known anybody who is gay or lesbian.
- Homosexuality is a biological defect or mental illness that should be treated.
- Homosexuality is seen as sinful in all religious traditions.
- Gay people seek to 'recruit' others into their lifestyle.

- Gays and lesbians are promiscuous and incapable of long-term relationships.
- Gay men molest children more frequently than heterosexual men.
- Lesbians hate men, want to be men, or haven't found the right man yet.
- Gay parents produce gay kids.
- Gays and lesbians could change if they really wanted to.
- Gays and lesbians are unreliable parents.
- AIDS is a gay plague.
- Lesbians and gays already have equal rights in society.
- Men become gay because of dominant mothers and absent fathers.
- Women become gay because of distant mothers.
- All gay people are obsessed with sex and seek to flaunt their sexuality.
- All lesbians are rough, manly, and butch, and all gay men are weak, effeminate, and passive.
- In gay or lesbian relationships, one partner always plays the man and the other plays the woman.
- Bisexuality doesn't really exist. Bisexuals are confused or 'closet' cases.

Strategies to Improve Medical School and Residency Training Programs

During interview and focus group discussions, gay and lesbian medical students identified six strategies to improve medical education and make it more responsive to the needs of lesbian, gay, and bisexual patients (Risdon et al., 2000).

Strategy 1: *Develop clinical and simulated patient problems that include gay or lesbian identity as a normal part of humanity's range.*
The curriculum should provide learning opportunities that are inclusive and encourage respect for diversity (see 13.2 for sample curriculum content). As many schools move to problem-based learning (PBL), curriculum planners must ensure that the problems presented represent the full diversity of the patients students will encounter in practice. For example:

- A simulated patient in the cardiovascular section of the curriculum could be a gay man with coronary artery disease. In addition to setting learning objectives in the clinical and basic sciences, students could set objectives relating to same-sex powers of attorney and sexual activity in the post MI period.
- A woman who brings a child in with an earache could be a lesbian who shares custody of her daughter with her female partner.

13.2 Sample Content for Lesbian and Gay Curriculum across Medical Training

Undergraduate

- Introduction to the patient/clinical medicine
- History and physical/patient interviewing
- Specific cases in problem-based learning (PBL)
- Small group sessions in family medicine, psychiatry, pediatrics, and other appropriate rotations

Postgraduate

- Grand rounds, small group teaching sessions (family medicine, psychiatry, pediatrics); HIV is often the springboard

CME

- Inclusion of gay, lesbian, and bisexual issues in CME programs

---

Strategy 2: *Enhance medical school and residency curricula on sexuality.*
Traditional medical education has failed to adequately address the health care needs of lesbians and gay men. At the current time, human sexuality is poorly taught (Murphy, 1992; Wallick et al., 1992; Wallick et al., 1995; Tesar & Susan, 1998). To train health professionals who have the sensitivity, skill, and knowledge to care for people from sexual minorities, schools need a more comprehensive human sexuality curriculum. Robinson and Cohen (1996) have drafted a framework for curriculum reform in medical schools that addresses both content and attitude. See 13.3 for content and relevant learning objectives and

13.4 and 13.5 for checklists that professionals can use to assess their own attitudes.

13.3 Curriculum on Gay and Lesbian Health Care: Educational Objectives

Knowledge

- Understanding of definitions, prevalence, and varieties of sexual orientation
- History of homosexuality: relationship to medicine and psychiatry
- Current theories on origins of sexual orientation and the bias inherent in this research
- Effects of homophobia, prejudice, and discrimination on gay men and lesbians
- Incidence and impact of antigay and antilesbian violence
- Normal social development of gay men and lesbians, including impact of sexual orientation on childhood and adolescence
- Coming out issues
- Challenges for gay families
- Cultural characteristics of gay and lesbian communities
- Clinical issues relevant to gay men and lesbians: preventive care, screening, treatment
- Barriers to health care for gay men and lesbians
- Legal issues for gays and lesbians: custody issues, employment, benefits, recognition of same-sex relationships
- Awareness of common 'myths' regarding gays and lesbians (see 13.1)

Skills

- Ability to take an age and gender-appropriate history using gender-neutral language
- Ability to take a comprehensive sexual history
- Ability to survey a clinical environment for examples of both inclusive and homophobic/heterosexist messages
- Ability to perform an appropriate physical examination, including comprehensive STD screening

- Ability to provide appropriate support and referral to a gay, lesbian, or bisexual youth about 'coming out'

Attitudes

Learners will demonstrate in their behavior and demeanor that they are:

- Aware of their own values and attitudes toward lesbians and gay men (see 13.4)
- Able to be respectful and caring toward gay and lesbian patients
- Committed to positive, ethical approaches to working with their gay and lesbian patients and colleagues (Townsend & Wallick, 1996).

From Stein, T.S. (1994). A curriculum for learning in psychiatric residencies about homosexuality, gay men, and lesbians. *Academic Psychiatry, 18,* 59–70.

13.4 Are You Homophobic? Assessing Personal Attitudes and Values

Homophobia may be defined as an unrealistic fear of or generalized negative attitude toward homosexual people. Homophobia may be experienced and expressed by lesbians and gay men as well as by nongays.

1. Do you stop yourself from doing or saying certain things because someone might think you're gay or lesbian? If yes, what things?
2. Do you ever intentionally do or say things so that people will think you're not gay?
3. Do you believe that gays or lesbians can influence others to become homosexual? Do you think someone could influence you to change your sexual and affectional preference?
4. If you are a parent, how would you (or do you) feel about having a lesbian daughter or a gay son?
5. How do you think you would feel if you discovered that one of your parents or parent figures, or a brother or sister, were gay or lesbian?

6. Are there any jobs, positions, or professions that you think lesbians and gays should be barred from holding or entering? If yes, why?

7. Would you go to a physician whom you knew or believed to be gay or lesbian if that person were of a different gender from you? If that person were of the same gender as you? If not, why not?

8. If someone you care about were to say to you, 'I think I'm gay,' would you suggest that the person see a therapist?

9. Have you ever been to a gay or lesbian bar, social club, or march? If not, why not?

10. Would you wear a button that says, 'How dare you presume I'm heterosexual'? If not, why not?

11. Can you think of three positive aspects of a gay or lesbian lifestyle? Can you think of three negative aspects of a straight lifestyle?

12. Have you ever laughed at a 'queer' joke?

From Cassidy, J., Poynter, I.L., & Schroer, S. (2002). *The safe on campus program resource manual.* www.salp.wmich.edu/lbg/GLB/manual/resource.html

---

13.5 Homophobic Scale: Index of Attitudes toward Gays and Lesbians

Purpose

This questionnaire is designed to measure the way you feel about working or associating with gays and lesbians.

Directions

Consider each item as accurately as you can, then place the number indicating your feelings next to each item. The numbers:

Strongly Agree	1
Agree	2
No Opinion	3
Disagree	4
Strongly Disagree	5

_____ 1. I would feel comfortable working with a gay/lesbian.

_____ 2. I would enjoy attending social functions at which gays/lesbians were present.

_____ 3. I would feel uncomfortable if I learned that my neighbor was gay/lesbian.

_____ 4. I would feel uncomfortable knowing I was attractive to members of my gender.

_____ 5. I would feel uncomfortable being seen in a gay bar.

_____ 6. I would be comfortable if I found myself attracted to a member of my gender.

_____ 7. I would feel disappointed if I learned that my child was gay/lesbian.

_____ 8. I would feel nervous being in a group of gays or lesbians.

_____ 9. I would feel comfortable knowing that my priest/pastor was gay/lesbian.

_____ 10. I would feel that I had failed as a parent if I learned that my child was gay/lesbian.

_____ 11. If I saw two men holding hands in public, I would feel disgusted.

_____ 12. I would feel comfortable if I learned that my daughter's teacher was a lesbian.

_____ 13. I would feel uncomfortable if I learned that my spouse or partner was attracted to members of his or her gender.

_____ 14. I would feel at ease talking with a gay man or lesbian at a party.

_____ 15. I would feel comfortable if I learned that my boss was a lesbian or gay man.

_____ 16. It would not bother me to walk through a predominantly gay section of town.

_____ 17. It would disturb me to find out that my doctor was lesbian or gay.

_____ 18. I would feel comfortable if I learned that the best friend of my gender was gay or lesbian.

_____ 19. I would feel uncomfortable knowing that my son's male teacher was gay.

_____ 20. I would feel comfortable working closely with a lesbian.

Scoring

For the following items, you must first reverse the scoring: 3, 5, 7, 8, 10, 11, 13, 15, 17, 19. To do so, change the number you wrote for the item as follows:

Change a: 1 to a 5
2 to a 4
3 remains the same
4 to a 2
5 to a 1

When you have written in these new numbers and crossed out the old numbers, add up your total number of points. From this total score subtract 20.
This is your score: _____.

The scale measures the degree to which you have fear or discomfort of being in close quarters to gays or lesbians. The minimum score is 0 and represents the least amount of discomfort. The maximum score is 80 and represents the greatest amount.

In general, if you score between 0 and 20 then you are probably accepting of homosexuality. If you score between 21 and 40 you are probably moderately accepting of homosexuality. A score of between 41 and 60 indicates that you are moderately homophobic, while a score of between 61 and 80 indicates that you are probably very homophobic.

Strategy 3: *Sponsor support groups that recognize the stresses of being gay or lesbian during medical training.*
Strategy 4: *Provide faculty role models and mentors for gay and lesbian physicians in training.*
These two strategies speak to the need for support. All students find medical education emotionally intensive and experience the stress of trying to balance competing demands from the training program, family, significant others, and their own values. For students who are in the process of consolidating their gay or lesbian identity, the stress can be that much greater. Lesbian and gay students may have tremendous difficulty accommodating and surviving the professionalization process (Townsend & Wallick, 1996; Risdon et al., 2000). They may also

encounter discrimination and homophobia that affects their safety and
their ability to learn (see 13.6). Support groups that are sponsored and
endorsed by the institution can help students cope with stress. Role
modeling is another powerful way to offer support to students dealing
with identity consolidation in a potentially unsupportive culture. Many
schools have established a formal student–faculty liaison for gay and
lesbian issues (Townsend et al., 1991).

13.6 The Experience of Gay and Lesbian Students and Residents

- In a focus group of Canadian gay and lesbian medical students
  in training, many reported choosing medicine as a strategy for
  compensating for the perceived 'flaw' of being gay. The same
  students reported spending a significant amount of energy
  assessing the safety of their learning environments, which displayed overt homophobia and provided few openly lesbian or
  gay role models (Risdon et al., 2000).
- While the majority of gay and lesbian applicants ranked being
  accepted as a homosexual as important when choosing a residency, more than half believed being 'out' would lower their
  application ranking (Oriel et al., 1996).
- A significant percentage of training directors report a tendency
  to rank known homosexual family practice residency applicants lower than other applicants (Oriel et al., 1996).
- Among psychiatry residency applicants, lesbians encounter a
  higher incidence of harassment and stigmatization and are more
  likely to have their professional commitment challenged and to
  be questioned inappropriately about their interpersonal relationships during the interview process (Townsend et al., 1993).
- The Women Physicians' Health Study (WPHS), a survey of
  4,501 women physicians aged 30 to 70, examined the prevalence of harassment among lesbian and heterosexual physicians during medical school, graduate medical education, and
  medical practice. The results confirmed the existence of harassment based on sexual orientation. Lesbian physicians were
  four times more likely than heterosexual physicians to report
  ever having experienced harassment based on sexual orientation in a medical setting (41% for lesbians vs. 10% for heterosexuals, $P<.0001$) (Brogan et al., 1999).

Strategy 5: *Develop written, broadly distributed policies condemning discrimination against gay and lesbian persons, with effective reporting and enforcement mechanisms.*
Strategy 6: *Take practical institutional measures to address homophobia and heterosexism.*
The last two strategies address the overall milieu of medical training. A recent survey of accredited U.S. medical schools revealed that 63% of the 97 schools that responded include sexual orientation as an institutionally protected category (Wallick et al., 1995). National medical organizations have moved considerably in the past ten years to pass sexual orientation and nondiscrimination policies (Schneider & Levin, 1999). The Society of Obstetricians and Gynecologists of Canada has published clinical practice guidelines on lesbian health needs, which are available online (www.sogc.medical.org).

However, first-person accounts collected by Risdon et al. (2000) attest to the fact that written policies are not enough to challenge the hidden curriculum, which continues to perpetuate negative stereotypes and assumptions about gay and lesbian patients. When these attitudes go unchallenged, gay and lesbian medical students are likely to experience their learning environment as 'unsafe.' Medical schools will need to be proactive to ensure behaviors are consistent with policies on anti-discrimination and respect for diversity. Gay and lesbian medical students provide an accurate barometer of the environment. Their input should be sought and acted upon.

The Practice Environment

The practice environment can be extremely difficult for lesbian, gay, and bisexual health care professionals. In a widely quoted survey of physicians in San Diego, 40% indicated that they would not refer patients to a gay colleague, 40% would discourage gay or lesbian medical students from being psychiatrists or pediatricians, and 30% would not admit an openly gay person to medical school (Mathews et al., 1986). However, physicians surveyed more recently in New Mexico were considerably more tolerant. Only 4.3% would refuse medical school admission to applicants known to be gay or lesbian; 11.8% would not refer patients to gay and lesbian obstetrician-gynecologists (Ramos et al., 1998).

A qualitative study conducted in the United Kingdom reported most gay practitioners had not openly declared their homosexuality because they thought disclosure would jeopardize their career prospects (Rose,

1994). The most extensive study of antigay discrimination in medicine was done by the American Association of Physicians for Human Rights (a forerunner to the Gay and Lesbian Medical Association) in a 1994 survey of over 700 gay, lesbian, and bisexual practicing physicians in North America (see 13.7) (Schatz & O'Hanlan, 1994). This study confirmed that even lesbians and gay men in a 'high-status' profession are not insulated from the discrimination, bigotry, and violence directed toward lesbian and gay people in our society.

13.7 Key Findings from Antigay Discrimination in Medicine Survey

Social Ostracism

- 34% of physicians and 51% of medical students reported being subjected to verbal harassment or insulted by their medical colleagues because of their orientation.
- 34% of physicians and 54% of medical students reported being socially ostracized because of their orientation.
- 14% reported being punched, kicked, spat upon, attacked with knives, bottles, or rocks, or run off the road because of their orientation.

Professional Respect

- 12% of physicians and medical students agreed that 'gay, lesbian, and bisexual physicians were accepted as equals in the medical profession,' while 64% disagreed.

Discrimination is not limited to professional colleagues. Patients have also expressed concern about having a gay or lesbian physician. In a telephone survey of 500 randomly chosen Canadians from a large urban center, 11.8% of respondents said they would refuse to see a gay or lesbian physician, fearing that a gay physician would be 'incompetent' or 'make them uncomfortable' (Druzin et al., 1998). The climate for bisexual, lesbian, and gay physicians has improved significantly over the past twenty years, but there is still a way to go. Burke et al. (2001) recently posed a series of questions that can be used to assess progress (or lack thereof) over the next twenty years:

- Do gay, lesbian, and bisexual doctors feel accepted in their professional life?
- Would they advise a homosexual or bisexual premedical student to choose medicine as a career?
- Would they themselves do it again?
- What changes in medicine would improve their well-being?
- Are most gay, lesbian, and bisexual doctors open about their sexual orientation to colleagues, office staff, and patients?
- What are the professional ramifications of a decision to be open?
- Are openly gay, lesbian, and bisexual doctors happier and more successful, and do they suffer more or less stress?
- How many employers of doctors include 'sexual orientation' in their nondiscrimination statement? How many offer benefits for same-sex partners?

See 13.8 for strategies to enhance the well-being of lesbian and gay physicians and residents.

13.8 Enhancing Well-Being of Bisexual, Lesbian, and Gay Medical Professionals and Trainees

For Professionals

- When possible, come out.
- Join a gay, lesbian, and bisexual organization. If none is available near you, form one.
- If you work for a hospital or doctor group, ask that 'sexual orientation' be added to its nondiscrimination statement – if not for yourself, then for your patients.
- Sponsor a booth at the local Gay Pride celebration.
- Join a gay, lesbian, and bisexual e-mail list, such as glb-medical. To join, send an e-mail message (listserv@listserv.utoronto.ca) and, in the body of the message, write: 'subscribe glb-medical-l (Your name).'
- If you live near a medical school, volunteer to speak as part of the homosexual and bisexual curriculum.
- Act as a mentor for a homosexual or bisexual medical student or resident.

For Residents

- Seek out out gay health providers. The Gay and Lesbian Medical Association (www.glma.org) is a good starting place.
- Choose a residency program in a city with an active and diverse gay life. These settings are also more likely to have other openly out lesbian or gay health professionals who may provide you with personal and career mentorship.
- As you get to know your colleagues, you will gradually develop the sense of who to come out to. It's important not to isolate yourself (or your partner) from potentially helpful sources of support.
- Do not feel obliged to let homophobic responses go unchecked. Respond firmly and calmly.
- Resist any tendency to overcompensate because you are lesbian or gay. If you are having trouble reconciling your personal and professional identities, seek psychotherapy from a gay-affirming counselor.

From Burke, Brian P., White, Jocelyn C., & Saunders, Daniel. (2001). Wellbeing of gay, lesbian, and bisexual doctors. *British Medical Journal, 322*, 422–5.

The Research Environment

Over the long term, advances in the care of lesbians and gay men will depend on a deeper understanding of the factors that enhance or diminish their health. As has been noted several times in this book, little research has been done to assess gay and lesbian health needs, and certain groups within the gay community (e.g., ethnoracial minorities, elders, Aboriginal people, disabled people) are completely absent from the research. See 13.9 and 13.10 for a proposed research agenda for lesbian and gay male health. These wish lists illustrate the vast research and – indirectly – the existing gaps. Although 13.9 was designed specifically to address the health needs of lesbians, many of the questions could be reworded to apply to gay men.

One of the priorities in the research agenda for gay men is addressing homophobia. Ultimately, the work of providing compassionate and skilled care to all patients – regardless of sexual orientation – is an act of defiance against homophobia. The benefits of addressing homophobia extend far beyond the gay community (see 13.11).

13.9 Proposed Research Agenda for Lesbian Health

- What is the impact of homophobia and heterosexism on physical and emotional health across the life span? What factors are 'protective'?
- What are the childbearing patterns of lesbians?
- To what extent are lesbians involved in a community of women similar to themselves, and what is the impact of that involvement on health?
- How are lesbian support systems mapped and maintained?

Life-Span Development

- What interventions could help lesbian adolescents address areas of risk (i.e., STDs, smoking, depression)?
- What helps and hinders the coming out process? How do we understand a 'healthy' coming out?
- What are the career paths of lesbians? How do they experience retirement?

Mental Health

- What is the prevalence of mental health disorders for lesbians?
- How is identity formed for women with more than one 'minority' status (i.e., lesbians from ethnic or racial minorities)?
- How do lesbians define family? What role does family play in mental health?
- What are effective psychotherapies for lesbians?
- What is the prevalence of violence and hate crimes against lesbians?

Diseases and Disorders

- Do lesbians have higher rates of breast cancer?
- What is the risk of transmission of HIV or STDs from sexual contact between women?
- What are the most effective treatments for substance use disorders among lesbians?

Service Delivery and Access to Service

- What models of care most effectively remove access barriers for lesbians?
- What is the basic standard of care for lesbian health?

From Solarz, A. (Ed). (1999). *Lesbian health: Current assessment and direction for the future*. Washington, DC: Institute of Medicine.

13.10 Proposed Research Agenda for Gay Men's Health

Aging

- risks for cardiovascular disease
- prostate health: cancer detection, screening, impact on sexuality
- social supports and social networks for aging gay men

STDs beyond HIV

- strategies for primary prevention/behavior change
- vaccinations: development and access for gay men
- screening rates
- rates of hepatitis vaccine use/strategies for improving uptake
- relationships between substance abuse and STDs

Anal Cancer

- effectiveness of anal Pap
- population-based education and uptake of anal Pap as screening tool
- identifying people at risk, use of registries, etc.
- HPV vaccine: effectiveness, availability

Mental Health

- longitudinal mental health issues for gay men over life cycle: self-esteem, depression, mid-life issues
- evaluating suicide prevention strategies
- 'club culture' – impact on self-esteem, risk-taking behavior

- eating disorders/body dysmorphic disorder: prevention, detection, treatment
- enhancing resilience of gay youth

Recreational Drug Use

- long-term effects
- relationship to identity and culture

Violence and Hate Crimes

- incidence/prevalence
- impact on global functioning
- origins of homophobia leading to violence
- primary prevention of homophobia
- impact of stress, stigma, discrimination on mental health

Other

- gay immigrants, impact of ethnicity on health status for gay men
- impact of gay-positive providers on health status
- gay male parenting style

Bisexuality Issues

- identity formation, emotional and psychosocial development
- health risks
- protective factors

13.11 How Homophobia Hurts Us All

You do not have to be gay, lesbian, or bisexual, or know someone who is, to be negatively affected by homophobia. Although homophobia actively oppresses gay men, lesbians, and bisexuals, it also hurts heterosexuals. Homophobia:

- Inhibits the ability of heterosexuals to form close, intimate relationships with members of their own sex, for fear of being perceived as gay, lesbian, or bisexual (GLB)

- Locks people into rigid, gender-based roles that inhibit creativity and self-expression
- Is often used to stigmatize heterosexuals; those perceived or labeled by others to be GLB; children of GLB parents; parents of GLB children; and friends of GLBs
- Compromises human integrity by pressuring people to treat others badly, actions that are contrary to their basic humanity
- Combined with sex-phobia, results in the invisibility or erasure of GLB lives and sexuality in school-based sex education discussions, keeping vital information from students; such erasures can kill people in the age of AIDS
- Is one cause of premature sexual involvement, which increases the chances of teen pregnancy and the spread of sexually transmitted diseases; young people, of all sexual identities, are often pressured to become heterosexually active to prove to themselves and others that they are 'normal'
- Prevents some GLB people from developing an authentic self-identity and adds to the pressure to marry, which in turn places undue stress and oftentimes trauma on themselves as well as their heterosexual spouses, and their children
- Inhibits appreciation of other types of diversity, making it unsafe for everyone because each person has unique traits not considered mainstream or dominant; we are all diminished when any one of us is demeaned.

By challenging homophobia, people are not only fighting oppression for specific groups of people but striving for a society that accepts and celebrates the differences in all of us. For more about this topic, see *Homophobia: How We All Pay the Price* (Blumenfeld, 1992).

CHAPTER FOURTEEN

Legal Issues

Denise and Ruth have been in a committed relationship for fourteen years. During that time, they have had no significant contact with Ruth's parents, who cut themselves off when they discovered their daughter's sexual orientation.

Ruth was in a serious motor vehicle accident, which caused a head injury that has affected her speech and short-term memory. She is found to be incapable of making financial and treatment decisions. Her parents appear on the scene and demand that she be transferred to a rehab facility close to where they live, 800 miles away. Denise's wishes are ignored.

Evan is a 37-year-old engineer who works in a mid-sized company. He has been HIV-positive for nine years. His infection has progressed to the point where he needs to consider taking antiviral medications. Evan is very concerned about submitting his prescriptions to his drug plan. He has not told anyone at work about his illness, and he fears his job security and progress in the company would be seriously threatened if anyone knew of his HIV status.

Because in most jurisdictions same-sex couples cannot legally enter into marriage, they are excluded from rights enjoyed by married couples and must take steps to protect themselves, their partners, and their families. Legal implications of this difference in rights may profoundly affect same-sex partners and their children (Gruskin, 1999). Differences in rights can also have a serious impact in health care settings. For example, in the absence of documented instructions, a same-sex partner may have no say in the selection of health care providers or treatment facilities and no role in treatment decisions. He or she may also be denied the right to visit his or her partner in hospital. When the number of visitors to an ICU is limited, the same-sex partner may be ranked after the partner's family of origin.

Health care providers have a responsibility to function as effective advocates for gay and lesbian patients within health care settings, helping them to secure equal treatment, access, and respect. Because of the impact of discrimination and other legal issues on health, clinicians should also ensure that lesbian and gay patients are aware of their rights and the legal protections available to them. To fulfill this role, practitioners should be aware of local and provincial/territorial/state laws and ensure that lesbian and gay patients are advised about any appropriate protective legal measures they should take. This chapter looks specifically at legal issues for gay and lesbian youth, reproductive issues, legal agreements between same-sex couples, legal agreements that take effect when a person is incapacitated, wills, immigration and refugee issues, HIV legal issues, and workplace discrimination.

Legal Issues for Gay and Lesbian Youth

Confidentiality and Consent to Treatment

Gay and lesbian minors may avoid seeking medical care or counseling because they assume their parents will be informed of either their homosexuality or their medical condition, and they fear negative consequences (Ryan & Futterman, 1998). To reassure young patients and encourage them to be forthcoming about their problems and concerns, clinicians should establish patient–provider trust at the first meeting and explain the teen's right to confidentiality. It is important that young patients understand that care providers are required to keep their information confidential except in a few exceptional circumstances: when the clinician has evidence that patients are at risk of imminent harm to themselves (suicide) or to others (homicide), or when the clinician suspects the patient is being abused by caring professionals.

Competence and Autonomy

When treating minors, practitioners should be well informed about legal rights and obligations in their jurisdictions and should ensure their adolescent patients understand both their rights as a patient and the limitations of their autonomy as a minor. It is generally accepted that teens who are at least 14 years old are capable of making their own decisions and, under certain conditions, are able to consent to treatment without parental involvement. Parental consent is also not required for teens who have been declared emancipated/mature minors, are married, have served in the military, have lived independently, or who support themselves financially. Adolescents are able to make their own medical decisions without parental consent for emergency care, STD treatment, substance abuse treatment, pregnancy or contraceptive services, HIV testing and treatment, mental health services, and sexual assault treatment. In certain jurisdictions, parents must be informed of any treatment or services their minor children access but are not required to give consent. For example, some U.S. states require that a minor's HIV-positive test result be disclosed to a parent or guardian.

Teens are capable of granting informed consent and of making treatment decisions. *Informed consent* means that there has been adequate disclosure of information by the health care provider, comprehension of this information by the patient, the patient is competent, and consent for treatment was voluntary. It is critical for clinicians to recognize the autonomy of adolescent patients and to respect the ethics of confidentiality. When treating lesbian and gay adolescents, practitioners should be aware of any personal biases they may have, particularly about teen competence. They should also avoid making the assumption that the teen's sexual orientation is transient or unfavorable (Sobocinski, 1990). Practitioners should keep on hand a list of teen-specific referral services.

Reproductive Issues

Lesbian women seeking alternative insemination may face a number of legal issues. For example, there have been documented cases in Canada and the United States of lesbians being denied access to fertility clinics and related procedures. Limiting access to insemination services is generally considered a discriminatory practice – motivated more by personal prejudice than medical ethics (Capen, 1997). If this situation arises, the patient should seek legal counsel.

Couples considering alternative insemination with a known donor and those who wish to co-parent a child can face legal issues, such as disagreements over child custody, and may wish to consider formalizing the arrangement either through a donor agreement or a co-parenting agreement. See Appendix B for sample contracts; a co-parenting agreement is also available online (www.lesbian.org/lesbian-moms/knwpr.html).

- A donor agreement is a contract between the sperm donor and recipient that outlines the conditions under which sperm is donated as well as the rights and obligations or exclusion of each party. For example, the agreement would protect the sperm donor from any attempt by the recipient to gain financial support for the child in the future, and it would protect the recipient and the child from any attempt by the donor to claim custody rights. The contract should be clearly worded, highly specific, and understood by both parties.
- A co-parenting agreement is a contract between the biological mother and her partner or intended co-parent. It acknowledges their intent to jointly conceive and raise a child and outlines the parental rights and obligations of the nonbiological parent. A co-parenting agreement should stipulate that both parties will share decision-making rights and responsibilities for the child, and it should also set out provisions for child support and visitation in the event that the parents' relationship ends. In addition, the agreement should discuss custody and guardianship of the child in the event of death of one or both of the parents.

Legal Agreements between Same-Sex Couples

Some same-sex couples want to formalize their relationships and avoid legal problems associated with death, separation, or divorce. Others seek agreements that will give them rights comparable to heterosexual married couples. There are three legal tools that same-sex couples may be able to use: domestic partnership, a cohabitation contract, or joint ownership.

Domestic Partnership

In some regions of the United States, same-sex partners may register as domestic partners and complete a domestic partnership, which is a contract that recognizes persons (heterosexual or homosexual) who are in a committed relationship and who are cohabiting but not married (Gruskin, 1999). A domestic partnership generally allows each partner to gain access to the other's health care and other economic benefits, to bereavement leave, and to family sick leave (Gruskin, 1999). Couples considering a domestic partnership should be aware of the following:

- Domestic partnerships are not recognized (Sobocinski, 1990) in all states, and those registered in one region may not have access to equal benefits and securities outside that region.
- The advantages of these agreements are limited because they are not recognized by the federal or all state governments. Even with a domestic partnership, therefore, partners will not be able to sponsor partners for immigration or to apply for green cards for noncitizen partners.

For up-to-date information on human rights groups seeking legitimacy for gay and lesbian marriage, see the following online sources: in Canada (www.samesexmarriage.ca); in the United States, the Human Rights Campaign (www.hrc.org).

Cohabitation Contract

A cohabitation contract is a legal agreement that sets out the rights of each partner in the relationship and what will happen to financial holdings and property if the relationship dissolves. It can be a comprehensive, blanket agreement applying to all aspects of a relationship, or it may cover only certain aspects, such as jointly or individually purchased homes (McCarthy & Redbord, 2000). When partners decide to include intimate/day-to-day aspects of a relationship, it is advisable for them to execute two separate cohabitation contracts: one dealing with personal issues and the other dealing with finances and property. This will ensure that only directly applicable details of the relationship are disclosed in court. It also avoids the situation where a single contract that includes intimate details appears frivolous or is rendered legally unenforceable. A cohabitation contract should encompass the following points:

- It should be executed using clear language, and its contents should be fully understood and agreed upon by both parties.
- All property should be listed, including any obtained before the relationship. Provisions should also be made for property acquired during the relationship.
- Spousal support rights consistent with provision or status laws should

be outlined, or the provision that neither party is obliged to provide spousal support should be included.

- The intent of property sharing should be indicated, including any specific holdings (pension, home, RSP, etc.) that are to be excluded from the agreement.
- The contract should be signed by both parties and witnessed.

Couples should be aware that improperly drafted cohabitation contracts may be legally invalid (in part or in whole), so it is not advisable to rely on them in matters of child custody or visitation rights. Joint custody orders or stepparent adoptions are more appropriate ways to address these issues. When partners prepare a cohabitation contract, they should determine whether the contract will apply upon death or if each partner will conduct his or her own estate planning. They should also be aware that this contract should not be relied upon in place of a last will and testament. Both parties should seek separate legal consultation when drawing up a cohabitation contract. Sample cohabitation agreements are included in Appendix B.

Joint Ownership

To avoid or minimize the expense of probating a will, it is often advisable for couples to enter into joint ownership of any property that the partners stand to inherit from one another. Joint ownership means that upon the death of one partner, the other is automatically fully entitled to the jointly held property, such as a home. Jointly owned property is also removed from each person's will, which means that it is out of the reach of family members in the event that they contest the will (Ettlebrick, 1996).

Couples can also arrange to have joint bank accounts and financial holdings. With these accounts, joint rights are not conditional. That means that either party to a joint account can access funds at any time (he or she does not require the signature of the other person).

Legal Agreements that Take Effect When Someone Is Incapacitated

Gays and lesbians can legally arrange for powers of attorney for both medical and financial decisions for one another, or for a conservatorship or guardianship in case they become incapacitated and are unable to make their own decisions.

Durable Power of Attorney (DPA)

When drawing up a power of attorney, couples have three choices: a general DPA, a limited DPA, and a power of attorney that is nondurable.

- A general DPA is a legal document that allows each partner in a couple to make financial decisions without limitation. Under its provisions, each partner is authorized to make decisions for the other, including when the other is incapacitated (see Appendix B).
- A limited DPA is similar to a general durable power of attorney. It permits a couple to make financial and legally binding decisions on each other's behalf, but it also allows each partner to limit the other's authority. For example, one partner may give the other authority to sell only particular belongings or property, or to do so only in order to cover medical expenses.
- A power of attorney that is executed as nondurable is an agreement that can be limited to certain situations. For example, it may be valid only during periods when the person is ill or hospitalized, or it can be drafted to expire upon the death of one partner.

Durable Medical Power of Attorney

A durable medical power of attorney is a legal document authorizing another person to make someone's medical decisions in the event that the person is unable to do so (see Appendix B). This includes but is not limited to dietary requirements, medications, surgery, changing health care providers, end-of-life treatment interventions, and relocation to another health care facility. It gives the designated person (i.e., the patient's partner) access to medical records and the right to visit the patient, both of which are often contested in conflicts between same-sex spouses and biological family members who do not recognize the relationship.

To ensure that the provisions of the medical power of attorney are respected, copies should be given to health care providers and placed in the patient's medical records. Clinicians then know who to contact if an emergency arises or a decision is required. Patients should also discuss the provisions of their durable medical power of attorney with their physicians and family members so that everyone is aware of their wishes (Ettlebrick, 1996).

Conservatorship / Guardianship

A conservatorship is the appointment of an individual to make personal and financial decisions on one's behalf when one becomes incapacitated or unable to care for one's self (Gruskin, 1999). This may be a less than ideal way to exercise power because all decisions made under provision of a conservatorship must receive court approval and become part of public record. The legal fees and related expenses required to finalize decisions make this an impractical care option for many couples. However, those who choose this route should be aware of the following:

- A guardian is usually appointed when a person is incapacitated. However, the person can sign a document of nomination in advance, identifying his or her chosen conservator or guardian.
- A nomination is less likely to be challenged if it is made before the person becomes ill or suffers any cognitive deterioration. This may be particularly important for same-sex couples because, in the absence of a prearranged document, courts generally appoint a biological family member rather than a same-sex partner as guardian, and any disputes are usually resolved in favor of blood family.
- Although the advance nomination of a conservator is not legally binding, it does put a gay man's or lesbian's partner in a stronger position than he or she would otherwise have been.

Will and Testament

A last will and testament allows an individual to stipulate what is to be done with his or her property and financial holdings in the event of death. A will allows a person to express wishes beyond how property will be distributed and his or her estate administered. For example:

- People can indicate who they wish to care for their children by nominating a guardian in their will – although this is not always legally binding.
- A person's wishes for funeral and burial arrangements can also be included in a will, which ensures that his or her wishes are respected. This may be particularly important for gay and lesbian clients if their wishes are contrary to those of their family or partner.

A will may be amended or revoked at any time and comes into effect only upon death. In the absence of a will, all property – potentially including any held jointly with a same-sex spouse in the absence of a joint ownership agreement – may be distributed to biological relatives. For this and other reasons, it is advisable for gays and lesbians to have wills, to make any revisions while of sound mind, and to avoid 'deathbed' wills that are more open to challenges (Ettlebrick, 1996). Lesbian and gay clients should also be aware that the sexual orientation of a testator and of a will's beneficiary cannot be used as a basis for overturning a will.

Immigration / Refugee Issues

People who are gay, lesbian, or transgendered may not be denied access to Canada or the United States on the basis of sexual orientation. However, openly gay or lesbian people are often subject to systemic discrimination, which makes cross-border travel more difficult. For example, when applying for immigration visas or asylum, gays and lesbians may be asked for documentation that is not required of heterosexual individuals or couples. In addition, U.S. immigration policy denies entry to all persons who are HIV-positive unless their condition is the grounds upon which they are seeking refugee status. Under select circumstances, temporary visas may be granted to people who are HIV-positive.

When considering immigration or applying for visas to other countries, gays and lesbians should be aware of the following:

- Spousal recognition for same-sex couples may not be granted. A same-sex couple may have to apply for status individually.
- In Canada and the United States, sexual orientation – specifically, the fear of prosecution as a result of one's sexual orientation – is accepted as grounds for seeking refugee status. Those applying for such status in the United States must do so within one year upon arrival. (No time restrictions exist in Canada.)
- In the case of both refugee and same-sex spousal reunification applications, persons will often be required to produce 'evidence' substantiating their sexual orientation. This is difficult for applicants who were not 'out' in their home country due to fear of prosecution. The testimony of a witness may be used as evidence. The Lesbian and

Gay Immigration Rights Task Force can assist in locating appropriate witnesses (www.lgirtf.org).

HIV Legal Issues

People living with HIV may have some unique legal issues, including discrimination based on their health status, patients' rights, and travel and immigration restrictions.

Discrimination Based on HIV Status

Under the Canadian Human Rights Act, HIV/AIDS is considered a disability, and therefore any discrimination against someone with HIV/AIDS is prohibited. The Canadian Charter of Rights and Freedoms and the Royal Commission on Aboriginal Peoples also prohibit discrimination on the basis of having HIV/AIDS. In addition, many levels of Canadian government and many employers have policies protecting people with HIV against discrimination in the workplace.

However, discrimination based on HIV status does occur. It may be motivated by ignorance or fear of the virus and of possible contagion; homophobia (including the assumption that an infected person is gay); prejudice against any type of disfigurement or visible disability; or the assumption that a person with HIV is a street drug user. Protective laws exist to combat this discrimination, and it is important that patients be aware of their rights. They should also be aware that the human rights codes in certain provinces and territories do not protect against antigay discrimination. Patients in these regions may be obligated to prove they were subject to discrimination based on their HIV status rather than their sexual orientation.

A person who is subject to discrimination has the right to obtain advice on whether a law has been broken and to file a complaint with the Human Rights Commission. No lawyer is required, and confidentiality is ensured. Some local AIDS organizations, community legal clinics, and legal aid offices will provide specialized legal assistance and referrals. These services and organizations may also help clients decide the most appropriate course of action. For information about how to deal with discrimination in the workplace, contact Canada Employment and Immigration offices or provincial/territorial departments of labor.

People with HIV Who Put Others at Risk

People who are HIV-positive and who deliberately transmit the virus to others may be subject to both criminal and civil prosecution. In the criminal justice system, they can be charged with common nuisance, negligence, assault, or attempted murder. Under civil law, they can be sued for monetary compensation by anyone who they have harmed. This course of action may be appropriate in certain cases of HIV transmission or exposure (CATIE, 1999).

In cases where HIV-positive patients refuse to modify behaviors that put others at risk (including informing partners of their serostatus), it is legal and ethical for a practitioner to notify any identifiable people at risk or to arrange for public health authorities to do so. Clinicians may also notify public health authorities in circumstances where a patient is putting unidentifiable people at risk, such as anonymous unsafe sexual encounters. Public health law generally requires the collection of health information and enforcement of health standards and sets out provisions for quarantine and compulsory treatment. These laws vary between jurisdictions, and health care providers should be familiar with the specific laws in their province or state.

Patients' Rights

Under mental health legislation, most jurisdictions have the authority to hospitalize people who are a risk to themselves or others. However, HIV-positive inpatients cannot be detained involuntarily simply as a means of protecting others from infection when discharge is otherwise clinically appropriate. Nor can they be forced to accept treatment.

- To justify forced hospitalization, a patient's high-risk behaviors must be the result of a specific mental illness with related potential for harm to self or others.
- HIV-positive patients have the right to refuse treatment provided they are able to communicate a fixed choice, understand they are ill and understand the nature of the illness, are aware of treatment options and effects, and understand the consequences of refusing treatment.

Because HIV disease is associated with mental and cognitive impairment, clinicians should discuss legal issues and precaution with their

HIV-positive patients during the early stages of illness – before there is any impairment in judgment. It may also be beneficial to request a psychiatric evaluation of a patient's capacity to execute legal documents, such as general and medical powers of attorney, living wills, and last wills and testaments, including funeral arrangements. (A sample living will is provided in Appendix B.) This is particularly important if patients suspect that relatives or acquaintances may challenge the validity of any of these documents. Having these legal documents in place can help patients feel more secure and may alleviate the perception of losing or relinquishing control.

Clinicians should also be aware of the following:

- Patients may not be denied psychiatric admission based on their HIV status.
- Mandatory HIV screening of patients, including psychiatric inpatients, is considered inappropriate because negative test results do not conclusively indicate seronegativity.
- Testing must be performed only when medically indicated, with a patient's informed consent, and when accompanied by pretest and posttest counseling.
- Under certain conditions (e.g., acute psychosis), psychiatric patients may not be capable of giving informed consent.
- Before asking about a patient's HIV status, psychiatrists should ensure the patient understands the limits of medical confidentiality or provide options for anonymous HIV testing.

14.1 Suicide and Euthanasia

Some patients with HIV, particularly those who are ill, may ask clinicians about suicide or euthanasia. At the current time, assisted suicide and euthanasia are prohibited in Canada and the United States. In Canada, it is not illegal for a person to take his or her own life, and others may be present without any legal repercussions as long as they do not actively intervene in the suicide. However, patients contemplating suicide should be aware that it may affect their life insurance benefits. For example, their beneficiaries may receive a lesser amount or may receive nothing at all. For more information, visit the site of the HIV-AIDS Legal Counsel of Ontario (www.halco.org).

Immigration and Travel Issues

Immigration policy specifies that anyone who immigrates to Canada must not pose a danger to public health and safety nor place excessive demand on the country's health care and social services systems. Because of their potential health care and support needs, people with HIV are considered 'medically inadmissible' (Jürgens & Palles, 1997). A similar situation exists in the United States where HIV-positive applicants are considered inadmissible because HIV is classified as a communicable disease of significant public health concern (Lesbian & Gay Immigration Rights Task Force, n.d.).

The issue then becomes: How do immigration officials know who is infected? Prospective immigrants to the United States can be required to undergo mandatory HIV screening, and Canada is considering a similar policy, which is designed to reduce the health costs incurred when the country admits someone with HIV. Many medical ethicists disagree with this policy on humanitarian grounds (Sommerville, 1989). At the current time, immigration officials cannot order mandatory HIV screening based on the person's country of origin, race, gender, or sexual orientation. The indications for mandatory HIV testing include but are not limited to: a history of receiving unscreened blood transfusions or products; a history of IV drug use; having an HIV-positive mother; a history of engaging in unsafe sexual practices with a partner who is or is suspected to be HIV-positive; or a current medical history or physical examination consistent with an AIDS-defining condition (Jürgens, 1997).

People with HIV who simply want to travel may be denied a visa to visit the United States unless they have obtained a waiver of the HIV ban. Waivers are available only for nonimmigrant visas. People seeking entry to the United States who attempt to conceal their HIV-positive status may be detained. Immigration officials are authorized to require a nonimmigrant visa holder to undergo HIV testing if they suspect the person of being HIV-positive.

Workplace Discrimination

For gays and lesbians, workplace cultures can be either significant sources of stress or support. Unless an employer is explicitly known to support diversity and to be gay-positive, lesbians, gay men, and bi-sexuals must often read between the lines to determine how safe it is to be 'out' in the workplace. In settings without explicit nondiscriminatory policies, lesbian or gay employees are often caught in a no-win position: to be open about their sexual orientation and risk both direct and indirect discrimination (Rubenstein, 1993), or to remain closeted and conceal part their personal life, which may also affect their success in the workplace (Shime, n.d.).

Certain professional or service-focused jobs may justify excluding gay or lesbian workers from opportunities or roles on the basis of 'honoring the preferences of the clients (or parents or patients).' This line of reasoning is often symbolic of significant homophobia within the workplace culture, which is conveniently displaced and labeled as the 'client's problem.' The assumption that the majority of people prefer (or even care) that a service provider be heterosexual is unfounded. Excluding openly gay people from sensitive positions, such as teaching, is often based on the myth that gay people are more likely than heterosexuals to molest children. It also ignores the benefit of having teachers who can provide positive role models for the significant minority of students who themselves are gay and struggling with their orientation.

A growing number of large private sector employers are offering same-sex benefits to their employees – a visible symbol of support for lesbian and gay workers. (The Canadian House of Commons extended such support to MPs and House of Commons employees in 1997.) The Canadian Human Rights Commission has clearly laid out guidelines for nondiscrimination in job interviews, what constitutes a bona fide 'occupational requirement,' and the exact provisions of the Employment Equity Act. It also publishes an annual summary of human rights litigation based on sexual orientation issues, which can be accessed online (www.chrc-ccdp.ca/). U.S.-based information may be found at (www.hrc.org). A useful tool for employers and human resource departments – 'Is My Workplace Heterosexist?' – is also available to help companies assess how inclusive their work settings are (www.mun.ca/the/BusinessTest.html).

Factors that May Indicate an Increase in Risk for Specific Diseases

Disease or Condition	Risk Factors
In gay men	
Gastrointestinal infections (including those caused by Giardia lamblia, Entomoeba histolytica, Shingella species, various species of Compylobacter, and hepatitis A)	Oral-anal sexual contact
STDs (including gonorrhea, chlamydia, syphilis, herpes, HIV, HPV, and HBV)	Anal-receptive sexual intercourse; oral-genital sexual intercourse
Colon cancer	Increased smoking; decreased frequency of screening
Anal cancer	Higher incidence of human papillomavirus (HPV), transmitted via anal-receptive sexual intercourse
Hepatocellular carcinoma	Hepatitis B virus (HBV) transmitted via anal-receptive sexual intercourse
Eating disorders	Subcultural attitudes toward thinness and beauty
In lesbians	
Breast cancer	Nulliparity, older age at first childbirth, no breast-feeding, smoking, increased alcohol use, higher body mass index (BMI), and fewer screening exams

Disease or Condition	Risk Factors
Ovarian cancer	Limited or absent use of oral contraceptive, nulliparity, smoking
Endometrial cancer	No oral contraceptive use, nulliparity, oligoparity
Colon cancer	Smoking, increased BMI, fewer screening exams
In both gay men and lesbians	
Stroke, coronary artery disease	Increased smoking, fewer screening exams
Lung cancer	Increased smoking
Alcoholism, depression, suicide	Increased stress from living in a homophobic society
Antigay violence, hate crimes	Being openly gay/lesbian; being perceived as gay

From Harrison, A.E. (1996). Primary care of lesbian and gay patients: Educating ourselves and our students. *Family Medicine, 28*(1), 10–23. Reprinted with permission.

Sample Legal Contracts

Sample contracts are reprinted with permission from *On Our Own Terms: A Practical Guide for Lesbian and Gay Relationships*, by Laurie Bell (Toronto: CLGRO, 1991). Please note these documents are provided for information purposes only. Patients should be advised to seek legal counsel to discuss relevant state/provincial legislation. Counselors and therapists may wish to review these documents for specific discussion within therapy sessions concerning life, health, and family transitions.

Sample Sperm Donation Agreement

This AGREEMENT is made this March 8th of (*year*), by and between *Jim Lee*, hereafter DONOR, and *Ann Parent*, hereafter RECIPIENT, who may also be referred to as parties.

NOW, THEREFORE, in consideration of the promises of each other, DONOR and RECIPIENT agree as follows:

1. Each clause of this AGREEMENT is separate and divisible from the others; should a court refuse to enforce one or more clauses of this AGREEMENT, the others are still valid and in full force.
2. DONOR has provided his semen to RECIPIENT for the purpose of artificial insemination.
3. In exchange, DONOR has received from RECIPIENT one dollar exactly ($1.00).
4. Each party is a single person who has never married.
5. Each party acknowledges and agrees that, through the procedure of artificial insemination, RECIPIENT has become pregnant.
6. Each party acknowledges and agrees that DONOR provided his

semen for purposes of said artificial insemination, and did so with the clear understanding that he would not demand, request, or compel any guardianship, custody, visitation rights with any child(ren) born from the artificial insemination procedure. Further, DONOR acknowledges he fully understood he would have no parental rights whatsoever with said child(ren).

7. Each party acknowledges and agrees that RECIPIENT has relinquished any and all rights that she might otherwise have to hold DONOR legally, financially, or emotionally responsible for any child(ren) resulting from the artificial insemination procedure.

8. Each party acknowledges and agrees that DONOR and RECIPIENT will remain in acquaintance with each other to the best of their abilities, and that each will always be apprised of the other's home address and home telephone; such information will remain the private knowledge of DONOR and RECIPIENT, and will be used at their discretion.

9. Each party acknowledges and agrees that when said child(ren) is/are of such age as to request information regarding the identity of DONOR, or when it is agreed that the child(ren) would benefit from such information, the child(ren) will be informed of the DONOR's identity; the child(ren) and the DONOR will then be able to develop a mutually agreeable, nonparental, voluntary relationship, provided that said relationship does not contravene the provisions of the AGREEMENT.

10. Each party acknowledges and agrees that the sole authority to name child(ren) resulting from the artificial insemination shall rest with RECIPIENT.

11. Each party acknowledges and agrees that there shall be no father named on the birth certificate of any child(ren) born from artificial insemination.

12. Each party relinquishes and releases any and all rights he or she may have to bring a suit to establish paternity.

13. Each party covenants and agrees that, in light of the expectations of each party, as stated above, RECIPIENT shall have absolute authority and power to appoint a guardian for her child(ren), and that the mother and guardian may act with sole discretion as to all legal, financial, medical, emotional needs of said child(ren) without any involvement with or demands of authority from DONOR.

14. Each party covenants and agrees that neither of them will identify

the DONOR as a parent of the child(ren), nor will either of them reveal the identity of the DONOR to any of their respective parents or relatives.

15. Each party acknowledges and agrees that the relinquishment of all rights, as stated above, is final and irrevocable. DONOR further understands that his waivers shall prohibit any action on his part for custody, guardianship, or right to visitation in any future situation, including the event of RECIPIENT's disability or death.

16. Each party covenants and agrees that any dispute pertaining to this AGREEMENT shall be submitted to binding arbitration according to:

 a) the request for arbitration may be made by either party and shall be in writing and delivered to the other party;

 b) pending the outcome of arbitration, there shall be no change made in the language of this AGREEMENT;

 c) arbitration panel that will resolve any disputes regarding this AGREEMENT shall consist of three persons: one person chosen by DONOR; one person chosen by RECIPIENT; and one person chosen by the other two panel members;

 d) within fourteen calendar days following the written arbitration request, the arbitrators shall be chosen;

 e) within fourteen calendar days following the selection of all members of the arbitration panel, the panel will hear the dispute between parties;

 f) within seven days subsequent to the hearing, the arbitration panel will make a decision and communicate it in writing to each party.

17. Each party acknowledges and understands that legal questions are raised by issues in this AGREEMENT which have not been settled by statute or prior to court decisions. Notwithstanding this, the parties choose to enter into this AGREEMENT.

18. Each party acknowledges and agrees that she or he signed this AGREEMENT voluntarily and freely, of his or her own choice, without any duress of any kind whatsoever.

19. This AGREEMENT contains the entire understanding of the parties. There are no promises, understandings, or agreements other than those stated herein.

Sample Agreement to Jointly Raise a Child

We, Ann Parent and Martha Jones, make this agreement to set out our rights and obligations regarding our child who will be born to us by Ann Parent. We realize that our power to contract, as far as a child is concerned, is limited by state/provincial law. We also understand that the law will recognize Ann Parent as the only mother of the child. With this knowledge, and in a spirit of cooperation and mutual respect, we state the following as our agreement:

1. It is our intention to parent jointly and equally, including providing support and guidance. We will do our best to share jointly the responsibilities involved in feeding, clothing, loving, raising, and disciplining our child.
2. Ann Parent will sign a Temporary Guardianship or Power of Attorney giving Martha Jones the power to make medical decisions she thinks are necessary for the child in Ann Parent's absence.
3. We both agree to be responsible for our child's support until she or he reaches the age of majority (or finishes college). We each agree to contribute to our child's support in proportion to our net incomes. This agreement to provide support is binding, whether or not we live together. If we dispute the amount of support our child needs, or the percentage that either of us is to pay, we agree to submit our dispute to binding arbitration, as laid out in paragraph 9.
4. Our child will be given the last name of Parent.
5. Ann Parent agrees to designate Martha Jones as guardian of Ann Parent's estate, and of the child, in her will. We understand that naming Martha Jones legal guardian of the child isn't legally binding, but believe it should be persuasive in Court.
6. Because of the possible trauma our separation might cause our child, we agree to participate in a jointly agreed-upon program of counseling if either considers separating.
7. If we separate, we will both do our best to see that our child grows up in a good and healthy environment. Specifically we agree that:

   a) We will do our best to see that our child maintains a close and loving relationship with each of us.
   b) We will share in our child's upbringing, and will share in our child's support, depending on our needs, our child's needs, and our respective abilities to pay.

c) We will make a good-faith effort to make jointly all major decisions affecting our child's health and welfare.

d) We will base all decisions upon the best interests of our child.

e) Should our child spend a greater portion of the year living with one of us, the person who has actual custody will take all steps to maximize the other's visitation and help make visitation as easy as possible.

f) If we disagree about what is in the best interests of our child, we will undergo jointly agreed-upon counseling with the hope that we'll work out our differences and avoid taking our problems to court.

g) If either of us dies, our child will be cared for and raised by the other, whether or not we were living together. We will each state this in our wills.

8. We intend that this agreement be binding not only between ourselves but between each of us and our child.

9. Should any dispute arise between us regarding this agreement, we agree to submit the dispute to binding arbitration, sharing the cost equally.

10. We agree that if any court finds any portion of this contract illegal or otherwise unenforceable, the rest of the contract is still valid and in full force.

Sample Cohabitation Agreement #1

Linda Lover and Pam Partner make the following agreement:

1. They are living together now and plan to continue doing so.

2. All property owned by either Linda Lover or Pam Partner as of the date of this agreement remains her property and cannot be transferred to the other unless the transfer is made in writing.

3. The income of each person, as well as any accumulations of property from that income, belongs absolutely to the person who earns the money; joint purchases are covered under the provisions of clause 7.

4. If Linda Lover and Pam Partner separate, neither has a claim against the other for any money or property, for any reason, with the exception of property covered under clause 7 below (the joint pur-

chase clause), or unless a subsequent written agreement specifically changes this contract.

5. Linda Lover and Pam Partner will keep separate bank accounts, credit accounts, etc., and neither is responsible for the debts of the other.

6. Living expenses, which include groceries, utilities, rent, and day-to-day household upkeep, will be shared equally. Linda Lover and Pam Partner agree to open a joint bank account into which each agrees to contribute $500 per month to pay for living expenses.

7. Linda Lover and Pam Partner may make joint purchases (such as a house, car, or boat). The joint ownership of each specific item will be reflected on any title slip to the property. If no title slip exists, or if it's insufficient to record all the details to their agreement, Linda Lover and Pam Partner will prepare a separate, written, joint-ownership agreement. Any such agreement will apply to the specific jointly owned property only, and won't create an implication that any other property is jointly owned.

8. This agreement sets forth Linda Lover and Pam Partner's complete understanding concerning real and personal property ownership and takes the place of any and all prior contracts or understanding whether written or oral.

9. This agreement can be added to or changed only by a subsequent written agreement.

10. Any provision in this agreement found to be invalid shall have no effect on the validity of the remaining provisions.

Sample Cohabitation Agreement #2

Pam Partner and Linda Lover agree that:

1. They are living together now and plan to continue doing so.

2. All property earned or accumulated prior to Pam Partner and Linda Lover's living together belongs absolutely to the person earning or accumulating it, and it cannot be transferred to the other unless it's done in writing.

3. All income earned by either Pam Partner or Linda Lover while they are living together and all property accumulated from that income belongs equally to both, and should they separate, all accumulated property will be divided equally.

4. Should either person receive real or personal property by gift or inheritance, the property belongs absolutely to the person receiving the inheritance or gift and it cannot be transferred to the other unless it's done in writing.
5. In the event that either Pam Partner or Linda Lover wishes to separate, all jointly owned property under clause 3 will be divided equally.
6. Once the jointly owned property is divided, neither party will have any claim to any money or property from the other for any reason.
7. This agreement represents the complete understandings of Pam Partner and Linda Lover regarding their living together and replaces any and all prior agreements, whether written or oral, and can be added to or changed only by a subsequent agreement.
8. Any provision in this agreement found to be invalid shall have no effect on the validity of the remaining provisions.

Sample General Power of Attorney

THIS GENERAL POWER OF ATTORNEY is given on November 22, (*year*) by Jane Smith, of the City of Toronto, in the Municipality of Metropolitan Toronto.

I APPOINT Mary Jones of the City of Toronto, in the Municipality of Metropolitan Toronto, to be my attorney in accordance with the Powers of Attorney Act and to do on my behalf anything that I can lawfully do by an attorney.

This Power of Attorney is subject to the following conditions and restrictions: NONE.

In accordance with the Powers of Attorney Act, I declare that this Power of Attorney may be exercised during any subsequent legal incapacity on my part. In accordance with the Powers of Attorney Act, I declare that, after due consideration, I am satisfied that the authority conferred on the attorney named in this Power of Attorney is adequate to provide for the competent and effectual management of all my estate in case I should become a patient in a psychiatric facility and be certified as not competent to manage my estate under the Mental Health Act. I therefore direct that in that event, the attorney named in this Power of Attorney may retain this Power of Attorney for the management of my estate by complying with subsection 38(2) of the Mental Health Act and in that case the Public Trustee shall not become committee of my estate as would otherwise be the case under clauses 38(1)(a) and (b) of that Act.

Sample Medical Power of Attorney

THIS GENERAL POWER OF ATTORNEY is given on June 1, (*year*) by Jane Client of the City of Toronto, in the Municipality of Metropolitan Toronto.

I APPOINT Susan Friend of the City of Toronto, in the Municipality of Metropolitan Toronto, to be my attorney in accordance with the Powers of Attorney Act and to do on my behalf anything that I can lawfully do by an attorney.

This Power of Attorney is limited to the following powers:

1. To authorize any and all diagnosis, medical treatment, or hospital care which any physician or dentist may deem advisable be rendered me.
2. To advise a treating physician, dentist, or other medical personnel as to any diagnosis, treatment, medical procedure, or care that might be under consideration for me.
3. To have first priority to visit me in any facility in the event of injury, illness, incapacity, or incarceration.
4. To receive into her possession any and all items of personal property and effects which may be recovered from or about my person by any hospital, police agency, or any other person at the time of my illness or disability.

In accordance with the Powers of Attorney Act, I declare that this Power of Attorney may be exercised during any subsequent legal incapacity on my part.

Sample Living Will

To My Family, My Physician, My Lawyer, and All Others Whom It May Concern:

Death is as much a reality as birth, growth, maturity, and old age – it is the one certainty of life. If the time comes when I can no longer take part in decisions for my own future, let this statement stand as an expression of my wishes and my directions, while I am still of sound mind.

If at some time the situation should arise in which there is no reasonable expectation of my recovery from extreme physical or mental disability, I direct that I be allowed to die and not be kept alive by medications, artificial means, or 'heroic measures.' I do, however, ask that medication be mercifully administered to me to alleviate suffering even though this may shorten my remaining life. This statement is made after careful consideration and is in accordance with my strong convictions and beliefs. I want the wishes and directions herein expressed carried out to the extent permitted by law. Insofar as they are not legally enforceable, I hope that those to whom this will is addressed will regard themselves as morally bound by these provisions.

1. I appoint James Doe to make binding decisions concerning my medical treatment. OR,
1. I have discussed my views as to life-sustaining measures with the following who understand my wishes: James Doe, John Smith, and Jane Friend.
2. Measures of artificial life support in the face of impending death that are especially abhorrent to me are:

   a) Electrical or mechanical resuscitation of my heart when it has stopped beating;
   b) Nasogastric tube feedings by machine when I am paralyzed and no longer able to swallow; and,
   c) Mechanical respiration by machine when my brain can no longer sustain my own breathing.

3. If it does not jeopardize the chance of my recovery to a meaningful and sentient life or impose an undue burden on my friends and family, I would like to live out my last days at home rather than in a hospital.

References

A comprehensive selection of online resources used throughout this book has been indexed by the authors and is available at www.glbcare.com.

1: Why a Clinical Guide on Lesbian and Gay Health?

American Medical Association, Council on Scientific Affairs. (1996). Health care needs of gay men and lesbians in the United States. *Journal of the American Medical Association, 275*(17), 1354–9.

Brotman, S., Peterkin, A., & Risdon, C. (2000). Unpublished questionnaire. Annual Meeting of the College of Family Physicians of Canada.

Brotman, S., Rowe, B., & Ryan, B. (2000). *Access to care: Exploring the health and well-being of gay, lesbian, bisexual, and two-spirit people in Canada.* McGill School of Social Work. http://www.arts.mcgill.ca/programs/socialwork/interact/interact.html [September 18, 2001].

Canadian AIDS Society. (1991). *Homophobia, heterosexism and AIDS: Creating a more effective response to AIDS.* Ottawa.

Dean, L., Meyer, I., Robinson, K., et al. (2000). *Lesbian, gay, bisexual and transgender health: Findings and concerns.* Conference Edition. Gay and Lesbian Medical Association. New York: Columbia University.

Friedman, R.C., & Downey, J.L. (1994). Homosexuality. *New England Journal of Medicine, 331*(14), 923–30.

GLMA–Columbia University White Paper. (2000). *LGBT health: Findings and concerns.* New York. http://www.glma.org/policy/whitepaper

Harrison, A. (1996). Primary care of lesbian and gay patients: Educating ourselves and our students. *Family Medicine, 28,* 10–23.

Jalbert, Y. (1999). *Gay health: Current knowledge and future actions.* (Literature review). Ottawa: Health Canada.

Jones, M.A., & Gabriel, M.A. (1999). Utilization of psychotherapy by lesbians, gay men, and bisexuals: Findings from a nationwide survey. *American Journal of Orthopsychiatry, 68*(2), 209–19.

Kaufman, H., Ford, P., Pranger, T., & Sankar-Mistry, P. (1997). Women who have sex with women: Linking HIV, Hepatitis B and C infection with risk behaviors. *Social Work, 65*(3), 77–86.

Millman, M. (1993). *Access to health care in America*. Washington, DC: National Academy Press.

O'Hanlan, K., Cabaj, R.B., Schatz, B., Lock, J., & Nemrow, P. (1997). A review of the medical consequences of homophobia with suggestions for resolution. *Journal of the Gay and Lesbian Medical Association, 1*(1), 25–40.

Peers, L., & Demczuk, I. (1998). Lorsque respect ne suffit pas: Intervenir auprès des lesbiennes. Sous la direction de Irene Demczuk, *Des droits à reconnaître – les lesbiennes face à la discrimination* (pp. 77–116). Montreal: Les éditions du Remue-ménage.

Rankow, E.J. (1995). Lesbian health issues for the primary care provider. *Journal of Family Practice, 40*(5), 486–93.

Robertson, A.E. (1998). The mental health experiences of gay men: A research study exploring gay men's health needs. *Journal of Psychiatric and Mental Health Nursing, 5*(1), 133–40.

Sell, R.L., Wells, J.A., & Wypij, D. (1995). The prevalence of homosexual behavior and attraction in the United States, the United Kingdom and France: Results of national population-based samples. *Archives of Sexual Behavior, 24*(3), 235–48.

2: Improving the Doctor–Patient / Provider–Client Relationship

Beckman, H.B., & Frankel, R.M. (1984). The effect of physician behavior on the collection of data. *Annals of Internal Medicine, 101*, 692–6.

Bradford, J., & Dye, J. (n.d.). *Physicians' readiness for providing cancer screening to lesbians*. Unpublished manuscript.

Brotman, S., Rowe, B., & Ryan, B. (2000). *Access to care: Exploring the health and well-being of gay, lesbian, bisexual, and two-spirit people in Canada*. McGill School of Social Work. http://www.arts.mcgill.ca/programs/socialwork/interact/interact.html [September 18, 2001].

Chaimowitz, G.A. (1991). Homophobia among psychiatric residents, family practice residents and psychiatric faculty. *Canadian Journal of Psychiatry, 36*, 206–9.

Ernst, R.S., & Houts, P.S. (1985). Characteristics of gay persons with sexually transmitted disease. *Sexually Transmitted Diseases, 12*(2), 59–63.

Gambrill, E.D., Stein, T.J., & Brown, C.E. (1984). Social services use and need among gay/lesbian residents of the San Francisco Bay area. *Journal of Social Work and Human Sexuality, 3*(1), 51–69.

Goodchilds, J., & Peplau, L. (1991). Issues in psychotherapy with lesbians and gay men: A survey of psychologists. *American Psychologist, 46*(9), 964–72.

Harrison, A. (1996). Primary care of lesbian and gay patients: Educating ourselves and our students. *Family Medicine, 28,* 10–23.

Kaplan, S.H., Greenfield, S., & Ware Jr, J.E. (1989). Assessing the effects of physician–patient interactions on the outcomes of chronic disease. *Medical Care, 27*(3), 110–27.

Kass, N.E., Faden, R.R., Fox, R., & Dudley, J. (1992). Homosexual and bisexual mens' perceptions of discrimination in health services. *American Journal of Public Health, 82*(9), 1277–9.

Mathews, W.M.C., Booth, M.W., Turner, J.D., et al. (1986). Physicians' attitudes toward homosexuality: Survey of a California county medical society. *Western Journal of Medicine, 144,* 106–10.

O'Hanlan, K., Cabaj, R.B., Schatz, B., Lock, J., & Nemrow, P. (1997). A review of the medical consequences of homophobia with suggestions for resolution. *Journal of the Gay and Lesbian Medical Association, 1*(1), 25–40.

Owen, W.F. (1996). Gay men and bisexual men and medical care. In Robert P. Cabaj & Terry S. Stein (Eds.), *Textbook of homosexuality and mental health* (pp. 673–85). Washington, DC: American Psychiatric Press.

Penn, R.E. (1997). *The Gay men's wellness guide.* New York: Henry Holt.

Randall, C.E. (1989). Lesbian phobia among BSN educators: A survey. *Journal of Nursing Education, 28,* 302–6.

Reagan, P. (1981). The interaction of health professionals and their lesbian clients. *Patient Counseling and Health Education, 3*(1), 21–5.

Riddle, D. (1994). The Riddle scale. In *Alone no more: Developing a school support system for gay, lesbian, and bisexual youth.* St Paul: Minnesota State Department.

Schatz, B., & O'Hanlan, K. (1994). *Anti-gay discrimination in medicine: Results of a national survey of lesbian, gay and bisexual physicians.* San Francisco: Gay and Lesbian Medical Association.

Stevens, P.E., & Hall, J.M. (1988). Stigma, health beliefs and experiences with health care in lesbian women. *Image: Journal of Nursing Scholarship, 20,* 69–73.

Tesar, C.M., & Rovi, S.L.D. (1998). Survey of curriculum on homosexuality/bisexuality in departments of family medicine. *Family Medicine, 30*(4), 283–7.

Wallik, M.N., et al. (1992). Homosexuality as taught in U.S. medical schools. *Academic Medicine, 67,* 601–3.

White, J.C., & Dull, V.T. (1998). Room for improvement: Communication between lesbians and primary care providers. In Christy M. Ponticelli (Ed.),

Gateways to improving lesbian health and health care: Opening doors (pp. 95–110). New York: Harrington Park Press.

Wright, Adams, & Bernat homophobia scale. (2000). http://www.pbs.org/ wgbh/pages/frontline/shows/assault/etc/quiz.html [August 24, 2001].

3: Lesbians' Physical and Sexual Health

Berger, B.J., et al. (1995). Bacterial vaginosis in lesbians: A sexually transmitted disease. *Clinical Infectious Diseases, 21*(6), 1402–5.

Blumstein, P., & Schwarz, P. (1983). *American couple: Money, work, sex.* New York: William Morrow and Company.

Brotman, S., Rowe, B., & Ryan, B. (2000). *Access to care: Exploring the health and well-being of gay, lesbian, bisexual, and two-spirit people in Canada.* McGill School of Social Work. http://www.arts.mcgill.ca/programs/socialwork/ interact/interact.html [September 18, 2001].

Carroll, N. (1999). Optimal gynecologic and obstetric care for lesbians. *Obstetrics and Gynecology, 93*(4), 611–13.

Cochran, S.D., & Mays, V.M. (1988). Disclosure of sexual preference to physicians by black lesbian and bisexual women. *Western Journal of Medicine, 149,* 616–19.

Degen, K., & Waitkevicz, H.J. (1982). Lesbian health issues. *British Journal of Sexual Medicine, 32,* 40–7.

Diamant, A.L., Schuster, M.A., McGuigan, K., & Lever, J. (1999). Lesbians' sexual history with men: Implications for taking a sexual history. *Archives of Internal Medicine, 159,* 2730–6.

Ferris, D.G., et al. (1996). A neglected lesbian health concern: Cervical neoplasia. *Journal of Family Practice, 43*(6), 581–4.

Geddes, V.A. (1994). Lesbian expectations and experiences with family doctors: How much does the physician's sex matter to lesbians? *Canadian Family Physician, 40,* 908–20.

Hall, M. (1978). Lesbian families. *Social Work, 23,* 380–5.

Harrison, A.E., & Silenzia, V.M.B. (1996). Comprehensive care of lesbian and gay patients and families. *Primary Care: Models of Ambulatory Care, 23*(1), 31–46.

Harvey, S.M., Carr, C., & Bernheine, S. (1989). Lesbian mothers: Health care experiences. *Journal of Nurse Midwifery, 34*(3), 115–19.

Haynes, S. (1995). Breast cancer risk: Comparisons of lesbians and heterosexual women. In D.J. Bowen (Ed.), *Cancer and cancer risks among lesbians.* Seattle: Fred Hutchinson Cancer Research Center Community Liaison Program.

Johnson, S.R., Smith, S.M., & Guenther, S.M. (1987). Comparison of gynecologic health care problems between lesbians and bisexual women: A
survey of 2,345 women. *Journal of Reproductive Medicine, 32*(11), 805–11.

Jussim, J. (2000). *Lesbians facing the gay baby boom with empty arms.* http://
www.gayhealth.com [September 18, 2001].

Kenney, J., & Tash, D. (1992). Lesbian childbearing couples' dilemmas and
decisions. *Health Care for Women International, 13,* 209–19.

Lemp, G.F., et al. (1995). HIV seroprevalence and risk behaviors among lesbians and bisexual women in San Francisco and Berkeley, California. *American
Journal of Public Health, 85,* 1549–52.

Marrazzo, J.M., Koutsky, L.A., Stine, K.L., et al. (1998). Genital human papillomavirus infection in women who have sex with women. *Journal of Infectious Diseases, 178*(6), 1604–9.

Moran, N. (1996). Lesbian health care needs. *Canadian Family Physician, 42,*
879–84.

Newman, F. (1999). *The whole lesbian sex book: A passionate guide for all of us.* San
Francisco: Cleis Press.

Patterson, C.J. (1996). Lesbian and gay families with children: Implications of
social science research for policy. *Journal of Social Issues, 52*(3), 29.

Rankow, E.J., & Tessero, I. (1998). Cervical cancer risk and papanicolaou
screening in a sample of lesbian and bisexual women. *Journal of Family
Practice, 47*(2), 139–43.

Reilly, T. (1996). Gay and lesbian adoptions: A theoretical examination of
policy-making and organizational decision making. *Journal of Sociology and
Social Welfare, 23*(4), 99–115.

Roberts, S.J., & Sorensen, L. (1995). Lesbian health care: A review and recommendations for health promotion in primary care settings. *Nurse Practitioner,
20*(6), 42–7.

Rounds, K. (1993). Are lesbians a high-risk group for breast cancer? *Ms.
Magazine, 3*(6), 44–5.

Ryan, C., & Bradford, J. (1993). The national lesbian health care survey: An
overview. In L.D. Garrets and D.C. Kimmel (Eds.), *Psychological Perspectives
on Lesbian and Gay Male Experiences. Between Men – Between Women: Lesbian
and Gay Studies* (pp. 541–56). New York: Columbia University Press.

Simkin, R. (1991). Lesbians face unique health care problems. *Canadian Medical
Association Journal, 145*(12), 1620–3.

Simkin, R. (1998). Not all patients are straight. *Journal of the American Medical
Association, 159*(4), 370–5.

Skinner, C.J., et al. (1996). A case-controlled study of the sexual health needs of
lesbians. *Genitourinary Medicine, 72*(4), 277–80.

Smith, E.M., Johnson, S.R., & Guenther, S.M. (1985). Health care attitudes and experiences during gynecologic care among lesbians and bisexuals. *American Journal of Public Health, 75*, 1085–7.

Solarz, A. (Ed.). (1999.) *Lesbian health: Current assessment and direction for the future.* Washington, DC: Institute of Medicine.

Stevens, P.E., & Hall, J.M. (1988). Stigma, health beliefs and experiences with health care in women. *Image: Journal of Nursing Scholarship, 20*, 69–73.

Ulstad, V.K. (1999). Coronary health issues for lesbians. *Journal of the Gay and Lesbian Medical Association, 3*(2), 59–67.

Walter, M.H., & Rector, W.G. (1986). Sexual transmission of Hepatitis A in lesbians. (Letter). *Journal of the American Medical Association, 56*, 594.

Whatley, M.H. (1992). Images of gays and lesbians in sexuality and health textbooks. *Journal of Homosexuality, 22*, 197–211.

White, J.C. (1997). HIV risk assessment and prevention in lesbians and women who have sex with women: Practical information for clinicians. *Health Care for Women International, 18*, 127–38.

White, J.C., & Dull, V.T. (1998). Room for improvement: Communication between lesbians and primary care providers. In Christy M. Ponticelli (Ed.), *Gateway to improving lesbian health and health care: Opening doors.* New York: Harrington Park Press.

4: Gay Men's Physical and Sexual Health

Barrie, A., et al. (1998). *Sexual meanings and safer sex practices.* Ottawa: Canadian AIDS Society.

Bell, R. (1999). ABC of sexual health: Homosexual men and women. Clinical Review. *British Medical Journal, 318*(13), 452–5.

Boden, D., Hurley, A., Zhang, L., Cao, Y., Guo, Y., Jones, E., Tsay, J., Ip, J., Farthing, C., Limoli, K., Parkin, N., & Markowitz, M. (1999). HIV-1 drug resistance in newly infected individuals. *Journal of the American Medical Association, 282*(12), 1135–41.

Breese, P.L., Judson, F.N., Penley, K.A., & Douglas, J.M. (1995). Anal human papilloma virus infection among homosexual and bisexual men: Prevalence of type-specific infection and association with human immunodeficiency virus. *Sexually Transmitted Diseases, 22*, 7–14.

Buchbinder, S.P., Holmberg, S.D., Scheer, S., Colfax, G., O'Malley, P., & Vittinghoff, E. (1999). Combination antiretroviral therapy and incidence of AIDS-related malignancies. *Journal of Acquired Immune Deficiency Syndrome, 21*(1), S23–6.

Canadian Male Sexual Health Council. (1999). *Education on erectile dysfunction.* Symposium Report: Pfizer (CD-ROM).

Canadian Medical Association. (1995). *Counseling guidelines for HIV testing from the expert working group on HIV testing*. Ottawa: CMA.

Centers for Disease Control and Prevention. (1996). (Published erratum, 1997, *Morbidity and Mortality Weekly Report, 46*(25), 588). Prevention of Hepatitis A through active or passive immunization: Recommendations of the Advisory Committee on Immunization Practices (ACIP). *Morbidity and Mortality Weekly Report, 45*(RR-15), 1–30.

Centers for Disease Control and Prevention. (1999). Cases of syphilis, gonorrhea on rise among gay men in Seattle area (Associated Press), September 10. http://www.egroups.com/message/glbthealth/145 [January 27, 2001].

Centers for Disease Control and Prevention. (1999). HIV/AIDS surveillance. *Morbidity and Mortality Weekly Report, 11*(1), midyear edition.

Centers for Disease Control and Prevention. (2000). HIV/AIDS among racial/ethnic minority men who have sex with men: United States, 1989–1998. *Morbidity and Mortality Weekly Report, 49*(1).

Chan, P. (2001). *Outpatient and primary care medicine* (2001 ed.). Laguna Hills, CA: Current Clinical Strategies Publishing.

Chapple, M.J., Kippax, S., & Smith, G. (1998). 'Semi-straight sort of sex': Class and gay community attachment explored within a framework of older homosexually active men. *Journal of Homosexuality, 35*(2), 65–83.

Cole, S.W., Kemeny, M.E., Taylor, S.E., & Visscher, B.R. (1996). Elevated physical health risk among gay men who conceal their homosexual identity. *Health Psychology, 15*, 243–51.

Coleman, E., Rosser, B.R.S., et al. (1992). Sexual and intimacy dysfunction in homosexual men and women. *Psychiatric Medicine, 10*, 257–71.

Daling, J.R., Weiss, N.S., Hislop, G., Maden, C., Coates, R.J., Sherman, K.J., Ashley, R.L., Beagrie, M., Ryan, J.A., & Corey, L. (1987). Sexual practices, sexually transmitted diseases, and the incidence of anal cancer. *New England Journal of Medicine, 317*, 973–7.

Dean, L., Meyer, I., Robinson, K., et al. (2000). *Lesbian, gay, bisexual and transgender health: Findings and concerns*. Conference Edition. Gay and Lesbian Medical Association. New York: Columbia University.

Dillon, B., Hecht, F.M., Swenson, M., et al. (2000). *Primary HIV infections associated with oral transmission*. Abstract of presentation 473. 7th Conference on Retroviruses and Opportunistic Infections, San Francisco, CA, January 30–February 2. http://www.retroconference.org/2000/abstracts473.htm

Elford, J., Bolding, G., Maguire, M., & Sherr, L. (1999). Sexual risk behavior among gay men in a relationship. *AIDS, 13*(11), 1407–11.

Goldie, S.J., Kuntz, K.M., Weinstein, M.C., Freedberg, K.A., Welton, M.L., & Palefsky, J.M. (1999). The clinical effectiveness and cost-effectiveness of screening for oral squamous intraepithelial lesions in homosexual and bisexual HIV-positive men. *Journal of the American Medical Association, 281*(19), 1822–9.

Goldstone, S. (1999). *The ins and outs of gay sex: A medical handbook for men.* New York: Random House.

Health Canada. (1997). *CPA, HIV and psychiatry: A training and resource manual.* Ottawa: Health Canada.

Hickson, F.C., Reid, D.S., Davies, P.M., Weatherburn, P., Beardsell, S., & Keogh, P.G. (1996). No aggregate change in homosexual HIV risk behavior among gay men attending the Gay Pride festivals, United Kingdom, 1993–1995. *AIDS, 10*(7), 771–4.

Hospers, H.K., & Kok, G. (1995). Determinants of safe and risk-taking sexual behavior among gay men: A review. *AIDS Education and Prevention, 7*(1), 74–96.

Jacques, T., et al. (1999). *The safe edge: SM 101.* Toronto: AIDS Committee of Toronto.

Jalbert, Y. (1999). *Gay health: Current knowledge and future actions.* (Literature review). Ottawa: Health Canada.

Kaul, D., Cinti, S.K., Carver, P.L., & Kaznjian, P.H. (1999). HIV protease inhibitors: Advances in therapy and adverse reactions, including metabolic complications. *Pharmacotherapy, 19*(3), 281–99.

Kelly, J.A., Hoffman, R.G., Rompa, D., & Gray, M. (1998). Protease inhibitor combination therapies and perceptions of gay men regarding AIDS severity and the need to maintain safer sex. *AIDS, 12*(10), F91–5.

Koblin, B.A., Hessol, N.A., Zauber, A.G., Taylor, P.E., Buchbinder, S.P., Katzh, M.H., & Stevens, C.E. (1996). Increased incidence of cancer among homosexual men, New York City and San Francisco, 1978–1990. *American Journal of Epidemiology, 144*, 916–23.

Leiblum, S.R., & Rosen, R.C. (2000). *Principles and practice of sex therapy* (3rd ed.). New York: Guildford Press.

Martin, J.N., Ganem, D.E., Osmond, D.H., Page-Shafer, K.A., Macrae, D., & Kedes, D.H. (1998). Sexual transmission and the natural history of human herpes virus and infection. *New England Journal of Medicine, 338*, 948–54.

Maurice, W.L. (1999). *Sexual medicine in primary care.* St Louis, MI: Mosby.

Nichols, M. (2000). *Sex therapy with minorities.* In S.R. Leiblum (Ed.), *Principles and practice of sex therapy.* New York: Guildford Press.

Nycum, B. (2000). *The XY survival guide.* San Diego: XY Publishing.

Ottawa–Carleton Health Department. (n.d.). *Protect yourself: Use a condom* (pamphlet).

Palefsky, J.M., Holly, E.A., Ralston, M.L., & Jay, N. (1998). Prevalence and risk factors for human papillomavirus infection of the anal canal in human immunodeficiency virus (HIV)-positive and HIV-negative homosexual men. *Journal of Infectious Diseases, 177*, 361–7.

Penn, R.E. (1997). *The gay men's wellness guide*. New York: Henry Holt.

Peterkin, A. (1998). Negotiating safer sex: Tips for men who have sex with men. *Toronto Star* (Toronto Star Lifeline).

Rosser, B.R., et al. (1997). Sexual difficulties, concerns and satisfaction in homosexual men: An empirical study with implications for HIV prevention. *Journal of Sex and Marital Therapy, 23*, 61–73.

Saddul, R.B. (1996). Coming out: An overlooked concept. *Clinical Nurse Specialist, 10*(1), 2–5.

Scarce, M. (1999). *Smearing the queer*. New York: Harrington Park Press.

Shalits, P. (1998). *Living well: The gay man's essential health guide*. Los Angeles: Alyson Books.

Tillman, P.S., & Pequegnat, W. (1996). *Interventions to prevent HIV risk behavior*. (Current Bibliographies in Medicine 96–7). Prepared in support of the National Institutes of Health Consensus Development Conference on Interventions to Prevent HIV Risk Behavior, Bethesda, MD, February 11–13, 1997. http://www.nih.gov

Ungvarski, P.J., & Grossman, A.H. (1999). Health problems of gay and bisexual men. *Nursing Clinics of North America, 34*(2), 313–31.

Vittinghoff, E., and Douglas, J. (1999). Per-contact risk of human immunodeficiency virus transmission between male sexual partners. *American Journal of Epidemiology, 150*(3), 311. http://www.groups.yahoo.com/group/glbthealth/message/308 [November 2, 2000].

Wolfe, D. (1999). *Men like us: The GMHC (Gay Men's Health Crisis Clinic) complete guide to gay men's sexual, physical and emotional wellbeing*. New York: Ballantine Books.

5: Gay, Lesbian, and Bisexual Adolescent Physical and Mental Health

Allen, L.B., Glicken, A.D., Beach, R.K., & Naylor, K.E. (1998). Adolescent health care experience of gay, lesbian, and bisexual young adults. *Journal of Adolescent Health, 23*, 212–20.

American Academy of Pediatrics. (1993). Homosexuality and adolescence. *Committee on Adolescence, 92*, 631–4.

Anderson, S.C. (1996). Substance abuse and dependency in gay men and lesbians. In K.J. Paterson (Ed.), *Health care for lesbians and gay men: Confronting homophobia and heterosexism*. New York: Harrington Park Press.

Basgara, O., et al. (1993). Human immunodeficiency virus type I replication in peripheral blood mononuclear cells in the presence of cocaine. *Journal of Infectious Diseases, 168*, 1157–64.

Blum, R.W., & Bearinger, L.H. (1990). Knowledge and attitudes of health professionals toward adolescent health care. *Journal of Adolescent Health, 23*, 191–3.

Boxer, A., & Haas, J. *Mental health care for lesbian, gay, and bisexual adolescents.* http://www.gayhealth.com/binary-data/GH-TEXT-BLOCK/attachment/1314.pdf

Brotman, S., Rowe, B., & Ryan, B. (2000). *Access to care: Exploring the health and well-being of gay, lesbian, bisexual, and two-spirit people in Canada.* McGill School of Social Work. http://www.arts.mcgill.ca/programs/socialwork/interact/interact.html [September 18, 2001].

Centers for Disease Control and Prevention. (1993). *HIV and substance abuse in the gay male community.* (Report). Atlanta: CDC.

Chitwood, D.D., & Comerford, M. (1990). Drugs, sex and AIDS risk. *American Behavioral Science, 33,* 465.

Coates, T.J., Faigle, M., & Stall, R.D. (1995). *Does HIV prevention work for men who have sex with men?* (Report). San Francisco: Office of Technology Assessment, University of California, Center for AIDS Prevention Studies.

Crosby, R.A., Newman, D., Kamb, M.L., et al. (2000). Misconceptions about STD-protective behavior. *American Journal of Preventive Medicine, 19*(3), 167–73.

D'Augelli, A.R. (1996). Lesbian, gay and bisexual development during adolescence and young adulthood. In R.P. Cabaj & T.S. Stein (Eds.), *Textbook of homosexuality and mental health.* Washington, DC: American Psychiatric Press.

D'Augelli, A.R., & Hershberger, S.L. (1993). Lesbian, gay and bisexual youth in community settings: Personal challenges and mental health problems. *American Journal of Community Psychology, 21*(4), 421–48.

Dean, L., Martin, J.L., & Wu, S. (1992). Trends in violence and discrimination against gay men in New York City: 1984–1990. In G.M. Herek and K.T. Berrill (Eds.), *Hate crimes: Confronting violence against lesbians and gay men.* Newbury Park, CA: Sage Publications.

Dean, L., Meyer, I., Robinson, K., et al. (2000). *Lesbian, gay, bisexual and transgender health: Findings and concerns.* Conference Edition. Gay and Lesbian Medical Association. New York: Columbia University.

Dempsey, C.L. (1994). Health and social issues of gay, lesbian, and bisexual adolescents. *Families in Society: The Journal of Contemporary Human Services, 75*(3), 160–7.

Durby, D.D. (1994). Gay, lesbian, and bisexual youth. *Journal of Gay and Lesbian Social Services, 1*(3/4), 1–37.

East, J.A., & Rayess, F. (1998). Pediatricians' approach to the health care of lesbian, gay, and bisexual youth. *Journal of Adolescent Health, 23,* 191–3.

Fisher, P., & Shaffer, D. (1990). Facts about suicide: A review of national mortality statistics and records. In M. Rotheram-Borus, J. Bradley, & K. Obalenshy (Eds.), *Planning to live: Suicidal youth in community settings*. Tulsa: University of Oklahoma Press:

Fontaine, D.H., & Hammond, N.L. (1996). Counseling issues with gay and lesbian adolescents. *Adolescence, 31*(124).

Fontaine, J.H. (1997). The sound of silence: Public school response to the needs of gay and lesbian youth. *Journal of Gay and Lesbian Social Services, 7*(4), 101–9.

Futterman, D., Hein, K., Reuben, N., Dell, R., & Shaffer, N. (1993). Human immunodeficiency virus-infected adolescents: The first 50 patients in a New York City program. *Pediatrics, 91,* 730.

Gibson, P. (1989). *U.S. Department of Health and Human Services Secretary's task force on youth suicide*. (Report). Washington, DC. http://www.hcqsa.virtualave.net/ref.html

Gochros, H., & Bidwell, R. (1996). Lesbian and gay youth in a straight world: Implications for health care workers. In K.J. Paterson (Ed.), *Health care for lesbians and gay men: Confronting homophobia and heterosexism* (pp. 1–17). New York: Harrington Park Press.

Goldsmith, M.P. (1993). Medical news and perspectives. *Journal of the American Medical Association, 270,* 16.

Herek, G.M. (1989). Hate crimes against lesbians and gay men. *American Psychologist, 44,* 948–55.

Herr, K. (1997). Learning lessons from school: Homophobia, heterosexism, and the construction of failure. *Journal of Gay and Lesbian Social Services, 7*(4), 51–64.

Hershberger, S.L., Pilkington, N.W., & D'Augelli, A.R. (1996). Categorization of lesbian, gay, and bisexual suicide attempters. In Christopher J. Alexander (Ed.), *Gay and lesbian mental health: A sourcebook for practitioners*. New York: Harrington Park Press.

Hetrick, E., & Martin, D. (1987). Developmental issues and their resolution for gay and lesbian adolescents. *Journal of Homosexuality*. http://www.hmi.org

Hoffman, N., & Ocepek, D. (1994). *Protocol for primary care of lesbian and gay adolescents*. Conference on the Primary Care Needs of Lesbian and Gay Adolescents. Washington, DC: Health Resource and Services Administration, December 5–6.

Jalbert, Y. (1999). *Gay health: Current knowledge and future actions*. (Literature review). Ottawa: Health Canada.

Kreiss, J.L., & Patterson, D.L. (1997). Psychosocial issues in primary care of lesbian, gay, bisexual, and transgender youth. *Journal of Pediatric Health Care, 11,* 266–74.

Kruks, G. (1991). Gay and lesbian homeless/street youth: Special issues and concerns. *Journal of Adolescent Health, 12*, 515–18.

Lock, J., & Steiner, H. (1999). Gay, lesbian, and bisexual youth risks for emotional, physical, and social problems: Results from a community-based survey. *Journal of American Academic Child and Adolescent Psychiatry, 38*(3), 297–304.

Massachusetts Governor's Commission on Gay and Lesbian Youth. (1993). *Making schools safe for gay and lesbian youth.* (Report). Boston.

Nelson, J.A. (1997). Gay, lesbian, and bisexual adolescents: Providing esteem-enhancing care to a battered population. *Nurse Practitioner, 22*(2), 94–109.

Nycum, B. (2000). Coming out, you're what? *The XY survival guide.* San Diego: XY Publishing.

Paroski, P.A. (1987). Health care delivery and concerns of gay and lesbian adolescents. *Journal of Adolescent Health Care, 8*, 188–92.

Philadelphia Lesbian and Gay Task Force. (1992). *Discrimination and violence toward lesbian women and gay men in Philadelphia and the Commonwealth of Pennsylvania.* (Report).

Price, J., & Telljohan, S. (1991). School counselors' perceptions of adolescent homosexuals. *Journal of School Health,* (December).

Remafedi, G. (1987). Male homosexuality: The adolescent's perspective. *Pediatrics, 79*, 326–30.

Remafedi, G., Farrow, J.A., & Deischer, R.W. (1991). Risk factors for attempted suicide in gay and bisexual youth. *Pediatrics, 87*, 869–75.

Rosario, M., Rotheram-Borus, M.J., & Reid, H. (1996). Gay-related stress and its correlates among gay and bisexual male adolescents of predominantly black and Hispanic background. *Journal of Community Psychology, 24*, 136–59.

Rosenberg, P.S., Biggar, R.J., & Goedert, J.J. (1994). Declining age at HIV infection in the United States. *New England Journal of Medicine, 330*, 789.

Ryan, B., & Frappier, J. (1993). Les difficultés des adolescents gais et lesbiennes. *Le Médecine du Québec, 28*(9), 71–6.

Ryan, C., & Futterman, D. (1998). *Lesbian and gay youth: Care and counseling.* New York: Columbia University Press.

Saulmier, C.F. (1998). Prevalence of suicide attempts and suicidal ideation among lesbian and gay youth. *Journal of Gay and Lesbian Social Services, 8*(3), 51–68.

Sears, J. (1992). Homosexuality and homosexual students: Are personal feelings related to professional beliefs? In K. Harbek (Ed.), *Coming out of the classroom closet.* New York: Harrington Park Press.

Shapiro, S. (1991). *Rethinking adolescent homosexuality, assessment and treatment considerations.* Paper presented at the American Academy of Child and Adolescent Psychiatry Conference. Toronto: CAMH, Clarke Division.

Stall, R., McKusick, L., Wiley, J., & Coates, T. (1986). Alcohol and drug use during sexual activity and compliance with safe sex guidelines for AIDS: The AIDS behavioral research project. *Health Education Quarterly, 13*(4), 359–71.

Traveler's Aid: Victim Services. (1991). *Streetwork Project Study.* San Francisco.

Troiden, R.R. (1989). The formation of homosexual identities. *Journal of Homosexuality, 17*(42), 43–73.

Young, V. (1995). *The equality complex: Lesbians in therapy – a guide to anti-oppressive practice.* London: Cassell.

6: Diagnosing and Treating Sexually Transmitted Diseases

Centers for Disease Control and Prevention. (1998). *Guidelines for the treatment of sexually transmitted diseases.* http://www.cdc.gov/nchstp/dstd/1998_STD_Guidlines/1998_guidelines_for_the_treatment.htm [December 6, 2000].

Centers for Disease Control and Prevention. (2001). Outbreak of syphilis among men who have sex with men. *Morbidity and Mortality Weekly Report, 50*(7), 117–20.

Epstein, R.M., Morse, D.S., Frankel, R.M., Frarey, L., Anderson, K., & Beckman, H.B. (1998). Awkward moments in patient–physician communication about HIV risk. *Annals of Internal Medicine, 128*, 435–42.

Erickson, P.I., Bastani, R., Maxwell, A.E., Marcus, A.C., Capell, F.J., & Yan, K.X. (1995). Prevalence of anal sex among heterosexuals in California and its relationship to other AIDS risk behaviors. *AIDS Education Prevention, 7*, 477–93.

Goldstone, S. (1999). *The ins and outs of gay sex: A medical handbook for men.* New York: Random House.

Grosskurth, H., Mosha, F., Todd, J., Mwijarubi, E., Klokke, A., Senkoro, K., Mayaud, P., Changalucha, J., Nicoll, A., et al. (1995). Impact of improved treatment of sexually transmitted diseases on HIV infection in rural Tanzania: Randomised control trial. *Lancet, 346*(8974), 530–6.

Halperin, D. (1999). Heterosexual anal intercourse: Prevalence, cultural factors, and HIV infection and other health risks (Part I). *AIDS Patient Care, 13*(12), 717–30.

Health Canada. (1998). *Canadian STD guidelines.* http://www.hc-sc.gc.ca/hpb/lcdc/publicat/std98/index.html [February 26, 2001].

Marrazzo, J.M., Koutsky, L., Stine, K., et al. (2000). *Bacterial vaginosis and vaginal lactobacilli in women who have sex with women.* Presented at the Joint

Meeting of the ASTDA and MSSVD Conference, STIs at the Millennium: Past, Present and Future. Baltimore, MD.

Ottawa–Carleton Health Department. (n.d.). *Specific considerations in approaching STD care in lesbians and gay men.*

Ralph, S.G., et al. (1999). Influence of bacterial vaginosis on conception and miscarriage in the first trimester: Cohort study. *British Medical Journal, 39,* 220–3.

Taha, T.E., et al. (1998). Bacterial vaginosis and disturbances of vaginal flora: Association with increased acquisition of HIV. *AIDS, 12,* 1699–706.

7: HIV Issues

Caldwell, S., Burnhaum, R., & Forstein, M. (Eds.). (1994). *Therapists on the front line: Psychotherapy with gay men in the age of AIDS.* Washington, DC: American Psychiatric Press.

Canadian Medical Association. (1995). *Counseling Guidelines for HIV testing from the expert working group on HIV testing.* Ottawa: CMA.

Canadian Medical Association. (1997). HIV postexposure prophylaxis: New recommendations. *Canadian Medical Association Journal, 156*(2).

Centers for Disease Control and Prevention. (1998). Management of possible sexual, injecting-drug-use, or other nonoccupational exposure to HIV, including considerations related to antiretroviral therapy. Public Health Service Statement. *Morbidity and Mortality Weekly Report, 47*(RR-17), 1–14.

Citron, K. (1999). *What next? Mental Health and HIV in the era of combination antiretroviral therapy.* Presentation to the Canadian Psychiatric Association, Toronto.

Dillon, B., Hecht, F.M., Swenson, M., et al. (2000). *Primary HIV infections associated with oral transmission.* Abstract of presentation 473. 7th Conference on Retroviruses and Opportunistic Infections, San Francisco, CA, January 30–February 2. http://www.retroconference.org/2000/abstracts473.htm

Elliott, R., & Jürgens, R. (2000). *Rapid HIV screening at the point of care: Legal and ethical questions.* Canadian HIV/AIDS Legal Network.

Fleming, D.T., & Wasserheit, J.N. (1999). From epidemiological synergy to public health policy and practice: The contribution of other sexually transmitted diseases to sexual transmission of HIV infection. *Sexually Transmitted Infections, 75,* 3–17.

Goldie, S.J., Kuntz, K.M., Weinstein, M.C., Freedberg, K.A., Welton, M.L., & Palefsky, J.M. (1999). The clinical effectiveness and cost-effectiveness of screening for anal squamous intraepithelial lesions in homosexual and bisexual HIV-positive men. *Journal of the American Medical Association, 281*(19), 1822–9.

Hecht, F.M., et al. (1999). Optimizing care for persons with HIV infection. *Annals of Internal Medicine, 131*, 136–43.

Palefsky, J.M., Holly, E.A., Ralston, M.L., Jay, N., Berry, J.M., & Darragh, T.M. (1998). High incidence of anal high-grade squamous intra-epithelial lesions among HIV-positive and HIV-negative homosexual and bisexual men. *AIDS, 12*(5), 495–503.

Peterkin, A. (1993). *Psychosocial issues in HIV primary care.* HIV Module: Adult Care. College of Family Physicians of Canada.

Quinn, T., Gray, R., Sewankambo, N., et al. (2000). *Therapeutic reductions of HIV viral load to prevent HIV transmission: Data from HIV discordant couples, Rakai, Uganda.* Program and abstracts of the 13th International AIDS Conference, July 9–14, 2000. Durban, South Africa. Abstract TuPeC3391.

Robert, L.M., & Bell, D.M. (1994). HIV transmission in the health-care setting: Risks to health-care workers and patients. *Infectious Disease Clinics of North America, 8*(2), 319–29.

Royce, R.A., Sena, A., Cates Jr, W., & Cohen, M.S. (1997). Sexual transmission of HIV. *New England Journal of Medicine, 336*, 1072–8.

Safer Sex Institute. (2000). http://www.safersex.org [November 12, 2001].

Schneider, J.S., & Levin, S. (1999). Uneasy partners: The lesbian and gay health care community and the AMA. *Medical Student Journal of the American Medical Association, 282*, 1287–8.

White, J.C. (1997). Risk assessment and prevention in lesbians and women who have sex with women: Practical information for clinicians. *Health Care for Women International, 18*, 127–38.

Williams, A., & Friedland, G. (1997). Aherence, compliance and HAART: Patient-focused strategies to increase medication adherence. *AIDS Clinical Care, 9*(7), 51–4, 58.

8: The Mental Health of Gays, Lesbians, and Bisexuals

Adam, B., et al. (1998). *Sexual meanings and safer sex practices.* Ottawa: Canadian AIDS Society.

Atkinson, J.H., Grant, I., Kennedy, C.J., et al. (1998). Prevalence of psychiatric disorders among men infected with HIV. *Archives of General Psychiatry, 45*, 859–64.

Bartholow, B.N., Doll, L.S., Joy, D., Douglas, J.M., et al. (1994). Emotional, behavioral, and HIV risks associated with sexual abuse among adult homosexual and bisexual men. *Child Abuse and Neglect, 18*(9), 747.

Bell, R. (1999). ABC of sexual health: Homosexual men and women. Clinical Review. *British Medical Journal, 318*(13), 452–5.

Berrill, K.T. (1992). Anti-gay violence and victimization in the United States:

An overview. In G.M. Herek & K.T. Berrill (Eds.), *Hate crimes: Confronting violence against lesbians and gay men*. Newbury Park, CA: Sage Publications.

Boden, D., Hurley, A., Zhang, L., et al. (1999). HIV-1 drug resistance in newly infected individuals. *Journal of the American Medical Association, 282*(12), 1135–41.

Breese, P.L., Judson, F.N., Penley, K.A., & Douglas, J.M. (1995). Anal human papilloma virus infection among homosexual and bisexual men: Prevalence of type-specific infection and association with human immunodeficiency virus. *Sexually Transmitted Diseases, 22*, 7–14.

Brotman, S., Rowe, B., & Ryan, B. (2000). *Access to care: Exploring the health and well-being of gay, lesbian, bisexual, and two-spirit people in Canada*. McGill School of Social Work. http://www.arts.mcgill.ca/programs/socialwork/interact/interact.html [September 18, 2001].

Buchbinder, S.P., Holmberg, S.D., Scheer, S., Colfax, G., O'Malley, P., & Vittinghoff, E. (1999). Combination antiretroviral therapy and incidence of AIDS-related malignancies. *Journal of Acquired Immune Deficiency Syndrome, 21*(1), S23–6.

Bureau of Justice Statistics. (1994). *National crime victimization survey*. Bureau of Justice Statistics Bulletin. Washington, DC.

Cabaj, R.P., & Stein, T.S. (Eds.). (1996). *Textbook of homosexuality and mental health*. Washington, DC: American Psychiatric Press.

Canadian Male Sexual Health Council. (1999). *Education on erectile dysfunction*. Symposium Report: Pfizer (CD-ROM).

Cass, V.C. (1979). Homosexual identity formation: A theoretical model. *Journal of Homosexuality, 4*, 219–35.

Centers for Disease Control and Prevention. (1996). (Published erratum, 1997, *Morbidity and Mortality Weekly Report, 46*(25), 588). Prevention of Hepatitis A through active or passive immunization: Recommendations of the Advisory Committee on Immunization Practices (ACIP). *Morbidity and Mortality Weekly Report, 45*(RR-15), 1–30.

Centers for Disease Control and Prevention. (1999). Cases of syphilis, gonorrhea on rise among gay men in Seattle area (Associated Press), September 10. http://www.egroups.com/message/glbthealth/145 [January 27, 2001].

Centers for Disease Control and Prevention. (1999). HIV/AIDS surveillance. *Morbidity and Mortality Weekly Report, 11*(1), midyear edition.

Centers for Disease Control and Prevention. (2000). HIV/AIDS among racial/ethnic minority men who have sex with men: United States, 1989–1998. *Morbidity and Mortality Weekly Report, 49*(1).

Chapple, M.J., Kippax, S., & Smith, G. (1998). 'Semi-straight sort of sex': Class and gay community attachment explored within a framework of older homosexually active men. *Journal of Homosexuality, 35*(2), 65–83.

Clark, D.H. (1987/1997). *The new loving someone gay.* Berkeley, CA: Celestial Arts.

Cochran, S.D., & Mays, V.M. (1988). Disclosure of sexual preference to physicians by black lesbian women. *Western Journal of Medicine, 149*(5), 616–19.

Cole, S.W., Kemeny, M.E., Taylor, S.E., & Visscher, B.R. (1996). Elevated physical health risk among gay men who conceal their homosexual identity. *Health Psychology, 15,* 243–51.

Coleman, E. (1996). Developmental stages of the coming out process. *Journal of Homosexuality, 7,* 31–43.

Comstock, G.D. (1991). *Violence against lesbians and gay men.* New York: Columbia University Press.

Daling, J.R., Weiss, N.S., Hislop, G., et al. (1987). Sexual practices, sexually transmitted diseases, and the incidence of anal cancer. *New England Journal of Medicine, 317,* 973–7.

D'Augelli, A.R., & Hershberger, S. (1993). Lesbian, gay, and bisexual youth in community settings: Personal challenges and mental health problems. *American Journal of Community Psychology, 21*(4), 421–48.

Davies, D., et al. (1996). *Pink therapy: A guide for counselors and therapists working with gay and bisexual clients.* Philadelphia: Open University Press.

Dean, L., Meyer, I., Robinson, K., et al. (2000). *Lesbian, gay, bisexual and transgender health: Findings and concerns.* Conference Edition. Gay and Lesbian Medical Association. New York: Columbia University.

Doll, L.S., Joy, D., Bartholow, B.N., Eliaszewicz, M., Pialoux, G., Fournier, S., & Feuillie, V. (1992). Self-reported childhood and adolescent sexual abuse among adult homosexual and bisexual men. *Child Abuse and Neglect, 16*(6), 855–64.

Elford, J., Bolding, G., Maguire, M., & Sherr, L. (1999). Sexual risk behavior among gay men in a relationship. *AIDS, 13*(11), 1407–11.

Ferguson, D.M., Horwood, L.J., & Beautrais, A.L. (1999). Is sexual orientation related to mental health problems and suicidality in young people? *Archives of General Psychiatry, 56,* 876–80.

Finn, P., & McNeil, T. (1987). *The response of the criminal justice system to bias crime.* Cambridge, MA: Abt Associates.

Garnets, L., Hancock, K.A., Cochran, S.D., Goodchilds, J., & Peplau, L.A. (1991). Issues in psychotherapy with lesbians and gay men. *American Psychologist, 46*(9), 964–72.

Garnets, L., Herek, G.M., & Levy, B. (1990). Violence and victimization of lesbians and gay men: Mental health consequences. *Journal of Interpersonal Violence, 5*(3), 366–82.

Glatto, M.F., et al. (1999). *The concise guide to psychiatry for primary care practitioners.* Washington, DC: American Psychiatric Press.

Herek, G.M., Gillis, J.R., Cogan, J.C., & Glunt, E.K. (1997). Hate crime victimization among lesbian, gay and bisexual adults: Prevalence, psychological correlates and methodological issues. *Journal of Interpersonal Violence, 12*(2) 195–215.

Herek, G.M., et al. (1999). Psychological sequelae of hate-crime victimization among lesbian, gay and bisexual adults. *Journal of Consulting and Clinical Psychology, 67*(6), 945–51.

Herman, J.L., & Hirschman, L. (1981). Families at risk for father–daughter incest. *American Journal of Psychiatry, 138*, 967–70.

Hershberger, S.L., Pilkington, N.W., & D'Augelli, A.R. (1996). Categorization of lesbian, gay, and bisexual suicide attemptes. In C.J. Alexander (Ed.), *Gay and lesbian mental health: A source book for practitioners.* New York: Harrington Park Press.

Hickson, F.C., Reid, D.S., Davies, P.M., Weatherburn, P., Beardsell, S., & Keogh, P.G. (1996). No aggregate change in homosexual HIV risk behavior among gay men attending the Gay Pride festivals, United Kingdom, 1993–1995. *AIDS, 10*(7), 771–4.

Hopcke, R. (1989). *Jung and homosexuality.* Boston: Shambhala.

Hospers, H.K., & Kok, G. (1995). Determinants of safe and risk-taking sexual behavior among gay men: A review. *AIDS Education and Prevention, 7*(1), 74–96.

Isay, R.A. (1995). *Being homosexual: Gay men and their development.* New York: Avon Books.

Jones, M.A., & Gabriel, M.A. (1999). Utilization of psychotherapy by lesbians, gay men, and bisexuals: Findings from a nationwide survey. *American Journal of Orthopsychiatry, 68*(2), 209–19.

Kalichman, S.C., & Rompa, D. (1995). Sexually coerced and noncoerced gay and bisexual men: Factors relevant to risk for human immunodeficiency virus (HIV) infection. *Journal of Sex Research, 32*(1), 45–50.

Kaul, S.K., et al. (1999). HIV protease inhibitors: Advances in therapy and adverse reactions, including metabolic complications. *Pharmacotherapy, 19*(3), 281–99.

Kelly, J.A., Hoffman, R.G., Rompa, D., & Gray, M. (1998). Protease inhibitor combination therapies and perceptions of gay men regarding AIDS severity and the need to maintain safer sex. *AIDS, 12*(10), F91–5.

King, M. (1990). Male rape: Victims need sensitive management. *British Medical Journal, 201*, 1345–6.

Knisley, E.R. (1992). Psychosocial factors relevant to homosexual men who were sexually abused as children and homosexual men who were not sexually abused as children: An exploratory-descriptive study. *Dissertation Abstracts International, 53*(6-B), 3157.

Koblin, B.A., Hessol, N.A., Zauber, A.G., Taylor, P.E., Buchbinder, S.P., Katzh, M.H., & Stevens, C.E. (1996). Increased incidence of cancer among homosexual men, New York City and San Francisco, 1978–1990. *American Journal of Epidemiology, 144*, 916–23.

Liddle, B.J. (1999). Recent improvement in mental health services to lesbian and gay men. *Journal of Homosexuality, 37*(4), 127–37.

Martin, J.N., Ganem, D.E., Osmond, D.H., Page-Shafer, K.A., Macrae, D., & Kedes, D.H. (1998). Sexual transmission and the natural history of human herpes virus and infection. *New England Journal of Medicine, 338*, 948–54.

McHenry, S., & Johnson, I. (1993). Homophobia in the therapist and gay or lesbian client: Conscious and unconscious collusion in self hate. *Psychotherapy, 301*(1), 141–9.

Meyer, I.H., & Dean, L. 1998. Internalized homophobia, intimacy, and sexual behavior among gay and bisexual men. In G.M. Herek (Ed.), *Stigma, prejudice, and violence against lesbians and gay men*. Newbury Park, CA: Sage Publications.

National Institutes of Health. (1997). Consensus statement. *Interventions to Prevent HIV Risk Behavior, 15*(2), 1–41.

Ottawa–Carleton Health Department. (n.d.). *Protect yourself: Use a condom* (pamphlet).

Palefsky, J.M., Holly, E.A., Ralston, M.L., & Jay, N. (1998). Prevalence and risk factors for human papillomavirus infection of the anal canal in human immunodeficiency virus (HIV)–positive and HIV-negative homosexual men. *Journal of Infectious Diseases, 177*, 361–7.

Penn, R.E. (1997). *The gay men's wellness guide*. New York: Henry Holt.

Peterkin, A. (1998). Negotiating safer sex: Tips for men who have sex with men. *Toronto Star* (Toronto Star Lifeline).

Ponse, B.R. (1977). Identities in the lesbian world. *Dissertation Abstracts International, 38*(n1-A), 504.

Remafedi, G. (1999). Sexual orientation and youth suicide. *Journal of the American Medical Association, 282*(13), 1291–2.

Remafedi, G., Farrow, J.A., & Deischer, R.W. (1991). Risk factors for attempted suicide in gay and bisexual youth. *Pediatrics, 87*, 869–75.

Rosario, M., Rotheram-Borus, M.J., & Reid, H. (1996). Gay-related stress and its correlates among gay and bisexual male adolescents of predominantly black and Hispanic background. *Journal of Community Psychology, 24*, 136–59.

Rothblum, E.D. (1994). 'I only read about myself on bathroom walls': The need for research on the mental health of lesbians and gay men. *Journal of Consulting and Clinical Psychology, 62*(2), 213–20.

Saddul, R.B. (1996). Coming out: An overlooked concept. *Clinical Nurse Specialist, 10*(1), 2–5.

Scarce, M. (1997). *Male on male rape.* New York: Plenum Press.

Shaffer, D., Fisher, P., Hicks, R.H., Parides, M., & Gould, M. (1995). Sexual orientation in adolescents who commit suicide. *Suicide and Life-Threatening Behavior, 25,* 64–71.

Sorenson, L., & Roberts, S.J. (1997). Lesbian users of and satisfaction with mental health services: Results from Boston Lesbian Health Project. *Journal of Homosexuality, 33*(1), 35–49.

Trippet, S.E., & Bain, J. (1990). Preliminary study of lesbian health concerns. *Health Values, 14*(6), 31–6.

Troiden, R.R. (1988). Homosexual identity development. *Journal of Adolescent Health Care, 9,* 105–13.

Tross, S., Hirsch, D., Rabkin, B., et al. (1987). Determinants of current psychiatric disorders in AIDS spectrum patients. In *Programs and Abstracts of the Third International Conference on AIDS.* Washington, DC, June 1–5.

Ungvarski, P.J., & Grossman, A.H. (1999). Health problems of gay and bisexual men. *Nursing Clinics of North America, 34*(2), 313–31.

Vittinghoff, E., & Douglas, J. (1999). Per-contact risk of human immunodeficiency virus transmission between male sexual partners. *American Journal of Epidemiology, 150*(3), 311. http://www.groups.yahoo.com/group/glbthealth/message/308 [November 2, 2000].

Williams, J., Rabkin, J., Remien, R., et al. (1991). Multidisciplinary baseline assessment of homosexual men with and without human immunodeficiency virus infection: Standardized clinical assessment of current and lifetime psychopathology. *Archives of General Psychiatry, 48,* 124–30.

Wise, M.G., & Rundell, J.R. (1994). *Concise guide to consultation psychiatry* (2nd ed.). Washington, DC: American Psychiatric Press.

Wolfe, D. (1999). *Men like us: The GMHC (Gay Men's Health Crisis Clinic) complete guide to gay men's sexual, physical and emotional wellbeing.* New York: Ballantine Books.

9: Substance Abuse

Amico, J. (1997). *Sharing the secret: The need for gay specific treatment.* National Association of Alcoholism and Drug Abuse Counselors.

Anderson, S.C. (1996). Substance abuse and dependency in gay men and lesbians. In K.J. Paterson (Ed.), *Health care for lesbians and gay men: Confronting homophobia and heterosexism.* New York: Harrington Park Press.

Bailey, J.M., Benishay, D.S., et al. (1993). HIV and substance abuse in the gay male community. *American Journal of Psychiatry, 150*(2), 272–7.

Bloomfield, K.L. (1993). A comparison of alcohol consumption between lesbians and heterosexual women in an urban population. *Drug and Alcohol Dependence, 33,* 257–69.

Buenting, J.A. (1992). Treating lesbians and bisexual women. *Health Care for Women International, 13,* 165–71.

Cabaj, R.P., & Stein, T.S. (Eds.). (1996). *Textbook of homosexuality and mental health.* Washington, DC: American Psychiatric Press.

Canadian AIDS Society. (1997). Under the influence: Making the connection between HIV/AIDS and substance use: A guide for ASO workers who provide support to persons living with HIV/AIDS. Ottawa: Canadian AIDS Society.

Ewing, J. (1984). Detecting alcoholism: The CAGE questionnaire. *Journal of the American Medical Association, 25*(30), 1905–7.

Expert Panel. (1995). Substance use disorders. *American Journal of Psychiatry, 152* (supplement).

Ferrando, S.J. (1997). Review of substance use disorder and HIV illness. *The Aids Reader, 7*(2), 57–64.

Gliatte, M.F. (1999). *Concise guide to psychiatry for primary care practitioners.* Washington, DC: American Psychiatric Press.

Howard, B.M., & Collins, B.E. (1997). Working with lesbian and gay men. In S. Harrison & V. Carver (Eds.), *A practical guide for counselors: Alcohol and drug problems* (2nd ed.). Toronto: Addiction Research Foundation.

Hughes, T.L., & Wilsnack, S.C. (1997). Use of alcohol among lesbians: Research and clinical implications. *American Journal of Orthopsychiatry, 1,* 20–36.

Isay, R.A. (1995). *Being homosexual: Gay men and their development.* New York: Avon Books.

Lacouture, Y. (1998). *La toxicomanie chez les personnes homosexuelles: Une recension des écrits.* Comité permanent de lutte à la toxicomanie. Gouvernement du Québec.

Lesbians on health care for lesbians and gay men. (1996). (Originally published by Howarth Press). Reprinted in *Journal of Gay and Lesbian Services, 5*(1), 59–76.

McKirnan, D.J., & Peterson, P.L. (1989). Alcohol and drug use among homosexual men and women: Epidemiology and population characteristics. *Addictive Behaviors, 14,* 545–53.

Neisen, J., & Sandall, H. (1996). Alcohol and other drug use in gay and lesbian populations: Related to victimization? *Journal of Psychology and Human Sexuality, 3*(1), 151–68.

Ogborne, A.C. (2000). Identifying and treating patients with alcohol-related problems. *Canadian Medical Association Journal, 162*(12), 27.

O'Hanlan, K., Cabaj, R.B., Schatz, B., Lock, J., & Nemrow, P. (1997). A review of the medical consequences of homophobia with suggestions for resolution. *Journal of the Gay and Lesbian Medical Association, 1*(1), 25–40.

Reyes, M. (1998). Latina lesbians and alcohol and other drugs: Social work implication. *Alcohol Treatment Quarterly, 6*(1/2), 179–92.

Skinner, W.F. (1994). The prevalence and demographic predictors of illicit and licit drug use among lesbians and gay men. *American Journal of Public Health, 84*(8), 1307–10.

Skinner, W.F., & Otis, M.D. (1996). Drug and alcohol use among lesbian and gay people in a Southern U.S. sample: Epidemiological, comparative, and methodological findings from the Trilogy Project. *Journal of Homosexuality, 30*(3), 59–92.

Stall, R.D., Greenwood, G.L., Acree, M., Paul, J., & Coates, T.J. (1999). Cigarette smoking among gay and bisexual men. *American Journal of Public Health, 89*(12), 1875–8.

Stall, R.D., & Wiley, J. (1988). A comparison of alcohol and drug use patterns of homosexual and heterosexual men. *The San Francisco Men's Health Study, 22*(1/2), 63–73.

Weathers, B. (1980). Alcoholism and the lesbian community. In C. Eddy & J. Fords (Eds.), *Alcoholism and women.* Dubuque, IA: Kendall/Hunt.

Weir, E. (2000). Raves: A review of the culture, the drugs and the prevention of harm. *Canadian Medical Association Journal, 162*(13), 1843.

White, J.C., & Dull, V.T. (1997). Health risk factors and health seeking behavior in lesbians. *Journal of Women's Health, 6*(1), 103–12.

10: The Body

Beren, S., Hayden, H., Wilfley, D., & Grilo, C. (1996). The influence of sexual orientation on body dissatisfaction in adult men and women. *International Journal of Eating Disorders, 20*(2), 135–41.

Brand, P.A., Rothblum, E.D., & Solomon, J.J. (1992). A comparison of lesbians, gay men, and heterosexuals on weight and restricted eating. *International Journal of Eating Disorders, 11*, 253–9.

Brown, L. (1987). Lesbians, weight, and eating: New analyses and perspectives. In Boston Lesbian Psychologies Collective (Eds.), *Lesbian psychologies: Explorations and challenges.* Chicago: University of Illinois Press.

Carlat, D.J., Camargo, C.A., & Herzog, D.B. (1997). Eating disorders in males: A report on 135 patients. *American Journal of Psychiatry, 154*(8), 1127–32.

Care of new tattoos. (2000). http://www.cs.ruu.nl/wais/html/na-dir/bodyart/tattoo-faq/part6.html [February 14, 2001].

Carr, A., & Cooper, D.A. (2000). Private. *Lancet, 356*(9239), 1423–30.

Centers for Disease Control and Prevention. (1996). *Hepatitis surveillance.* Report No. 56.

Centers for Disease Control and Prevention. (1997). Estimated incidence of AIDS and deaths of persons with AIDS, adjusted for delays in reporting, by quarter-year of diagnosis/death, United States, January 1985 through June 1997. *The HIV/AIDS Surveillance Report, 9*(1).

French, S.A., Story, M., Remafedi, G., Resnick, M.D., & Blum, R.W. (1996). Sexual orientation and prevalence of body dissatisfaction and eating disordered behaviors: A population-based study of adolescents. *International Journal of Eating Disorders, 19*(2), 119–26.

Gettleman, T.E., & Thompson, J.K. (1993). Actual differences versus stereotypical perceptions of body image and eating disturbance: A comparison of male and female heterosexual and homosexual samples. *Sex Roles, 29*, 545–62.

Guzman, R. (2000). Circuit parties. *Focus, 15*(4) (published by AIDS Health Project, University of California, San Francisco).

Hadigan, C., et al. (2000). Metformin use in the HIV lipodystrophy syndrome: A randomized controlled trial. *Journal of the American Medical Association, 284*(4), 472–7.

Health Canada. (1999). Infection prevention and control practices for personal services: Tattooing, ear/body piercing and electrolysis. *Canadian Communicable Disease Report, 25*, S3.

Hefferman, K. (1994). Sexual orientation as a factor in risk for binge eating and bulimia nervosa: A review. *International Journal of Eating Disorders, 16*(4), 335–47.

Hefferman, K. (1996). Eating disorders and weight concern among lesbians. *International Journal of Eating Disorders, 19*, 127–38.

Herzog, D.B., Newman, K.L., Yeh, C.J., & Warshaw, M. (1992). Body image satisfaction in homosexual and heterosexual women. *International Journal of Eating Disorders, 11*, 391–6.

Jackson, L.A., Sullivan, L.A., & Rostker, R. (1988). Gender, gender role, and body image. *Sex Roles, 19*, 429–43.

Levins, P. (2000). *About our tattoo procedures.* http://www.tattooartist.com/procedures.html [July 21, 2001].

Ludwig, M.R., & Brownell, K.D. (1999). Lesbians, bisexual women, and body image: An investigation of gender roles and social group affiliation. *International Journal of Eating Disorders, 25*, 89–97.

Popkow, S. (2000). *Tattoo removal.* http://www.tatooremoval.org

Rothblum, E.D. (1994). Lesbians and physical appearance: Which model applies? In B. Green & G.M. Herek (Eds.), *Lesbian and gay psychology: Theory, research, and clinical applications.* Thousand Oaks, CA: Sage Publications.

Schultheiss, D. (1998). Uncircumcision: A historical review of preputial resto-ration. *Plastic Reconstructive Surgery, 101*(7), 1990–8.

Siever, M.D. (1994). Sexual orientation and gender as factors in socioculturally acquired vulnerability to body dissatisfaction and eating disorders. *Journal of Consulting and Clinical Psychology, 62,* 252–60.

Signorile, M. (1997). *Life outside.* New York: HarperCollins.

Silberstein, L.R., Mishkind, M., Streigel-Moore, R.H., et al. (1989). Men and their bodies: A comparison of homosexual and heterosexual men. *Psychoso-matic Medicine, 51*(3), 337–46.

Weir, E. (2001). Navel gazing: A clinical glimpse at body piercing. *Canadian Medical Association Journal, 164*(6), 864.

Woog, D. (1999, December 21). Plastic made perfect. *The Advocate.*

11: Relationships

Allen, N., & Burrel, N. (1996). Comparing the impact of homosexual and heterosexual parents on children: Meta-analysis of existing research. *Journal of Homosexuality, 32*(2), 19–35.

Barret, R.L., & Robinson, B.E. (1990). *Gay fathers.* http://www.domani.net/richard/cotk.html

Baum, M. (1996). Gays and lesbians choosing to be parents. In C. Alexander (Ed.), *Gay and lesbian mental health: A sourcebook for practitioners.* New York: Harrington Park Press.

Bernstein, F. (1998). This child does have two mothers ... and a sperm donor with visitation. *NYU Review of Law and Social Change, 22*(1).

Brotman, S., Rowe, B., & Ryan, B. (2000). *Access to care: Exploring the health and well-being of gay, lesbian, bisexual, and two-spirit people in Canada.* McGill School of Social Work. http://www.arts.mcgill.ca/programs/socialwork/interact/interact.html [September 18, 2001].

Clunis, D.M. (1988). *The lesbian couple.* Seattle: Seal Press.

Cowan, C.P., & Cowan, P.A. (1999). *The division of child care and housework: Implications for parents' and children's adaptation.* Paper presented at a Na-tional Institute of Health Workshop: New Approaches to Research on Sexual Orientation, Mental Health and Substance Abuse. Rockville, MD.

Craven, N.H. (1998). Relationship abuse: Stopping the cycle. *Canadian Journal of Continuing Medical Education,* (September), 69–75.

Davies, D., et al. (1996). *Pink therapy: A guide for counselors and therapists working with gay and bisexual clients.* Philadelphia: Open University Press.

Dean, L., Meyer, I., Robinson, K., et al. (2000). *Lesbian, gay, bisexual, and transgender health: Findings and concerns.* Conference Edition. Gay and Lesbian Medical Association. New York: Columbia University.

Deevey, S. (2000). Cultural variation in lesbian bereavement: Experiences in Ohio. *Journal of the Gay and Lesbian Medical Association,* 4(1), 9–17.

519 Community Resource Centre (Toronto). (1998). Abuse in lesbian relationships.

Frederiksen, K.L. (1999). Family caregiving responsibilities among lesbians and gay men. *Social Work,* 44(2), 142–55.

Friedman, R.C., & Downey, J. (1994). Homosexuality. *New England Journal of Medicine,* 331(14), 92.

Gay, D. (1996). Balancing autonomy and intimacy in lesbian and gay relationships. In G. Alexander (Ed.), *Gay and lesbian mental health: A sourcebook for practitioners.* New York: Harrington Park Press.

Gold, M.A., Perrin, E.C., Futterman, D., & Friedman, S.B. (1994). Children of gay or lesbian parents. *Pediatric Review,* 15(9), 354–8.

Golombok, S., Tasker, F., & Murray, C. (1997). Children raised in fatherless families from infancy: Family relationships and the socio-emotional development of children in lesbian and single heterosexual mothers. *Journal of Child Psychology and Psychiatry,* 38(7), 783–91.

Harvey, S.M., Carr, C., & Bernheine, S. (1989). Lesbian mothers: Health care experiences. *Journal of Nurse Midwifery,* 34(3), 115–19.

Havemann, J. (1997, December 18). New Jersey allows gays to adopt jointly; activists say settlement puts unmarried couples on equal footing. *Washington Post,* p. A1.

Island, D. (1991). *Men who beat them, men who love them: Battered gay men and domestic violence.* New York: Harrington Park Press.

Klinger, R. (1996). *Lesbian couples.* In R.P. Cabaj & T.S. Stein (Eds.), *Textbook of homosexuality and mental health.* Washington, DC: American Psychiatric Press.

Lasenza, S. (1999). The big lie: Lesbian bed death. *The Family,* (April).

Levy, E.F. (1996). Reproductive issues for lesbians. *Journal of Gay and Lesbian Social Services,* 5(1), 49–58.

Mason, M. (2001). *Census figures on same-sex couples.* http://www.speakout.com. [August 8, 2001].

McWhirter, D., & Mathieson, A. (1996). Male couples. In R.P. Cabaj & T.S. Stein (Eds.), *Textbook of homosexuality and mental health.* Washington, DC: American Psychiatric Press.

Patterson, C.J. (1996). Lesbian and gay families with children: Implications of social science research for policy. *Journal of Social Issues,* 52(3), 29.

Patterson, C.J., & Chan, R.W. (1996). Gay fathers and their children. In R.P.

Cabaj, & T.S. Stein (Eds.), *Textbook of Homosexuality and Mental Health.*
Washington, DC: American Psychiatric Press.

Reilly, T. (1996). Gay and lesbian adoptions: A theoretical examination of
policy-making and organizational decision making. *Journal of Sociology and
Social Welfare*, 23(4), 99–115.

Same-sex couples: More similarities than differences. (n.d.). Educational Pamphlet.
McGill University Student Health Services.

Schernoff, M. (1998). Gay widowers, grieving in relation to trauma and social
supports. *Journal of the Gay and Lesbian Medical Association*, 2(1), 27–33.

Shernoff, M. (1996). Gay men choosing to be fathers. In M. Shernoff (Ed.),
Human services for gay people: Clinical and community practice. New York:
Harrington Park Press.

Simon, G. (1996). Working with people in relationships. In D. Davies, et al.
(Eds.), *Pink therapy: A guide for counselors and therapists working with gay and
bisexual clients.* Philadelphia: Open University Press.

Slezak, M. (2000). *Coming out at work.* http://www.gayhealth.com/iowa-
robot/society/?record=32 [June 6, 2001].

12: Special Populations

Adams, C.L., & Kimmel, D.C. (1997). Exploring the lives of older African
American gay men. In B. Greene (Ed.), *Ethnic and cultural diversity among
lesbians and gay men: Psychological perspectives on lesbians and gay men* (3rd
ed.). Thousand Oaks, CA: Sage Publications.

Amico, J., & Neisen, J. (1997). Sharing the secret: The need for gay specific
treatment. *The Counselor*, (May/June), 12–15.

Anderson, S.C. (1996). Substance abuse and dependency in gay men and
lesbians. In K.J. Paterson (Ed.), *Health care for lesbians and gay men: Confronting homophobia and heterosexism.* New York: Harrington Park Press.

Auger, J.A. (1990). Lesbians and aging: Triple trouble or tremendous thrill? In
S.D. Stone (Ed.), *Lesbians in Canada.* Toronto: Between the Lines Press.

Beeler, J.A., Rawls, T.W., Herdt, G., & Cohler, B.J. (1999). The needs of older
lesbians and gay men in Chicago. *Journal of Gay and Lesbian Social Services*,
9(1), 31–49.

Berger, R.M. (1982). *Gay and gray: The older homosexual man.* New York:
Haworth Press.

Berger, R.M., & Kelly, J.J. (1986). Working with homosexuals of the older population: Social casework. *Journal of Contemporary Social Work*, 67(4), 203–10.

Berger, R.M., & Kelly, J.J. (1996). Gay men and lesbians growing older. In R.P.

Cabaj & T.S. Stein (Eds.), *Textbook of homosexuality and mental health*. Washington, DC: American Psychiatric Press.

Bonneau, M. (1998). L'affirmation lesbienne en milieu régional: Une visibilité problématique. Sous la direction de Irene Demczuk, *Des droits à reconnaître – les lesbiennes face à la discrimination*. Montreal: Les éditions du Remue-ménage.

Brotman, S., & Kraniou, S. (1999). Ethnic and lesbian: Understanding identity through the life-history approach. *Affilia, 14*(4), 417–38.

Brotman, S., Rowe, B., & Ryan, B. (2000). *Access to care: Exploring the health and well-being of gay, lesbian, bisexual, and two-spirit people in Canada*. McGill School of Social Work. http://www.arts.mcgill.ca/programs/socialwork/interact/interact.html [September 18, 2001].

Brown, L.B. (1999). Women and men, not-men and not-women, lesbians and gays: Gender style alternatives. *Journal of Gay and Lesbian Social Services, 9*(4), 5–20.

Coalition for Lesbian and Gay Rights in Ontario. (1997). *Systems failure*. CLGRO Project Affirmation. Toronto.

Cody, P.J., & Welch, P.L. (1997). Rural gay men in Northern New England: Life experiences and coping styles. *Journal of Homosexuality, 33*(1), 51–67.

Connolly, L. (1996). Long-term care and hospice: The special needs of older gay men and lesbians. In K.J. Paterson (Ed.), *Health care for lesbians and gay men: Confronting homophobia and heterosexism*. New York: Harrington Park Press.

Crow, L., Wright, J.A., & Brown, L.B. (1997). Gender selection in American Indian tribes. *Journal of Gay and Lesbian Social Services, 6*(2), 21–8.

Deevey, S. (1990). Older lesbian women – an invisible minority. *Journal of Gerontological Nursing, 16*(5), 35–9.

Dworkin, S.H. (1997). Female, lesbian and Jewish: Complex and invisible. In B. Greene (Ed.), *Ethnic and cultural diversity among lesbians and gay men: Psychological perspectives on lesbians and gay men* (3rd ed.). Thousand Oaks, CA: Sage Publications.

Ehrenberg, M. (1996). Aging and mental health: Issues in the gay and lesbian community. In C.J. Alexander (Ed.), *Gay and lesbian mental health: A source book for practitioners*. New York: Harrington Park Press.

Faria, G. (1997). The challenge of health care social work with gay men and lesbians. *Social Work in Health Care, 25*(1/2), 65–72.

Foster, S.J. (1997). Rural lesbians and gays: Public perceptions, worker perceptions, and service delivery. *Journal of Gay and Lesbian Social Services, 7*(3), 23–35.

Gonzalez, F.J., & Espin, O.M. (1996). Latino men, Latino women, and homosexuality. In R.P. Cabaj & T.S. Stein (Eds.), *Textbook of homosexuality and mental health*. Washington, DC: American Psychiatric Press.

Icard, L.D., Longres, J.F., & Williams, J.H. (1996). An applied research agenda for homosexually active men of color. *Journal of Gay and Lesbian Social Services*, 5(2/3), 139–64.

Jackson, K., & Brown, L.B. (1996). Lesbians of African heritage: Coming out in the straight community. *Journal of Gay and Lesbian Social Services*, 5(4), 53–67.

Jacobs, M.A., & Brown, L.B. (1997). American Indian lesbians and gays: An exploratory study. *Journal of Gay and Lesbian Social Services*, 6(2), 29–41.

Jacobs, R.J., Rasmussen, L.A., & Hohman, M.M. (1999). The social support needs of older lesbians, gay men, and bisexuals. *Journal of Gay and Lesbian Social Services*, 9(1), 1–30.

Kertzner, R.M., & Sved, M. (1996). Midlife gay men and lesbians: Adult development and mental health. In R.P. Cabaj & T.S. Stein (Eds.), *Textbook of homosexuality and mental health*. Washington, DC: American Psychiatric Press.

Kochman, A. (1997). Gay and lesbian elderly: Historical overview and implications for social work practice. *Journal of Gay and Lesbian Social Services*, 6(1), 1–10.

Lindhorst, T. (1997). Lesbians and gay men in the country: Practice implications for rural social workers. *Journal of Gay and Lesbian Social Services*, 7(3) 1–11.

Lombardi, E. (2001). Enhancing transgender health care. *American Journal of Public Health*, 91(6), 869–71.

Lopez, R.A., & Traung, L.B. (1998). Social supports among Vietnamese American gay men. *Journal of Gay and Lesbian Social Services*, 8(2), 29–50.

McDougall, G.J. (1993). Therapeutic issues with gay and lesbian elders. *Clinical Gerontologist*, 14(1), 45–57.

Mellor, M.J. (1996). Special populations among older persons. *Journal of Gerontological Social Work*, 25(1/2), 1–10.

Meyer, F. (n.d.). *The two-spirit papers: The impact of heterosexism and homophobia on Inuit and First Nations people's lives*. Research report submitted to the School of Social Work, Faculty of Graduate Studies, and research for the Master's degree in social work. McGill University.

Oriel, K.A. (2000). Medical care of transsexual patients. *Journal of the Gay and Lesbian Medical Association*, 4(4), 185–94.

O'Rourke, J. (1997). Negotiating HIV infection in rural America: Breaking through the isolation. In M. Forstein (Ed.), *Therapists on the frontline*. Washington, DC: American Psychiatric Press.

Otis, M.D., & Skinner, W.F. (1996). The prevalence of victimization and its effect on mental wellbeing among lesbian and gay people. *Journal of Homosexuality*, 30(3), 93–121.

Quam, J.K., & Whitford, G.S. (1992). Adaptations and age-related expectations of older gay and lesbian adults. *Gerontologist*, 32(3), 367–74.

Rodriguez, R. (1998). Clinical and practice considerations in private practice with lesbians and gay men of color. *Journal of Gay and Lesbian Social Services,* 8(4), 59–75.

Ryan, C., & Futterman, D. (1998). *Lesbian and gay youth: Care and counseling.* New York: Columbia University Press.

Simkin, R. (1998). Not all patients are straight. *Journal of the American Medical Association, 159*(4), 370–5.

Swigonski, M.E. (1995). For the white social worker who wants to know how to work with lesbians of color. *Journal of Gay and Lesbian Social Services, 3*(2), 7–21.

Tafoya, T.N. (1997). Native gay and lesbian issues: The two-spirited. In B. Greene (Ed.), *Ethnic and cultural diversity among lesbians and gay men: Psychological perspectives on lesbians and gay men* (3rd ed.). Thousand Oaks, CA: Sage Publications.

University of Ottawa. (1999). *Assume nothing.* Ottawa: University of Ottawa Pride Centre.

Urban versus rural: Life outside. (1998). *Hero Magazine,* (Fall).

Van Kestefen, P.J.M., Asscherman, H., Megena, J.A.J., et al. (1997). Mortality and morbidity in transsexual subjects treated with cross-sex hormones. *Clinical Endocrinology, 47,* 337–42.

Wahler, J., & Gabbay, S.G. (1997). Gay male aging: A review of the literature. *Journal of Gay and Lesbian Social Services, 6*(3), 1–20.

Walters, K.L. (1997). Urban lesbian and gay American Indian identity: Implications for mental health service delivery. *Journal of Gay and Lesbian Social Services, 6*(2), 43–65.

Williams, W.L. (1984). *The spirit and the flesh: Sexual diversity in American Indian culture.* Boston: Beacon Press.

Wright, J.A., Lopez, M.A., & Zumwalt, L.L. (1997). That's what they say: The implications of American Indian gay and lesbian literature of social service workers. In L.B. Brown (Ed.), *Two-spirited people: American Indian lesbian women and gay men.* New York: Harrington Park Press.

Zamora-Hernandez, C.E., & Patterson, D.G. (1996). Homosexually active Latino men: Issues for social work practice. *Journal of Gay and Lesbian Social Services, 5*(2/3), 69–91.

13: Professional and Training Issues

Blumenfeld, W.J. (1992). *Homophobia: How we all pay the price.* Boston: Beacon Press.

Brogan, D.J., Frank, E., Elon, L., Sivanesan, O., & O'Hanlan, K.A. (1999). Harassment of lesbians as medical students and physicians. *Journal of the American Medical Association, 282*(13), 1290–2.

Burke, B.P., White, J.C., & Saunders, D. (2001). Wellbeing of gay, lesbian, and bisexual doctors. *British Medical Journal, 322,* 422–5.

Cassidy, J., Poynter, I.L., & Schroer, S. (2002). *The safe on campus program resource manual.* http://www.salp.wmich.edu/lbg/GLB/manual/resource.html [July 17, 2002].

Druzin, P., et al. (1998). Discrimination against gay, lesbian and bisexual family physicians by patients. *Canadian Medical Association Journal, 158*(50), 593–7.

Mathews, W.M.C., Booth, M.W., Turner, J.D., et al. (1986). Physicians' attitudes toward homosexuality: Survey of a California county medical society. *Western Journal of Medicine, 144,* 106–10.

Murphy, B.C. (1992). Educating mental health professionals about gay and lesbian issues. *Journal of Homosexuality, 22*(2–4), 229–46.

Oriel, K.A., Madlon-Ka, D.J., Govaker, K., & Mersy, D.J. (1996). Gay and lesbian physicians-in-training: Family practice program directors' attitudes and students' perceptions of bias. *Family Medicine, 28,* 720–5.

Ramos, M.M., Tellez, C.M., Palley, T.B., Umland, B.E., & Skipper, B.J. (1998). Attitudes of physicians practicing in New Mexico toward gay men and lesbians in the profession. *Academic Medicine, 73*(4), 436–8.

Risdon, C., Cook, D.J., & Wilms, D. (2000). Gay and lesbian physicians in training: A qualitative study. *Canadian Medical Association Journal, 162*(3), 331–4.

Robinson, G., & Cohen, M. (1996). Gay, lesbian and bisexual health care issues and medical curricula. *Canadian Medical Association Journal, 155*(6), 709–11.

Rose, L. (1994). Homophobia among doctors. *British Medical Journal, 308,* 586–7.

Schatz, B., & O'Hanlan, K.A. (1994). *Antigay discrimination in medicine: Results of a national survey of lesbian, gay and bisexual physicians.* San Francisco: Gay and Lesbian Medical Association.

Schneider, J.S., & Levin, S. (1999). Uneasy partners: The lesbian and gay health care community and the AMA. *Medical Student Journal of the American Medical Association, 282,* 1287–8.

Solarz, A. (Ed.). (1999). *Lesbian health: Current assessment and direction for the future.* Washington, DC: Institute of Medicine.

Stein, T.S. (1994). A curriculum for learning in psychiatric residencies about homosexuality, gay men and lesbians. *Academic Psychiatry, 18,* 59–70.

Tesar, C.M., & Susan, L.D. (1998). Survey of curriculum on homosexuality/bisexuality in departments of family medicine. *Family Medicine, 30*(4), 283–7.

Townsend, M.H., Wallick, M., & Cambre, K.M. (1991). Support services for homosexual students at U.S. medical schools. *Academic Medicine, 66,* 361–3.

Townsend, M.H., Wallick, M., & Cambre, K. (1993). Gay and lesbian issues in residency training at U.S. psychiatry programs. *Academic Psychiatry, 17*(2), 67–72.

Townsend, M.H., & Wallick, M. (1996). Gay, lesbian and bisexual issues in medical schools. In R.P. Cabaj & T.S. Stein (Eds.), *Textbook of homosexuality and mental health*. Washington, DC: American Psychiatric Press.

Wallick, M.M., Cambre, K.M., & Townsend, M.H. (1992). How the topic of homosexuality is taught at U.S. medical schools. *Academic Medicine, 67*(9), 601–3.

Wallick, M.M., Townsend, M.H., & Cambre, K.M. (1995). Sexual orientation and non-discrimination policies. *Academic Medicine, 70,* 2.

14: Legal Issues

Bell, L. (1991). *On our own terms: A practical guide for lesbian and gay relationships*. Toronto: CLGRO.

Capen, K. (1997). Lesbians, artificial insemination, and human rights: Can doctors place limits on their medical practices? *Canadian Medical Association Journal, 156*(6), 839–40.

CATIE. (1999). *Managing your health: A guide for people living with HIV and AIDS*. Toronto: Canadian AIDS Treatment and Information Exchange.

Ettlebrick, P.L. (1996). Legal issues in health care for lesbians and gay men. *Journal of Gay and Lesbian Social Services, 5*(1), 93–109.

Gruskin, E.P. (1999). *Treating lesbians and bisexual women*. Thousand Oaks, CA: Sage Publications.

Jürgens, R. (1997). Immigration policy may be reviewed to require routine HIV testing of immigrants. *Canadian HIV/AIDS Policy and Law Newsletter, 3*(2/3).

Jürgens, R., & Palles, M. (1997). *HIV testing and confidentiality*. Montreal: Canadian HIV/AIDS Legal Network and Canadian AIDS Society.

Lesbian and Gay Immigration Rights Task Force and Lambda Legal Defense and Education Fund. (n.d.). *LGBT immigrants and the law: Frequently asked questions*. http://www.lgirtf.org/faq.html

McCarthy, M., & Redbord, J. (2000). Contracting love: New laws make relationship agreements very handy. *Xtra!*, March 9 issue.

Nolo Legal Encyclopedia. (1998). *Living together contracts*. http://www.nolo.com/lawcenter/ency/article.cfm/objectID/E354BF5F-A357-40DA-BAF2A0F4093A8BE8 [September 17, 2000].

Rubenstein, W.B. (1993). Employment discrimination: A survey of gay men and women. In W.B. Rubenstein (Ed.), *Lesbians, gay men and the law*. New York: New Press.

Ryan, C., & Futterman, D. (1998). *Lesbian and gay youth: Care and counseling.* New York: Columbia University Press.

Shime, P. (n.d.). *Homophobia in the law: The experiences of lesbians and gay men in the legal profession.* Unpublished paper, University of Toronto.

Sobocinski, M.R. (1990). Ethical principles in the counseling of gay and lesbian adolescents: Issues of autonomy, competence, and confidentiality. *Professional Psychology: Research and Practice, 20*(4), 240–7.

Sommerville, M.A. (1989). The case against HIV: Antibody testing refugees and immigrants. *Canadian Medical Association Journal, 141,* 889–94.

See www.glbcare.com for links to online resources used in the preparation of this book.

Index